Pathogenesis and Targeted Therapy of Epilepsy

Pathogenesis and Targeted Therapy of Epilepsy

Editor

Prosper N'Gouemo

MDPI • Basel • Beijing • Wuhan • Barcelona • Belgrade • Manchester • Tokyo • Cluj • Tianjin

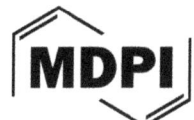

Editor
Prosper N'Gouemo
Howard University
USA

Editorial Office
MDPI
St. Alban-Anlage 66
4052 Basel, Switzerland

This is a reprint of articles from the Special Issue published online in the open access journal *Biomedicines* (ISSN 2227-9059) (available at: https://www.mdpi.com/journal/biomedicines/special_issues/Therapy_of_Epilepsy).

For citation purposes, cite each article independently as indicated on the article page online and as indicated below:

LastName, A.A.; LastName, B.B.; LastName, C.C. Article Title. *Journal Name* **Year**, *Volume Number*, Page Range.

ISBN 978-3-0365-6436-4 (Hbk)
ISBN 978-3-0365-6437-1 (PDF)

© 2023 by the authors. Articles in this book are Open Access and distributed under the Creative Commons Attribution (CC BY) license, which allows users to download, copy and build upon published articles, as long as the author and publisher are properly credited, which ensures maximum dissemination and a wider impact of our publications.

The book as a whole is distributed by MDPI under the terms and conditions of the Creative Commons license CC BY-NC-ND.

Contents

Prosper N'Gouemo
Pathogenesis and Targeted Therapy of Epilepsy
Reprinted from: *Biomedicines* **2022**, *10*, 3134, doi:10.3390/biomedicines10123134 1

**Julia L. Ergina, Dmitry V. Amakhin, Tatyana Y. Postnikova, Elena B. Soboleva
and Aleksey V. Zaitsev**
Short-Term Epileptiform Activity Potentiates Excitatory Synapses but Does Not Affect Intrinsic
Membrane Properties of Pyramidal Neurons in the Rat Hippocampus In Vitro
Reprinted from: *Biomedicines* **2021**, *9*, 1374, doi:10.3390/biomedicines9101374 3

Miracle Thomas, Mark Simms and Prosper N'Gouemo
Activation of Calcium-Activated Chloride Channels Suppresses Inherited Seizure Susceptibility
in Genetically Epilepsy-Prone Rats
Reprinted from: *Biomedicines* **2022**, *10*, 449, doi:10.3390/biomedicines10020449 21

**Willian Lazarini-Lopes, Gleice Kelli Silva-Cardoso, Christie Ramos Andrade Leite-Panissi
and Norberto Garcia-Cairasco**
Increased TRPV1 Channels and FosB Protein Expression Are Associated with Chronic Epileptic
Seizures and Anxiogenic-like Behaviors in a Preclinical Model of Temporal Lobe Epilepsy
Reprinted from: *Biomedicines* **2022**, *10*, 416, doi:10.3390/biomedicines10020416 37

**Irina B. Fedotova, Natalia M. Surina, Georgy M. Nikolaev, Alexandre V. Revishchin
and Inga I. Poletaeva**
Rodent Brain Pathology, Audiogenic Epilepsy
Reprinted from: *Biomedicines* **2021**, *9*, 1641, doi:10.3390/biomedicines9111641 57

Ji-Eun Kim and Tae-Cheon Kang
Blockade of TASK-1 Channel Improves the Efficacy of Levetiracetam in Chronically Epileptic
Rats
Reprinted from: *Biomedicines* **2022**, *10*, 787, doi:10.3390/biomedicines10040787 71

Ji-Eun Kim, Duk-Shin Lee, Hana Park, Tae-Hyun Kim and Tae-Cheon Kang
AMPA Receptor Antagonists Facilitate NEDD4-2-Mediated GRIA1 Ubiquitination by
Regulating PP2B-ERK1/2-SGK1 Pathway in Chronic Epilepsy Rats
Reprinted from: *Biomedicines* **2021**, *9*, 1069, doi:10.3390/biomedicines9081069 87

Ji-Eun Kim, Duk-Shin Lee, Hana Park, Tae-Hyun Kim and Tae-Cheon Kang
Inhibition of AKT/GSK3β/CREB Pathway Improves the Responsiveness to AMPA Receptor
Antagonists by Regulating GRIA1 Surface Expression in Chronic Epilepsy Rats
Reprinted from: *Biomedicines* **2021**, *9*, 425, doi:10.3390/biomedicines9040425 109

Ying Wang, Pedro Andrade and Asla Pitkänen
Peripheral Infection after Traumatic Brain Injury Augments Excitability in the Perilesional
Cortex and Dentate Gyrus
Reprinted from: *Biomedicines* **2021**, *9*, 1946, doi:10.3390/biomedicines9121946 131

**Xavier Ekolle Ndode-Ekane, Riikka Immonen, Elina Hämäläinen, Eppu Manninen,
Pedro Andrade, Robert Ciszek, Tomi Paananen, et al.**
MRI-Guided Electrode Implantation for Chronic Intracerebral Recordings in a Rat Model of
Post−Traumatic Epilepsy—Challenges and Gains
Reprinted from: *Biomedicines* **2022**, *10*, 2295, doi:10.3390/biomedicines10092295 155

Gaku Yamanaka, Fuyuko Takata, Yasufumi Kataoka, Kanako Kanou, Shinichiro Morichi, Shinya Dohgu and Hisashi Kawashima
The Neuroinflammatory Role of Pericytes in Epilepsy
Reprinted from: *Biomedicines* **2021**, *9*, 759, doi:10.3390/biomedicines9070759 . . . . **191**

An Buckinx, Dimitri De Bundel, Ron Kooijman and Ilse Smolders
Targeting the Ghrelin Receptor as a Novel Therapeutic Option for Epilepsy
Reprinted from: *Biomedicines* **2022**, *10*, 53, doi:10.3390/biomedicines10010053 . . . . **207**

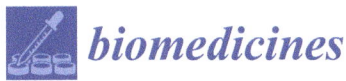

Editorial

Pathogenesis and Targeted Therapy of Epilepsy

Prosper N'Gouemo

Department of Physiology and Biophysics, Howard University College of Medicine, Washington, DC 20059, USA; prosper.ngouemo@howard.edu; Tel.: +1-202-806-9708

Citation: N'Gouemo, P. Pathogenesis and Targeted Therapy of Epilepsy. *Biomedicines* 2022, 10, 3134. https://doi.org/10.3390/biomedicines10123134

Received: 22 November 2022
Accepted: 1 December 2022
Published: 5 December 2022

Publisher's Note: MDPI stays neutral with regard to jurisdictional claims in published maps and institutional affiliations.

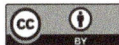

Copyright: © 2022 by the author. Licensee MDPI, Basel, Switzerland. This article is an open access article distributed under the terms and conditions of the Creative Commons Attribution (CC BY) license (https://creativecommons.org/licenses/by/4.0/).

The *Biomedicines* Special Issue (BSI) of "Pathogenesis and Targeted Therapy of Epilepsy" seeks papers providing new insights into the roles of voltage-gated and ligand-gated ion channels and their related signaling in the pathogenesis and pathophysiology of acquired epilepsy and inherited epilepsy. We are pleased that several renowned researchers have contributed to this first edition of BSI, comprising seven original articles and four reviews. Topics in this BSI include the identification of altered postsynaptic glutamate receptors as a potential mechanism underlying epileptogenesis in the hippocampus using the 4-aminopyridine in vitro model of epileptiform activity [1]. Another report suggests the activation of Ca^{2+}-activated chloride channels as a novel cellular mechanism for suppressing acoustically evoked generalized tonic-clonic seizures in the strain of the genetically epilepsy-prone rats exhibiting moderated seizure severity [2]. Using another model of acoustically evoked seizures (Wistar Audiogenic Rat, WAR), Lazarini-Lopes et al. [3] report that TRPV1 channels might contribute to the cellular mechanism underlying epileptogenesis and anxiety-like behavior following repetitive episodes of seizures. Furthermore, a comprehensive review discusses the relationship between acoustically evoked seizure susceptibility and post-ictal catalepsy and motor hyperactivity [4]. In another token, Kim and Kang [5] provide evidence of an upregulation of tandem of the P domain in weak inwardly rectifying K^+ channels (TWIK)-related acid-sensitive K^+-1 (TASK-1) channels in hippocampal CA1 astrocytes in the pilocarpine post-status epilepticus model of temporal lobe epilepsy. Another report from the same group reveals that co-treatment with an elective TASK-1 inhibitor and levetiracetam (LEV) reduced the severity of LEV refractory seizures. Additional studies from Kim et al. [6] provide evidence that dysregulation of AKT/GSK3b/CREB-mediated glutamate ionotropic receptor AMPA type 1 subunit (GRIA1) surface expression may contribute to AMPA receptor antagonists' refractory seizures in the pilocarpine model of temporal lobe epilepsy. Similarly, dysregulation of PP2B-ERK1/2-SGK1-NEDD4-2-mediated GRIA1 ubiquitination may also contribute to AMPA receptor antagonists' refractory seizures [7]. In a model of traumatic brain injury (TBI), Wang et al. [6] report that peripheral infection after TBI increases neuronal excitability and facilitates post-traumatic epileptogenesis in the pentylenetetrazole model of seizures [8]. Furthermore, Ndoke-Ekane et al. [9] provide evidence that magnetic resonance imaging (MRI) improves the placement accuracy of intracerebral electrode implantation and that chronically implanted electrodes do not increase cortical and hippocampal atrophy in a rat model of post-traumatic epilepsy. A review by Yamanaka et al. [10] discusses the neuroinflammatory role of brain pericytes in epilepsy. Finally, another study by Bucknix et al. [11] examines the potential mechanisms underlying the anticonvulsant effects mediated by the orexigenic peptide ghrelin.

Epilepsies are disorders of neuronal excitability characterized by the occurrence of spontaneous, repeated episodes of seizures, and their incidence rate continues to increase yearly. Although many antiseizure medications (ASM) are available, about 30% of epileptic patients have ASM-refractory seizures. Thus, there is a need to develop new therapies to mitigate epileptogenesis and ASM-refractory seizures based on novel molecular targets for controlling neuronal hyperexcitability that leads to seizures. This first edition of BSI provides evidence of novel molecular targets for controlling epileptogenesis, generalized tonic-clonic seizures, and ASM-refractory seizures.

Funding: This research was funded partially by the National Institute of Alcoholism and Alcohol Abuse (R01 AA027660) at the National Institutes of Health. The National Institute of Alcoholism and Alcohol Abuse had no further role in the decision to publish.

Conflicts of Interest: The author declares no conflict of interest.

References

1. Ergina, J.L.; Amakhin, D.V.; Postnikova, T.Y.; Soboleva, E.B.; Zaitsev, A.V. Short-term epileptiform activity potentiates excitatory synapses but does not affect intrinsic membrane properties of pyramidal neurons in the rat hippocampus in vitro. *Biomedicines* **2021**, *9*, 1374. [CrossRef] [PubMed]
2. Thomas, M.; Simms, M.; N'Gouemo, P. Activation of calcium-activated chloride channels suppresses inherited seizure susceptibility in genetically epilepsy-prone rats. *Biomedicines* **2022**, *10*, 449. [CrossRef] [PubMed]
3. Lazarini-Lopes, W.; Silva-Cardoso, G.K.; Leite-Panissi, C.R.A.; Garcia-Cairasco, N. Increased TRPV1 channels and FosB protein expression are associated with chronic epileptic seizures and anxiogenic-like behaviors in a Preclinical model of temporal lobe epilepsy. *Biomedicines* **2022**, *10*, 416. [CrossRef]
4. Fedotova, I.B.; Surina, N.M.; Nikolaev, G.M.; Revishchin, A.V.; Poletaeva, I. Rodent brain pathology, audiogenic epilepsy. *Biomedicines* **2021**, *9*, 1641. [CrossRef]
5. Kim, J.-E.; Kang, T.-C. Blockade of TASK-1 channel improves the efficacy of levetiracetam in chronically epileptic rats. *Biomedicines* **2022**, *10*, 787. [CrossRef]
6. Kim, J.-E.; Lee, D.-S.; Park, H.; Kim, T.-H.; Kang, T.-C. AMPA receptor antagonists facilitate NEDD4-2-mediated GRIA1 ubiquitination by regulating PP2B-ERK1/2-SGK1 pathway in chronic epilepsy rats. *Biomedicines* **2021**, *9*, 1069. [CrossRef]
7. Kim, J.-E.; Lee, D.-S.; Park, H.; Kim, T.-H.; Kang, T.-C. Inhibition of AKT/GSK3b/CREB pathway improves the responsiveness to AMPA receptor antagonists by regulating GRIA1 surface expression in chronic epilepsy rats. *Biomedicines* **2021**, *9*, 425. [CrossRef] [PubMed]
8. Wang, Y.; Andrade, P.; Pitkanen, A. Peripheral infection after traumatic brain injury augments excitability in the perilesional cortex and dentate gyrus. *Biomedicines* **2021**, *9*, 1946. [CrossRef] [PubMed]
9. Ndode-Ekane, X.E.; Immonen, R.; Hamalainen, E.; Manninen, E.; Andrade, P.; Ciszek, R.; Paananen, T.; Grohn, O.; Pitkanen, A. MRI-guided electrode implantation for chronic intracerebral recording in a rat model of post-traumatic epilepsy—Challenges and gains. *Biomedicines* **2022**, *10*, 2295. [CrossRef] [PubMed]
10. Yamanaka, G.; Takata, F.; Kataoka, Y.; Kanou, K.; Morichi, S.; Dohgu, S.; Kawashima, H. The neuroinflammatory role of pericytes in epilepsy. *Biomedicines* **2021**, *9*, 759. [CrossRef] [PubMed]
11. Buckinx, A.; De Bundel, D.; Kooijman, R.; Smolders, I. Targeting the ghrelin receptors as a novel therapeutic option for epilepsy. *Biomedicines* **2022**, *10*, 53. [CrossRef] [PubMed]

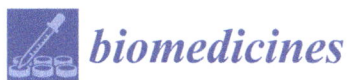

Article

Short-Term Epileptiform Activity Potentiates Excitatory Synapses but Does Not Affect Intrinsic Membrane Properties of Pyramidal Neurons in the Rat Hippocampus In Vitro

Julia L. Ergina, Dmitry V. Amakhin, Tatyana Y. Postnikova, Elena B. Soboleva and Aleksey V. Zaitsev *

Sechenov Institute of Evolutionary Physiology and Biochemistry of RAS, 44, Toreza Prospekt,
194223 Saint Petersburg, Russia; for.mail.ergin@gmail.com (J.L.E.); dmitry.amakhin@gmail.com (D.V.A.);
tapost2@mail.ru (T.Y.P.); soboleva.elena.1707@gmail.com (E.B.S.)
* Correspondence: aleksey_zaitsev@mail.ru

Abstract: Even brief epileptic seizures can lead to activity-dependent structural remodeling of neural circuitry. Animal models show that the functional plasticity of synapses and changes in the intrinsic excitability of neurons can be crucial for epileptogenesis. However, the exact mechanisms underlying epileptogenesis remain unclear. We induced epileptiform activity in rat hippocampal slices for 15 min using a 4-aminopyridine (4-AP) in vitro model and observed hippocampal hyperexcitability for at least 1 h. We tested several possible mechanisms of this hyperexcitability, including changes in intrinsic membrane properties of neurons and presynaptic and postsynaptic alterations. Neither input resistance nor other essential biophysical properties of hippocampal CA1 pyramidal neurons were affected by epileptiform activity. The glutamate release probability also remained unchanged, as the frequency of miniature EPSCs and the paired amplitude ratio of evoked responses did not change after epileptiform activity. However, we found an increase in the AMPA/NMDA ratio, suggesting alterations in the properties of postsynaptic glutamatergic receptors. Thus, the increase in excitability of hippocampal neural networks is realized through postsynaptic mechanisms. In contrast, the intrinsic membrane properties of neurons and the probability of glutamate release from presynaptic terminals are not affected in a 4-AP model.

Keywords: temporal lobe epilepsy; hippocampus; 4-aminopyridine; epilepsy model; long-term potentiation; AMPA receptor

Citation: Ergina, J.L.; Amakhin, D.V.; Postnikova, T.Y.; Soboleva, E.B.; Zaitsev, A.V. Short-Term Epileptiform Activity Potentiates Excitatory Synapses but Does Not Affect Intrinsic Membrane Properties of Pyramidal Neurons in the Rat Hippocampus In Vitro. *Biomedicines* **2021**, *9*, 1374. https://doi.org/10.3390/biomedicines9101374

Academic Editor: Prosper N'Gouemo

Received: 16 September 2021
Accepted: 30 September 2021
Published: 1 October 2021

Publisher's Note: MDPI stays neutral with regard to jurisdictional claims in published maps and institutional affiliations.

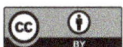

Copyright: © 2021 by the authors. Licensee MDPI, Basel, Switzerland. This article is an open access article distributed under the terms and conditions of the Creative Commons Attribution (CC BY) license (https://creativecommons.org/licenses/by/4.0/).

1. Introduction

A significant number of cases of temporal lobe epilepsy in humans develop in healthy people as a result of injury or disease. Acquired epilepsy is often a progressive disease that is resistant to pharmacological treatment [1]. Therefore, it is crucial to know the initial molecular and cellular abnormalities specific to epileptogenesis. Based on this knowledge, more promising therapeutic strategies for the prevention of acquired temporal lobe epilepsy can be developed [2,3].

In vitro brain tissue preparations allow the simple and accessible study of brain networks and provide an opportunity to understand the brain's molecular and cellular mechanisms of functioning in health and disease with detail that is unattainable in vivo. Therefore, in vitro brain slices are generally recognized as an optimal model for studying epileptiform activity in the brain tissue [4]. Among multiple in vitro models, many researchers utilized a 4-aminopyridine (4-AP)-based model to successfully induce epileptiform activity in the hippocampus and cortical areas [5–8]. 4-AP blocks voltage-gated potassium channels Kv1.1, Kv1.2, and Kv1.4, which are particularly important for action potential repolarization. This, in turn, promotes the enhanced release of glutamate and, therefore, an overactivation of glutamate receptors [9]. At the same time, GABA-mediated transmission paradoxically facilitates neuronal hyperexcitation in 4-AP-based epilepsy models [8]. Ultimately, both pyramidal neurons and interneurons seem to contribute to the generation of 4-AP-induced epileptiform activity [10–12].

Even relatively short seizures can lead to activity-dependent structural remodeling of neural circuits, resulting in increased network excitability. Although most mesial temporal lobe structures are highly susceptible to seizures, the hippocampal area demonstrates the heaviest damage in response to seizure activity [13,14]. Several mechanisms can provoke changes in the excitability of neuronal networks, including changes in intrinsic neuronal excitability [15–17], potentiation of excitatory synaptic contacts [9,18–21], changes in synaptic inhibition [22–25], and cell loss and sprouting of axons [26–28]. However, relatively little is known about the precise mechanisms of the network excitability increase resulting from a brief episode of epileptic activity—what specific changes occur at presynaptic and postsynaptic levels, and how these changes affect hippocampal circuit functioning.

In the present study, using a 4-aminopyridine model of epileptiform activity in vitro, we experimentally investigated mechanisms involved in the increased neuronal excitability in the CA1 hippocampal area. We focused on the alternations that persist 1 h after the short-term epileptiform activity.

2. Materials and Methods

2.1. Animals and Brain Slice Preparation

Juvenile Wistar rats (postnatal days 21–23) were used in this study. All the experiments were carried out according to the Guidelines on the Treatment of Laboratory Animals effective at the Sechenov Institute of Evolutionary Physiology and Biochemistry of the Russian Academy of Sciences. These guidelines comply with Russian and international standards.

Acute brain slices were obtained as previously described [29]. In brief, rats were decapitated and the brains were quickly removed and placed in ice-cold oxygenated (95% O_2: 5% CO_2) artificial cerebrospinal fluid (ACSF) containing (in mM) 126 NaCl, 24 $NaHCO_3$, 2.5 KCl, 2 $CaCl_2$, 1.25 NaH_2PO_4, 1 $MgSO_4$, and 10 dextrose. Horizontal entorhinal-hippocampal brain slices (300–350 µm) were prepared with Microm HM 650V vibratome (Microm, Dreieich, Germany) and allowed to recover for 1 h before electrophysiological experiments began.

2.2. Induction of Short-Term Epileptiform Activity In Vitro

Epileptiform activity was induced by an epileptogenic low-magnesium solution with the voltage-gated potassium ion channel inhibitor 4-AP. The solution contained the following (in mM): 120 NaCl, 8.5 KCl, 1.25 NaH_2PO_4, 0.25 $MgSO_4$, 2 $CaCl_2$, 24 $NaHCO_3$, 10 dextrose, and 0.05 4-AP. This solution induced epileptiform activity in the slice with a delay of 3–5 min. The brain slices were kept in this solution for 20 min at 30 °C. After that, the slices were washed in ACSF for 1 h. All solutions were oxygenated (95% O_2/5% CO_2).

2.3. Field Excitatory Postsynaptic Potential (fEPSP) Recordings

Field EPSPs were registered from the CA1 stratum radiatum using a glass microelectrode (0.2–1.0 MΩ) filled with ACSF. Synaptic responses were evoked by local extracellular stimulation of the Schaffer collaterals using a bipolar twisted stimulating electrode made of insulated nichrome wire (0.7 mm in diameter). The stimulating electrode was placed in the stratum radiatum at the CA1–CA2 border at 1 mm from the recording electrode. The dependence of fEPSP amplitude and the fiber volleys (FVs) amplitude on stimulation strength was determined by increasing the current intensity from 25 to 300 µA with a step of 25 µA via an A365 stimulus isolator (World Precision Instruments, Sarasota, FL, USA). Responses were recorded with the Model 1800 Microelectrode AC Amplifier (A-M Systems, Carlsborg, WA, USA). They were digitized with ADC/DAC NI USB-6211 (National Instruments, Austin, TX, USA) using WinWCP v5 software (University of Strathclyde, Glasgow, UK). As previously described [17], the maximum rise slope of the input–output

(I/O) relationships (fEPSP amplitude vs. FV amplitude) was calculated for every slice by fitting with a sigmoidal Gompertz function:

$$f\left[I; a, k, I_{infl}\right] = ae^{-e^{(-k(I-I_{infl}))}} \quad (1)$$

where e is Euler's number (e = 2.71828 ...), a is the asymptote of the maximum response amplitude, I_{infl} is the inflection current (in pA), which was the value of the stimulation current at which the maximum slope of the curve was observed, and k is the positive number that determines the slope of the curve. The maximum slope of the curve (in Hz/pA) was calculated as a × k/e.

2.4. Patch-Clamp Experiments

CA1 hippocampal pyramidal neurons were identified using a Zeiss Axioscop 2 microscope (Zeiss; Oberkochen, Germany) equipped with differential interference contrast optics and the video camera PointGrey Grasshopper3 GS3-U3-23S6M-C (FLIR Integrated Imaging Solutions Inc., Wilsonville, OR, USA). Signals were recorded using a Multiclamp 700B (Molecular Devices, Sunnyvale, CA, USA) patch-clamp amplifier and an NI USB-6343 A/D converter (National Instruments, Austin, TX, USA) using WinWCP 5 software (University of Strathclyde, Glasgow, UK).

Patch pipettes with tip resistance 2–5 MΩ were pulled from borosilicate filamented glass capillaries (World Precision Instruments, Sarasota, FL, USA) using a P-1000 Micropipette Puller (Sutter Instrument; Novato, CA, USA). The intracellular patch pipette solution for whole-cell recordings contained (in mM) 136 K-Gluconate, 10 NaCl, 5 EGTA, 10 HEPES, 4 ATP-Mg, and 0.3 GTP; pH was adjusted to 7.25 with KOH. A cesium-methanesulfonate-based intracellular patch pipette solution was used for the recordings of the AMPAR- and NMDAR-mediated currents; the composition, in mM, was 127 $CsMeSO_4$, 10 NaCl, 5 EGTA, 10 HEPES, 6 QX314, 4 ATP-Mg, and 0.3 GTP; pH was adjusted to 7.25 with CsOH. Access resistance was typically 10–15 MΩ and remained stable during the experiments (< 30% increase) for all cells included in the analysis.

The synaptic responses were evoked with a bipolar stimulating electrode placed at 100–200 μm from the recorded neuron. To evaluate the dependence of the AMPAR-mediated response amplitude from the stimulation current, the AMPAR-mediated EPSCs were recorded in the presence of an NMDAR channel blocker MK-801 (10 μM, Alomone Labs, Jerusalem, Israel) at the holding potential of −56 mV, which is equal to the reversal potential of GABAaR-mediated currents as it was found in our previous studies utilizing the same pipette and extracellular solutions [12,21,30].

The dependence of the evoked EPSC (eEPSC) amplitude on stimulation strength was determined by increasing the current intensity from 0 to 1000 μA via an A365 stimulus isolator (WPI Inc., Blacksburg, VA, USA). The obtained dependence was fitted with a sigmoid Gompertz function (Equation (1)).

In order to investigate the AMPA/NMDA ratio, the AMPAR-mediated EPSCs were recorded at the holding potential of −80 mV in the presence of bicuculline (20 μM), a GABAa receptor blocker. NMDAR-mediated EPSCs were recorded at +40 mV, in the presence of bicuculline and DNQX (10 μM, Tocris Bioscience, Bristol, UK), an AMPAR antagonist. The AMPA/NMDA ratio was calculated as a peak amplitudes ratio. Data were analyzed with Clampfit 10.0 software (Molecular Devices, Sunnyvale, CA, USA).

Recordings of miniature EPSCs (mEPSCs) were done in the presence of tetrodotoxin (TTX, 0.5 μM; Alomone Labs) and GABAR blockers (picrotoxin, 50 μM and bicuculline, 10 μM, Tocris Bioscience). Miniature events were detected and analyzed using Clampfit 10 software (Molecular Devices, Sunnyvale, CA, USA). The mEPSC amplitudes were determined from the baseline to the peak.

Intrinsic membrane properties of neurons were evaluated from the voltage responses to the series of 1500-ms current steps with 10–20 pA increments using custom scripts written in Wolfram Mathematica 10 (Wolfram Research, Champaign, IL, USA). Only neurons with the typical regular-spiking pattern were included.

The resting membrane potential (V_{rest}, in mV) was measured as an averaged potential before the current step application. The input resistance (R_{input}; in MΩ) was calculated as the voltage–current (V–I) curve slope. The membrane time constant (τ_m; in ms) was estimated by fitting a single exponential function to the voltage transient induced by the −25 pA current step.

The firing rate–current (f/I) curves were used to describe the firing properties of neurons. The firing rate was estimated as the number of action potentials per current step. The rising part of the f/I curve was fitted with a sigmoidal Gompertz function (Equation (1)).

2.5. Data Analysis and Statistics

The data were processed with Statistics 8 (StatSoft Inc., Tulsa, OK, USA), OriginPro 8 (OriginLab Corporation, Northampton, MA, USA), and Sigmaplot 12.5 (Systat Software Inc., San Jose, CA, USA). Statistical significance was assessed using the Student's *t*-test and ANOVA as stated in the text. All data are presented as the mean with the standard error of the mean. $p < 0.05$ was considered statistically significant.

3. Results

3.1. Epileptiform Activity in Entorhinal-Hippocampal Slices

This study investigated the short-term (within 1 h) effects of epileptiform activity on synaptic and nonsynaptic plasticity in the hippocampus. Epileptiform activity in rat entorhinal-hippocampal slices was induced by 20-min exposure to the 4-AP-containing bath solution with altered extracellular ion concentrations (8.5 mM K^+; 0.25 mM Mg^{2+}). As we have shown previously, this epileptogenic solution reliably induced discharges in the rat entorhinal cortex approximately 7–10 min after application [30]. In the CA1 hippocampal area, the first discharges emerged even earlier, in 3–5 min (Figure 1). Thus, the total duration of epileptiform activity in the hippocampal network was about 15 min.

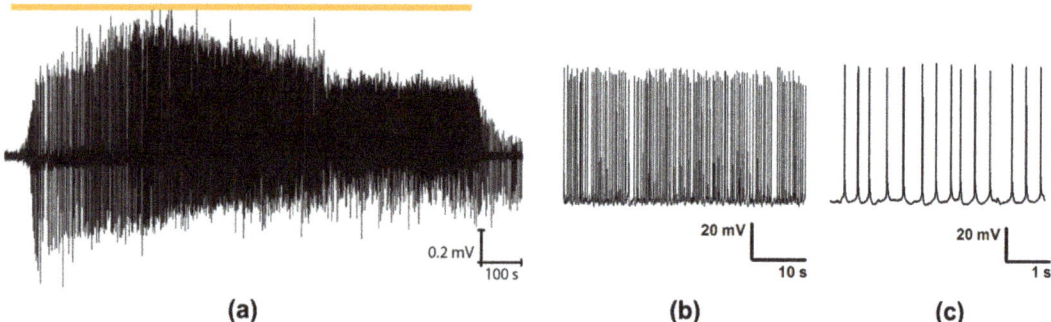

Figure 1. Epileptiform activity in rat brain slices. (**a**) Representative recording of epileptiform activity in the CA1 hippocampal area induced by the epileptogenic solution (local field potential (LFP) recording). (**b**,**c**) The interictal discharges registered in CA1 pyramidal cells (whole-cell current-clamp recordings at different time scale).

3.2. Epileptiform Activity Increases the Gain of Input–Output Relationship in CA3-CA1 Synapses

One hour after washing the sections in Ringer's solution, we examined the properties of synaptic transmission in the hippocampal CA3-CA1 synapses. This time interval is sufficient to trigger intracellular signaling cascades and induce plasticity [31].

We registered fEPSPs in response to extracellular stimulation of Shaffer collaterals at a range of current intensities (Figure 2a). Even in one hour, the 4-AP-treated slices (4-AP slices) exhibited significantly increased excitability compared with the control. Although the threshold of fEPSP initiation was similar in both groups (Figure 2b, control: 52 ± 2 μA, $n = 11$; 4-AP–slices: 46 ± 4 μA; $n = 6$; t-test = 1.49, $p = 0.16$), the amplitude of fEPSP increased significantly faster with increasing stimulation current strength (Figure 3a, repeated-measures ANOVA: $F_{7,105} = 4.3$, $p < 0.001$). In addition, the threshold of population spike generation was much lower than that in the control slices (Figure 2c, control: 150 ± 21 μA, $n = 11$; 4-AP–slices: 58 ± 5 μA; $n = 6$; t-test = 3.18, $p < 0.01$).

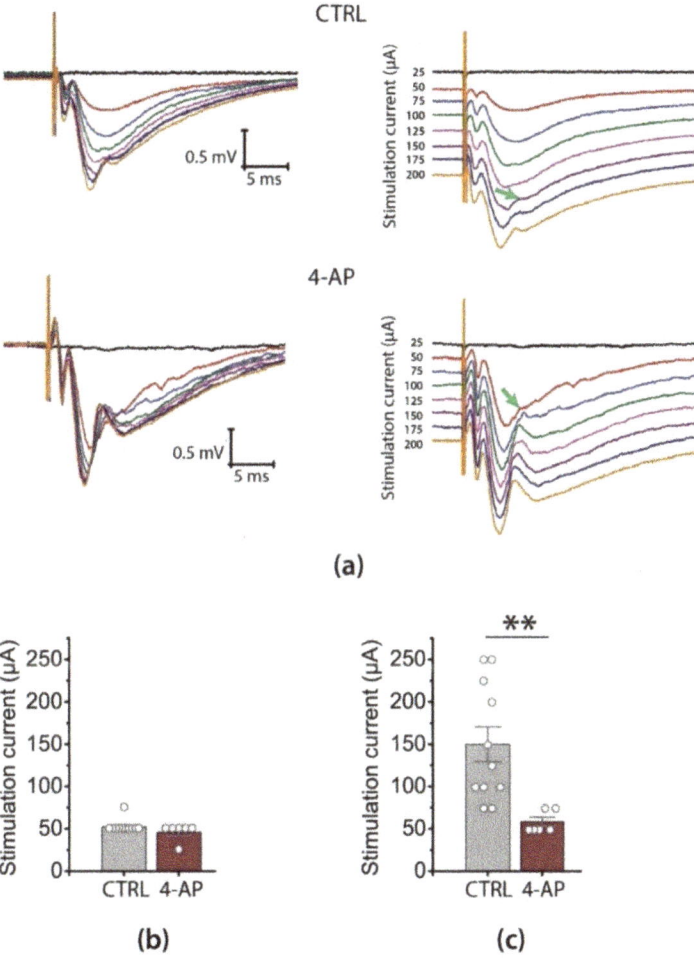

Figure 2. The effect of the short-term epileptiform activity on the basic synaptic transmission at CA3-CA1 hippocampal synapses. (**a**) Examples of local field excitatory postsynaptic potentials (fEPSP) recorded in stratum radiatum in control (CTRL) and after the period of the short-term epileptiform activity (4-AP). On the right, the same recordings are shown with the shift. The arrows point to the notches corresponding to the population spikes in the fEPSP recordings. Diagrams show the threshold of fEPSP initiation (**b**) and the threshold of population spike generation (**c**). All the data are presented as mean ± standard error of the mean, and each dot represents an individual value. ** $p < 0.01$: A significant difference versus the control group (t-test).

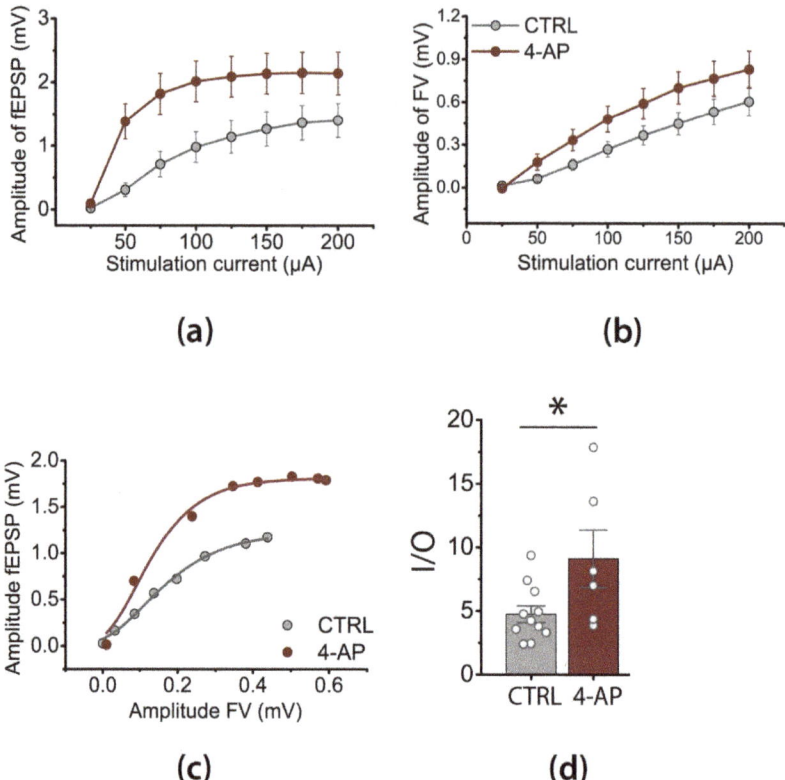

Figure 3. The effect of the short-term epileptiform activity on the basic synaptic transmission at CA3-CA1 hippocampal synapses. (**a**) Stimulation response relationships for fEPSP amplitudes, and (**b**) presynaptic fiber volley (FV), accordingly. (**c**,**d**) Changes in the maximal I/O slope after the period of the short-term epileptiform activity * $p < 0.05$, a significant difference versus the control group according to the Student's *t*-test.

To determine whether this increase in synaptic strength could result from enhanced presynaptic excitability, we have plotted the relationships between FV amplitude, a measure of presynaptic axon depolarization, and stimulus strength in control and 4-AP–slices (Figure 3b). We found that these relationships did not differ between the groups (effect of epileptiform activity: $F_{1,105} = 3.4$, $p = 0.08$), suggesting that the excitability of presynaptic axons was not affected.

To estimate the efficacy of basal synaptic transmission, we assessed the average slope of I/O curves plotted as fEPSP amplitudes vs. FV amplitudes (Figure 3c,d). Using a sigmoidal Gompertz function [17] to determine the maximum rise slope of the curves, we found that this value was significantly larger in 4-AP–slices (9 ± 2) than in control ones (4.8 ± 0.7, $t = 2.35$, $p = 0.03$; Figure 3d).

Together, these data suggest that short-term epileptiform activity increases neuronal excitability in the CA1 hippocampal area by increasing the synaptic efficacy in the CA3–CA1 synapses.

Next, we performed a similar experiment using the patch-clamp recording technique (Figure 4). We determined the relationships between the amplitude AMPAR-mediated eEPSCs and the stimulation current magnitude and then fitted them with the Gompertz function (Figure 4a,b).

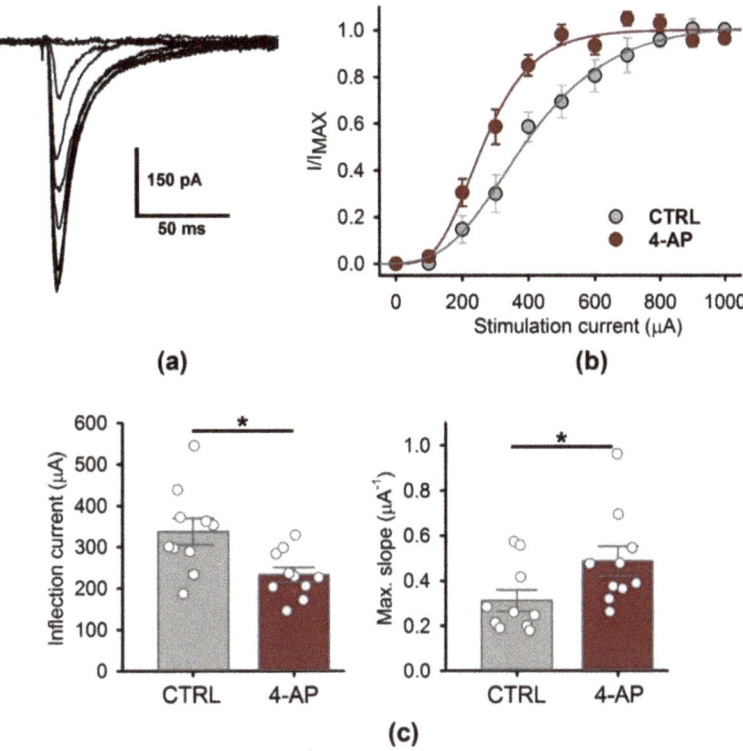

Figure 4. The effect of a period of epileptiform activity on the AMPAR-mediated eEPSC. (**a**) A representative set of 11 AMPAR-mediated eEPSCs, induced by the stimulation current of the increasing magnitude (from 0 to 1000 μA with the step of 100 μA). (**b**) The peak amplitude of AMPAR-mediated response vs. stimulus strength in control conditions and following a period of epileptiform activity (n = 10 for both cases). The data were normalized to the maximal response and fitted with the Gomperz function (Equation (1)). (**c**) The parameters of the Gompertz function under control conditions and following a period of epileptiform activity. A decrease in the inflection current (left) and an increase in the maximal slope of the curve (right) were detected; * $p < 0.05$, a significant difference versus the control group according to the Student's t-test.

In the presence of intact GABAergic transmission, we saw that following a period of epileptiform activity, the inflection current was decreased, and the slope of the curve was increased compared to the control (Figure 4c). These results indicate that smaller stimulation currents could evoke the same amplitude AMPAR-mediated eEPSCs (Figure 4).

Several factors can potentially contribute to the increased excitability of pyramidal neurons following epileptiform activity. This may be due to an increase in the probability of glutamate release, the number of receptors on the postsynaptic membrane, or the input resistance of the membrane. The latter would result in increased membrane depolarization for the same amount of incoming current through the synaptic receptors.

3.3. Biophysical Properties of CA1 Pyramidal Neurons

The change in membrane properties may explain the fact that we observed a significant increase in the amplitude of fEPSPs, but saw more minor changes in postsynaptic currents. To estimate the effect of short-term epileptiform activity on biophysical properties of hippocampal neurons, we recorded the responses of CA1 pyramidal neurons to current steps (from −50 to +25 pA with an increment of 25 pA). We evaluated input resistance, resting membrane potential, and membrane time constant (Figure 5). With the intact inhibitory synaptic transmission, only a slight increase of the resting membrane potential from −61.8 ± 0.5 mV to −60.1 ± 0.5 mV was detected following a period of seizures (Figure 5b; *t*-test, *p* = 0.03), while the other two parameters were unaltered. No significant changes in any of these parameters were detected in the presence of bicuculline, a GABAa receptor blocker (Figure 5c). The observed depolarizing effect of GABAergic transmission may indicate that changes in the driving force of Cl$^-$ ions that occur during epileptiform activity [24] persist for at least one hour. Thus, epileptiform activity had almost no effect on the subthreshold properties of the CA1 pyramidal neurons.

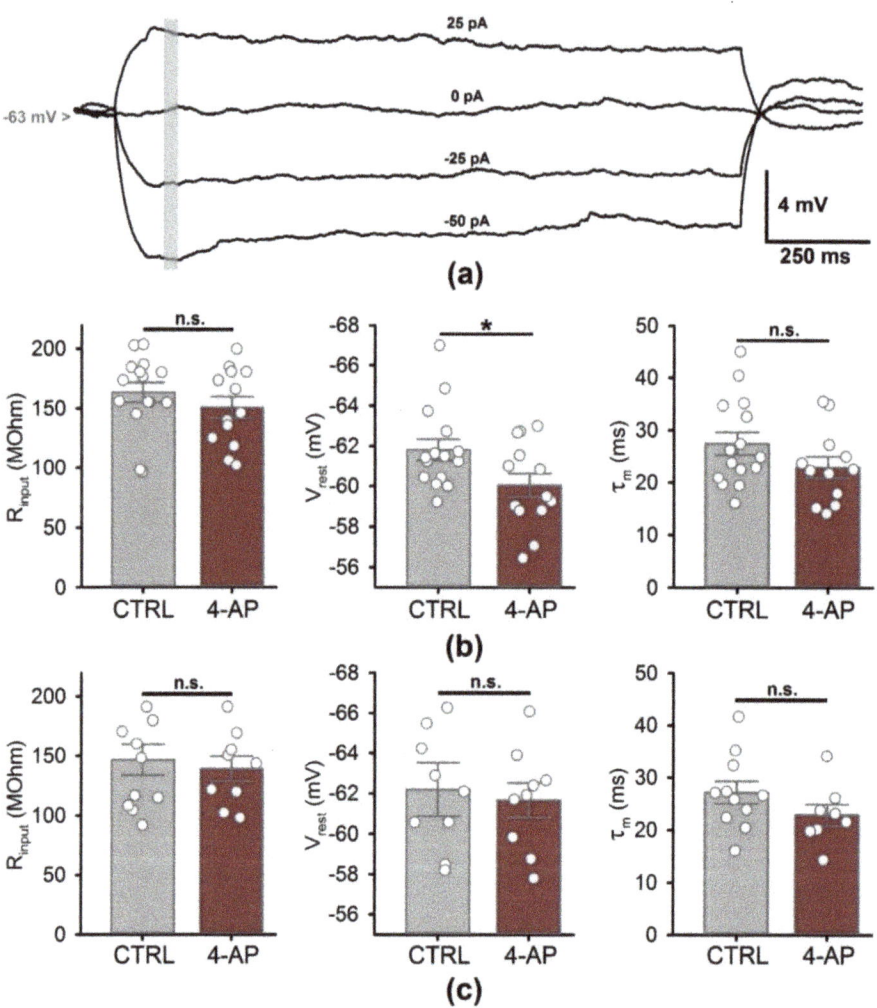

Figure 5. Changes of the subthreshold membrane properties of the neurons following a period of epileptiform activity induced by 4-aminopyridine-containing solution (4-AP). (**a**) A representative set of subthreshold responses to current steps from −50 to +25 pA. The gray bar indicates the time interval used to obtain the average values of membrane potential for the estimation of the input resistance. (**b**) Comparison of the membrane properties with the intact GABAergic synaptic transmission. (**c**) The exact comparisons in the presence of bicuculline, a GABAa receptor blocker. Data are presented as the mean with standard error of the mean. Each circle represents a value obtained in an individual neuron. * $p < 0.05$, a significant difference versus the control group according to the Student's *t*-test.

Additionally, we investigated whether epileptiform activity affected the firing properties of hippocampal neurons (Figure 6). We fitted the rising parts of the f/I curve with the Gompertz equation (Equation (1)) and investigated whether the obtained parameters were altered after epileptiform activity (Figure 6a,b). We detected no significant changes in the maximal slope, inflection current, and the maximal frequency of the AP generation, both with intact GABAergic inhibition (Figure 6c) and in the presence of bicuculline (Figure 6d). Taken together, these results indicate that a period of epileptiform activity did not change the intrinsic excitability of CA1 neurons.

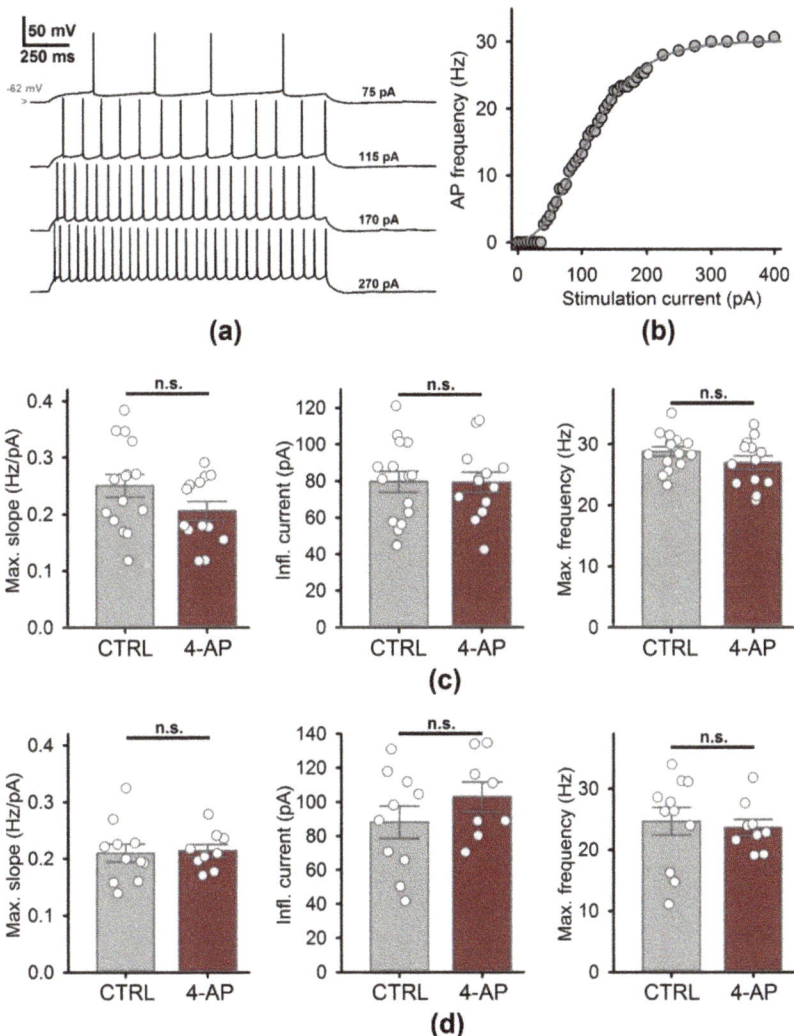

Figure 6. The firing properties of CA1 neurons do not change following a period of epileptiform activity induced by a 4-aminopyridine-containing solution (4-AP). (**a**) A representative set of voltage responses to depolarizing current steps was used to obtain the f/I curve (**b**). The data were fitted with the Gompertz function. (**c**) The comparisons of the parameters of the f/I curves, obtained with the intact GABAergic synaptic transmission. (**d**) Same comparisons in the presence of bicuculline, a GABAa receptor blocker. In both cases, no significant changes were detected (*t*-test was used for all comparisons).

3.4. Presynaptic Properties of CA1 Pyramidal Neurons 1 H after the Epileptiform Activity

To assess possible changes in the probability of glutamate release, we measured the frequency of mEPSCs and the paired-pulse ratio of eEPSCs. These parameters are traditionally employed to evaluate the transmitter release probability [32].

The registration of mEPSCs was carried out in the presence of tetrodotoxin (0.5 µM) and GABAa receptor blockers (picrotoxin, 50 µM and bicuculline, 10 µM; Figure 5a). Neither frequency (control: 0.21 ± 0.05 Hz; $n = 7$ vs. 4-AP–group: 0.18 ± 0.03 Hz; $n = 7$; t-test = 0.55, $p = 0.60$) nor amplitude (control: 20.3 ± 1.0 pA; $n = 7$ vs. 4-AP–group: 22.6 ± 1.7 pA; $n = 7$; t-test = 1.17, $p = 0.26$) differed significantly from control values (Figure 7).

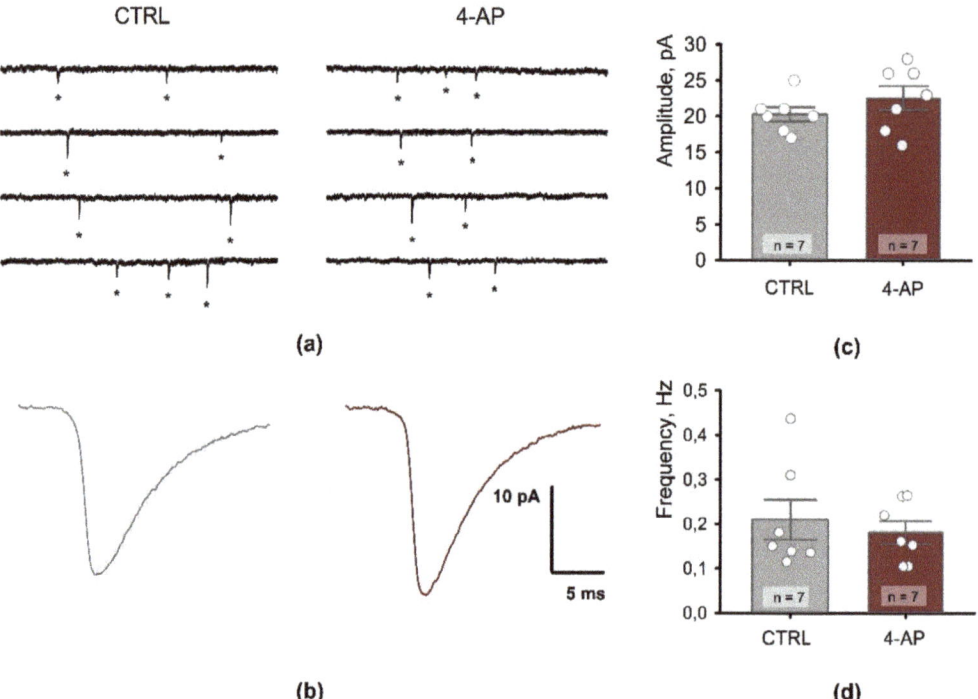

Figure 7. Properties of miniature excitatory postsynaptic currents (mEPSCs) 1 h after the period of short-term epileptiform activity. (**a**) Miniature EPSCs registered in the CA1 pyramidal neuron in the control (left) and 1 h after epileptiform activity (right). $V_{hold} = -80$ mV. (**b**) Representative examples of averaged mEPSCs from control (black) and 4-AP (red) pyramidal neurons. Graphs showing amplitude (**c**) and frequency (**d**) of mEPSCs in control (CTRL) and 1 h after epileptiform activity (4-AP). Data are presented as the mean with standard error of the mean. Each circle represents a value obtained in an individual neuron. No significant difference was detected between the control and 4-AP groups.

The eEPSC responses to paired stimuli are shown in Figure 8. There was no significant change in PPR following epileptiform activity (control: 1.72 ± 0.09; $n = 11$ vs. 4-AP group: 1.73 ± 0.11; $n = 9$; t-test for independent samples = 0.02, $p = 0.98$).

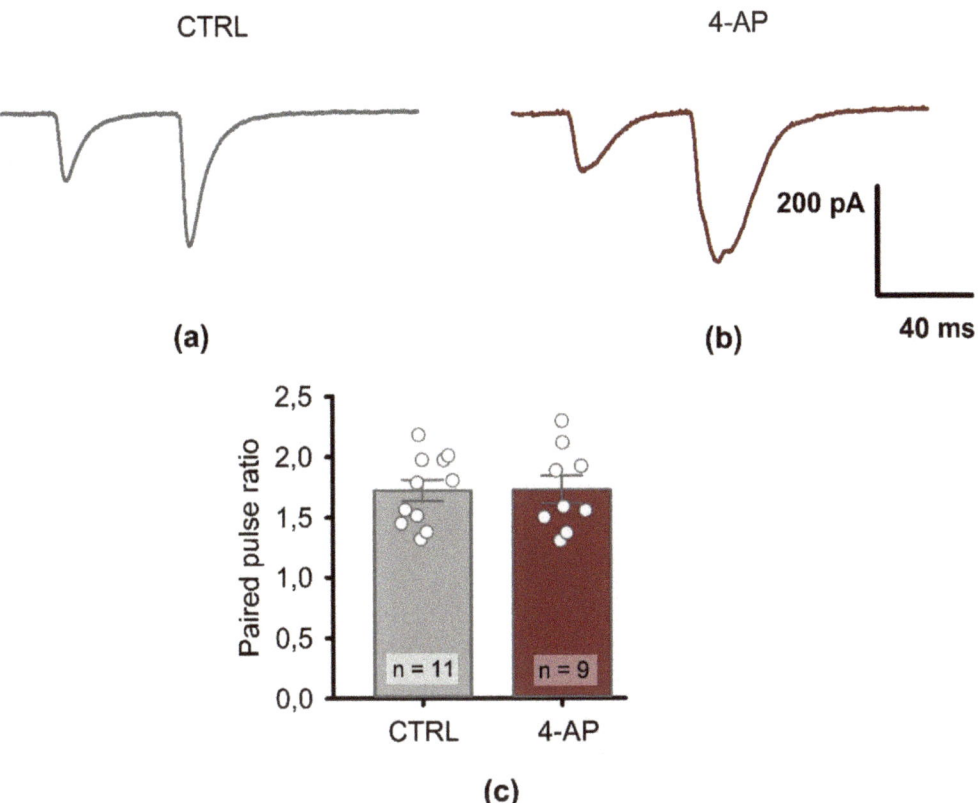

Figure 8. The paired-pulse amplitude ratio (PPR) of eEPSC recorded in the CA1 region of rat hippocampus in control and 1 h after short-term epileptiform activity. Representative examples of CA1 pyramidal neuron responses to a paired stimulus (inter-stimulus interval = 50 ms) in control (**a**) and 1 h after EA (**b**). (**c**) The bar graph shows PPR in control (CTRL) and 1 h after epileptiform activity (4-AP). Data are presented as the mean with standard error of the mean. Each circle represents a value obtained in an individual neuron. No significant difference was detected between the control and 4-AP groups.

The absence of differences in the frequency of mEPSCs and PPR indicates that the probability of glutamate release from presynaptic terminals has not changed.

3.5. Postsynaptic Properties of CA1 Pyramidal Neurons

As shown above, in this model, epileptiform activity strongly enhances AMPAR-mediated neurotransmission. Therefore, we tested whether epileptiform activity alters the contribution of AMPAR- and NMDAR-mediated currents at the postsynaptic membrane. We found that epileptiform activity leads to a significant increase in the AMPA/NMDA ratio (Figure 9, control: 2.61 ± 0.20; $n = 10$ vs. 4-AP group: 3.91 ± 0.34; $n = 9$; t-test for independent samples = 3.39, $p < 0.01$). These results indicate the incorporation of new AMPARs into the postsynaptic membrane.

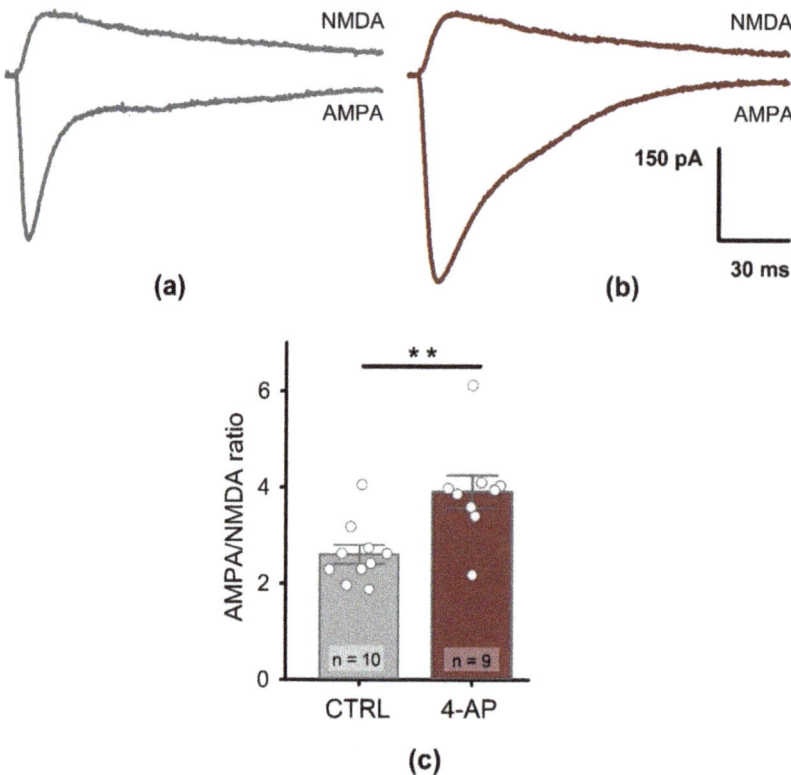

Figure 9. Postsynaptic properties of CA1 pyramidal neurons before and after the period of short-term epileptiform activity induced by 4-aminopyridine-containing solution (4-AP). Representative examples of AMPAR- or NMDAR-mediated currents in control (**a**) and 1 h after the period of short-term epileptiform activity induced by 4-AP (**b**). AMPAR-mediated responses were recorded −80 mV in the presence of bicuculline (20 µM), a GABAa receptor blocker. NMDAR-mediated EPSCs were recorded at +40 mV in the presence of bicuculline and DNQX (10 µM), an AMPAR antagonist. (**c**) The bar graph shows the AMPA/NMDA amplitude ratio increase after the period of the short-term epileptiform activity. Data are presented as the mean with standard error of the mean. Each circle represents a value obtained in an individual neuron. ** $p < 0.01$: A significant difference with the control group (t-test).

4. Discussion

A brief period of epileptiform activity increased hippocampal excitability, as demonstrated by the change in the I/O ratio of the fEPSPs. We tested several possible mechanisms, including changes in intrinsic membrane properties of neurons, and pre- and postsynaptic alterations. Neither input resistance nor other essential biophysical properties of hippocampal CA1 pyramidal neurons were affected by epileptiform activity. Furthermore, we did not detect any differences in the PPR of eEPSC amplitudes nor the frequency of mEPSC, leading us to conclude that 4-AP-induced epileptiform activity did not affect glutamate release probability. The absence of changes in the amplitude of fiber volley also indicates that presynaptic properties of glutamatergic transmission are not responsible for the observed increase in excitability. However, epileptiform activity in the 4-AP model increased the AMPA/NMDA ratio, suggesting that the alterations in the properties of postsynaptic glutamatergic receptors are the most likely explanation for the enhancement of basic synaptic transmission.

Our data are consistent with results obtained in other studies focused on the effects of short-term epileptiform activity in vitro. The 10-min perfusion of hippocampal slices with high K$^+$ (10 mM) solution changed the slope of fEPSP recorded in the stratum radiatum of CA1. The observed potentiation reached its maximum level about 30 min after washout and was still detectable 60 min after washout [33]. Similar results were obtained in two other studies: (1) The potentiation of the fEPSPs was observed 50 min after the washout of high-K$^+$-containing solution [34] and (2) at least 40 min after the washout of 4-AP (200 µM) [9]. Interestingly, even a brief period of epileptiform activity (40 s) has been observed to potentiate the amplitudes of fEPSPs (20 min after the washout), albeit hippocampal slices were exposed to very high levels of extracellular K$^+$ (50 mM KCl) [18]. Organotypic hippocampal slice cultures demonstrated potentiation at CA3-CA1 synapses in response to a very brief period of epileptiform activity (0.5–3 min) induced either by bicuculline or by Mg^{2+}-free solution. Potentiation of the fEPSP amplitude lasted at least 15 min after the washout of Mg^{2+}-free solution and at least 30 min after the washout of bicuculline-containing solution [19]. In another study, using a high K$^+$ model, the potentiation of the fEPSP slope in the CA1 area was reported, while the amplitude of FV was not affected [35].

The blockade of GABAaR-mediated inhibition and subsequent epileptiform activity has also been shown to lead to persisting changes in the properties of fEPSPs recorded in CA3 stratum radiatum/moleculare. Potentiation, defined as at least a 20% increase in the rising phase slope of fEPSPs, has been seen as long as 120 min after the washout of penicillin (2000 IU/mL) and cessation of spontaneous bursting [36].

Several mechanisms of increased excitability of hippocampal neural networks after epileptiform activity have been elucidated. For instance, a change in the neuronal network activity level can alter the intrinsic membrane properties of neurons [37–39]. Input resistance, especially, demonstrates close ties with mechanisms of homeostatic and non-homeostatic plasticity [40]. It should be noted that 4-AP alters the intrinsic membrane properties of neurons by inhibiting voltage-gated potassium ion channels, expanding action potentials [41]. However, in our experiments, we measured the membrane properties of neurons as early as one hour after washout of 4-AP, so this effect of 4-AP can be neglected.

In patients with pharmacoresistant epilepsy, neuronal loss in the CA1 region is frequently observed [42], suggesting that CA1 pyramidal neurons are among the most vulnerable cells to seizures. In this study, we found no significant effect of epileptiform activity on the passive membrane properties or firing properties of CA1 hippocampal neurons, although some studies have shown such changes. For example, 4-AP-induced epileptiform activity in the neocortex increased input resistance of parvalbumin-expressing neurons and reduced the action potential threshold for parvalbumin-expressing and pyramidal neurons both [43]. Apart from the 4-AP model, an increase in input resistance has been observed in the CA1 neurons of genetically epilepsy-prone rats [44], kindled rats [45], and in the pentylenetetrazole model [17]. However, after acute kainate-induced status epilepticus, there were no changes in input resistance in CA1 neurons [46], and the resting membrane potential and input resistance in piriform cortex neurons were not affected by abnormal activity induced by repeatedly applied tetanic stimulation [47]. In the lithium-pilocarpine model, seizures decreased the input resistance in entorhinal neurons [16]. As for other biophysical properties, there had been a decrease demonstrated in the membrane time constant in entorhinal and prefrontal neurons [16], significant membrane depolarization in CA1 neurons of kindled rats [45], latency of action potentials was prolonged, and the action potential half-width was increased 3–4 h after acute kainate-induced SE [46]. The exposure of immature hippocampal-cultured neurons to tetrodotoxin (0.5 µM) for 7–9 days, which led to spontaneous discharges, also affected the biophysical properties of cultured neurons. Neurons exhibited action potential broadening, lack of afterhyperpolarization, and had higher firing rates long after the medium was returned to standard composition [48]. The abnormal neuronal activity has also been shown to decrease A-type potassium currents [15] and hyperpolarization-activated currents [49,50], and increase T-type calcium channel-mediated currents [51,52] and persistent sodium currents [53]—the alternations mentioned above all have an impact on passive and active neuronal properties. Thus, changes in membrane properties depend primarily on the model used and the duration of epileptic activity. Likely, the short period of epileptiform activity in the model used was not sufficient to affect the membrane properties of neurons. Therefore, this mechanism is not involved in increasing the excitability of hippocampal neural networks.

In the presented work, we did not reveal presynaptic changes after epileptiform activity. The application of 4-AP affects the paired-pulse ratio, and during continuous perfusion of brain slices with 4-AP paired-pulse facilitation, turns into paired-pulse depression [9,54,55], suggesting an increase in neurotransmitter release probability. The frequency of mEPSCs was also significantly elevated during 4-AP-induced epileptiform activity, supporting that idea [9]. However, the duration of this effect remains unclear. In a model using overnight incubation in the bicuculline (50 µM), an increase in the frequency of mEPSC was detected. However, this is probably not due to changes in the probability of neurotransmitter release since no differences in the paired-pulse ratio were observed. Instead, this can be caused by the conversion of silent synapses into functional synapses [56].

We believe that postsynaptic changes are the primary mechanism of increased excitability of hippocampal neural networks. An increase in the AMPA/NMDA ratio is in favor of this assumption. It indicates that epileptiform activity led to the incorporation of AMPARs into the postsynaptic membrane. The incorporation of AMPARs is a well-known mechanism of synaptic plasticity that mediates activity-dependent synaptic changes during learning and memory [57]. The regulation of AMPAR trafficking to and from synapses involves lateral diffusion [58] and vesicular trafficking [59]. When on the membrane, AMPARs usually rapidly diffuse, while upon long-term potentiation (LTP), AMPARs get trapped at postsynaptic sites [58,60]. As confirmed recently, receptor trapping and clustering occur selectively opposite presynaptic release sites to ensure optimal receptor activation on neurotransmitter release [61,62].

AMPAR-mediated plasticity during epileptiform activity is rapid and often involves the incorporation of calcium-permeable AMPARs. The change in AMPAR-mediated transmission can be triggered by a 10–20-min period of epileptiform activity, as demonstrated in the in vitro epilepsy model [62] and pilocarpine model [63]. Peak AMPAR-mediated responses have been increased 2-fold during 4-AP-induced epileptiform activity in the entorhinal cortex, remained potentiated 15 min after short-term epileptiform activity in vitro, and this potentiation was shown to be NMDAR-dependent and at least partly mediated by the incorporation of calcium-permeable AMPARs [21]. There are multiple reports of changes in AMPAR protein expression levels and AMPAR subunit phosphorylation in the hippocampus several hours after seizures. The phosphorylation of 2 GluR1 subunit sites (S831 and S845) has been detectable 1 h after hypoxia-induced seizures and reached its maximum of 24 h after seizures [64]. Another study reports that surface expression of the GluA1 subunit was increased 60 min after the beginning of pilocarpine-induced SE [65]. A different pattern of AMPAR protein expression has been seen 3 h after pilocarpine-induced seizures. Reduced expression of GluA1, GluA3, and GluA4 subunits has been reported, in parallel with an elevation of GluA2 subunit expression [66].

Many studies also noted that epileptiform activity alters the AMPA/NMDA ratio and mEPSC in the hippocampus. In organotypic hippocampal slice cultures, an overnight incubation in the bicuculline (50 µM) increased the amplitude of mEPSCs and the AMPA/NMDA ratio. The addition of the NMDAR blocker CPP to the incubation solution prevented the changes in the AMPA/NMDA ratio and properties of miniature EPSC, pointing to the NMDAR-mediated nature of discussed changes [56]. Potentiation of AMPAR-mediated currents was noted 1 h after hypoxia-induced seizures in postnatal day 10 rats. Amplitudes of mEPSCs were elevated 1 h after seizures [64]. Amplitudes of mEPSCs recorded from CA1 pyramidal neurons were also increased in slices obtained from animals that had undergone pilocarpine-induced status epilepticus [65].

In our study, the amplitude of mEPSC remained indistinguishable from control levels. The difference in the effect of seizures on the amplitude of mEPSCs and eEPSCs in our experiments may arise because miniature events reflect the sheer broadness of the efferents CA1 receives from other areas. In contrast, the stimulation of Shaffer collaterals only provides CA3 input. Furthermore, it has been shown recently that spontaneous and synchronous transmitter release are distinct processes [67–69].

Overall, our data emphasize that AMPARs play a crucial role in seizure-induced synaptic plasticity. Considering that even a brief episode of epileptiform activity resulted in significant postsynaptic changes, the therapeutic strategies that rely on pharmacological modulation of postsynaptic glutamatergic receptors appear to have a good chance at alleviating damage associated with seizures or even preventing epileptogenesis.

Author Contributions: Formal analysis, J.L.E., D.V.A., T.Y.P. and A.V.Z.; investigation, J.L.E., D.V.A., T.Y.P. and E.B.S.; methodology, J.L.E., D.V.A. and A.V.Z.; project administration, A.V.Z.; writing—original draft, J.L.E., D.V.A., T.Y.P., E.B.S. and A.V.Z.; writing—review and editing, J.L.E., D.V.A. and A.V.Z. All authors have read and agreed to the published version of the manuscript.

Funding: This research was funded by the Russian Foundation for Basic Research (RFBR), project number 19-34-90122.

Institutional Review Board Statement: The study was conducted according to the EU Directive 2010/63/EU for animal experiments and approved by the Ethics Committee of the Sechenov Institute of Evolutionary Physiology and Biochemistry of the Russian Academy of Sciences (Ethical permit number 13-k-a, 15 February 2018).

Informed Consent Statement: Not applicable.

Data Availability Statement: The data presented in this study are available on request from the corresponding author.

Conflicts of Interest: The authors declare no conflict of interest.

References

1. Pitkänen, A.; Sutula, T.P. Is epilepsy a progressive disorder? Prospects for new therapeutic approaches in temporal-lobe epilepsy. *Lancet Neurol.* **2002**, *1*, 173–181. [CrossRef]
2. Herman, S.T. Epilepsy after brain insult: Targeting epileptogenesis. *Neurology* **2002**, *59*, S21–S26. [CrossRef]
3. Arzimanoglou, A.; Hirsch, E.; Nehlig, A.; Castelnau, P.; Gressens, P.; De Vasconcelos, A.P. Epilepsy and neuroprotection: An illustrated review. *Epileptic Disord.* **2002**, *4*, 173–182.
4. Dulla, C.G.; Janigro, D.; Jiruska, P.; Raimondo, J.V.; Ikeda, A.; Lin, C.K.; Goodkin, H.P.; Galanopoulou, A.S.; Bernard, C.; de Curtis, M. How do we use in vitro models to understand epileptiform and ictal activity? A report of the TASK 1- WG 4 group of the ILAE / AES Joint Translational Task Force. *Epilepsia Open* **2018**, *3*, 460–473. [CrossRef]
5. Martin, E.D.; Pozo, M.A. Valproate Reduced Synaptic Activity Increase Induced by 4-Aminopyridine at the Hippocampal CA3-CA1 Synapse. *Epilepsia* **2004**, *45*, 436–440. [CrossRef]
6. Heuzeroth, H.; Wawra, M.; Fidzinski, P.; Dag, R.; Holtkamp, M. The 4-Aminopyridine Model of Acute Seizures in vitro Elucidates Efficacy of New Antiepileptic Drugs. *Front. Neurosci.* **2019**, *13*, 677. [CrossRef] [PubMed]
7. Avoli, M.; Jefferys, J.G. Models of drug-induced epileptiform synchronization in vitro. *J. Neurosci. Methods* **2016**, *260*, 26–32. [CrossRef] [PubMed]
8. Perreault, P.; Avoli, M. Physiology and pharmacology of epileptiform activity induced by 4-aminopyridine in rat hippocampal slices. *J. Neurophysiol.* **1991**, *65*, 771–785. [CrossRef]
9. Gu, Y.; Ge, S.-Y.; Ruan, D.-Y. Effect of 4-aminopyridine on synaptic transmission in rat hippocampal slices. *Brain Res.* **2004**, *1006*, 225–232. [CrossRef]
10. Ziburkus, J.; Cressman, J.R.; Barreto, E.; Schiff, S.J. Interneuron and Pyramidal Cell Interplay During In Vitro Seizure-Like Events. *J. Neurophysiol.* **2006**, *95*, 3948–3954. [CrossRef]
11. Amakhin, D.V.; Smolensky, I.V.; Soboleva, E.B.; Zaitsev, A.V. Paradoxical Anticonvulsant Effect of Cefepime in the Pentylenetetrazole Model of Seizures in Rats. *Pharmaceuticals* **2020**, *13*, 80. [CrossRef] [PubMed]
12. Chizhov, A.V.; Amakhin, D.; Zaitsev, A.V. Computational model of interictal discharges triggered by interneurons. *PLoS ONE* **2017**, *12*, e0185752. [CrossRef] [PubMed]
13. McCormick, D.A.; Contreras, D. On The Cellular and Network Bases of Epileptic Seizures. *Annu. Rev. Physiol.* **2001**, *63*, 815–846. [CrossRef] [PubMed]
14. Thom, M. Review: Hippocampal sclerosis in epilepsy: A neuropathology review. *Neuropathol. Appl. Neurobiol.* **2014**, *40*, 520–543. [CrossRef] [PubMed]
15. Bernard, C.; Anderson, A.; Becker, A.; Poolos, N.P.; Beck, H.; Johnston, D. Acquired Dendritic Channelopathy in Temporal Lobe Epilepsy. *Science* **2004**, *305*, 532–535. [CrossRef]
16. Smirnova, E.Y.; Amakhin, D.; Malkin, S.L.; Chizhov, A.V.; Zaitsev, A.V. Acute Changes in Electrophysiological Properties of Cortical Regular-Spiking Cells Following Seizures in a Rat Lithium–Pilocarpine Model. *Neuroscience* **2018**, *379*, 202–215. [CrossRef]

17. Postnikova, T.Y.; Amakhin, D.V.; Trofimova, A.M.; Smolensky, I.V.; Zaitsev, A.V. Changes in Functional Properties of Rat Hippocampal Neurons Following Pentylenetetrazole-induced Status Epilepticus. *Neuroscience* **2019**, *399*, 103–116. [CrossRef]
18. Fleck, M.W.; Palmer, A.M.; Barrionuevo, G. Potassium-induced long-term potentiation in rat hippocampal slices. *Brain Res.* **1992**, *580*, 100–105. [CrossRef]
19. Debanne, D.; Thompson, S.M.; Gähwiler, B.H. A Brief Period of Epileptiform Activity Strengthens Excitatory Synapses in the Rat Hippocampus in Vitro. *Epilepsia* **2006**, *47*, 247–256. [CrossRef]
20. Postnikova, T.Y.; Amakhin, D.V.; Trofimova, A.M.; Zaitsev, A.V. Calcium-permeable AMPA receptors are essential to the synaptic plasticity induced by epileptiform activity in rat hippocampal slices. *Biochem. Biophys. Res. Commun.* **2020**, *529*, 1145–1150. [CrossRef]
21. Amakhin, D.; Soboleva, E.; Ergina, J.L.; Malkin, S.; Chizhov, A.; Zaitsev, A.V. Seizure-Induced Potentiation of AMPA Receptor-Mediated Synaptic Transmission in the Entorhinal Cortex. *Front. Cell. Neurosci.* **2018**, *12*, 486. [CrossRef]
22. Gibbs, I.J.W.; Sombati, S.; DeLorenzo, R.J.; Coulter, D.A. Physiological and Pharmacological Alterations in Postsynaptic GABAA Receptor Function in a Hippocampal Culture Model of Chronic Spontaneous Seizures. *J. Neurophysiol.* **1997**, *77*, 2139–2152. [CrossRef] [PubMed]
23. Joshi, S.; Rajasekaran, K.; Hawk, K.M.; Brar, J.; Ross, B.M.; Tran, C.A.; Chester, S.J.; Goodkin, H. Phosphatase inhibition prevents the activity-dependent trafficking of GABAA receptors during status epilepticus in the young animal. *Epilepsia* **2015**, *56*, 1355–1365. [CrossRef] [PubMed]
24. Burman, R.J.; Selfe, J.S.; Lee, J.H.; Berg, M.V.D.; Calin, A.; Codadu, N.K.; Wright, R.; E Newey, S.; Parrish, R.R.; A Katz, A.; et al. Excitatory GABAergic signalling is associated with benzodiazepine resistance in status epilepticus. *Brain* **2019**, *142*, 3482–3501. [CrossRef] [PubMed]
25. Zaitsev, A.V. The Role of GABAergic Interneurons in the Cortex and Hippocampus in the Development of Epilepsy. *Neurosci. Behav. Physiol.* **2017**, *47*, 913–922. [CrossRef]
26. Feng, Y.; Duan, C.; Luo, Z.; Xiao, W.; Tian, F. Silencing miR-20a-5p inhibits axonal growth and neuronal branching and prevents epileptogenesis through RGMa-RhoA-mediated synaptic plasticity. *J. Cell. Mol. Med.* **2020**, *24*, 10573–10588. [CrossRef] [PubMed]
27. Curia, G.; Lucchi, C.; Vinet, J.; Gualtieri, F.; Marinelli, C.; Torsello, A.; Costantino, L.; Biagini, G. Pathophysiogenesis of Mesial Temporal Lobe Epilepsy: Is Prevention of Damage Antiepileptogenic? *Curr. Med. Chem.* **2014**, *21*, 663–688. [CrossRef] [PubMed]
28. Dingledine, R.; Varvel, N.H.; Dudek, F.E. When and How Do Seizures Kill Neurons, and Is Cell Death Relevant to Epileptogenesis? In *Issues in Clinical Epileptology: A View from the Bench*; Springer: Dordrecht, The Netherlands, 2014; Volume 813, pp. 109–122.
29. Amakhin, D.V.; Malkin, S.L.; Ergina, J.L.; Kryukov, K.A.; Veniaminova, E.A.; Zubareva, O.E.; Zaitsev, A.V. Alterations in Properties of Glutamatergic Transmission in the Temporal Cortex and Hippocampus Following Pilocarpine-Induced Acute Seizures in Wistar Rats. *Front. Cell. Neurosci.* **2017**, *11*, 264. [CrossRef]
30. Amakhin, D.; Ergina, J.L.; Chizhov, A.; Zaitsev, A.V. Synaptic Conductances during Interictal Discharges in Pyramidal Neurons of Rat Entorhinal Cortex. *Front. Cell. Neurosci.* **2016**, *10*, 233. [CrossRef]
31. Citri, A.; Malenka, R.C. Synaptic Plasticity: Multiple Forms, Functions, and Mechanisms. *Neuropsychopharmacology* **2007**, *33*, 18–41. [CrossRef] [PubMed]
32. Zucker, R.S.; Regehr, W.G. Short-Term Synaptic Plasticity. *Annu. Rev. Physiol.* **2002**, *64*, 355–405. [CrossRef] [PubMed]
33. Morgan, S.L.; Teyler, T.J. Epileptic-like activity induces multiple forms of plasticity in hippocampal area CA1. *Brain Res.* **2001**, *917*, 90–96. [CrossRef]
34. Iyengar, S.S.; Mott, D.D. Neuregulin blocks synaptic strengthening after epileptiform activity in the rat hippocampus. *Brain Res.* **2008**, *1208*, 67–73. [CrossRef]
35. Lopantsev, V.; Both, M.; Draguhn, A. Rapid plasticity at inhibitory and excitatory synapses in the hippocampus induced by ictal epileptiform discharges. *Eur. J. Neurosci.* **2009**, *29*, 1153–1164. [CrossRef]
36. Schneiderman, J. The role of long-term potentiation in persistent epileptiform burst-induced hyperexcitability following GABAA receptor blockade. *Neuroscience* **1997**, *81*, 1111–1122. [CrossRef]
37. Sourdet, V.; Russier, M.; Daoudal, G.; Ankri, N.; Debanne, D. Long-Term Enhancement of Neuronal Excitability and Temporal Fidelity Mediated by Metabotropic Glutamate Receptor Subtype 5. *J. Neurosci.* **2003**, *23*, 10238–10248. [CrossRef]
38. Desai, N.S.; Rutherford, L.C.; Turrigiano, G.G. Plasticity in the intrinsic excitability of cortical pyramidal neurons. *Nat. Neurosci.* **1999**, *2*, 515–520. [CrossRef]
39. Cudmore, R.; Turrigiano, G.G. Long-Term Potentiation of Intrinsic Excitability in LV Visual Cortical Neurons. *J. Neurophysiol.* **2004**, *92*, 341–348. [CrossRef] [PubMed]
40. Beck, H.; Yaari, Y. Plasticity of intrinsic neuronal properties in CNS disorders. *Nat. Rev. Neurosci.* **2008**, *9*, 357–369. [CrossRef] [PubMed]
41. Mitterdorfer, J.; Bean, B.P. Potassium Currents during the Action Potential of Hippocampal CA3 Neurons. *J. Neurosci.* **2002**, *22*, 10106–10115. [CrossRef] [PubMed]
42. Blümcke, I.; Thom, M.; Aronica, E.; Armstrong, D.D.; Bartolomei, F.; Bernasconi, A.; Bernasconi, N.; Bien, C.G.; Cendes, F.; Coras, R.; et al. International consensus classification of hippocampal sclerosis in temporal lobe epilepsy: A Task Force report from the ILAE Commission on Diagnostic Methods. *Epilepsia* **2013**, *54*, 1315–1329. [CrossRef] [PubMed]
43. Codadu, N.K.; Graham, R.T.; Burman, R.J.; Jackson-Taylor, R.T.; Raimondo, J.V.; Trevelyan, A.J.; Parrish, R.R. Divergent paths to seizure-like events. *Physiol. Rep.* **2019**, *7*, e14226. [CrossRef] [PubMed]

44. Verma-Ahuja, S.; Pencek, T.L. Hippocampal CA1 neuronal properties in genetically epilepsyprone rats: Evidence for increased excitation. *Epilepsy Res.* **1994**, *18*, 205–215. [CrossRef]
45. Ghotbedin, Z.; Janahmadi, M.; Mirnajafi-Zadeh, J.; Behzadi, G.; Semnanian, S. Electrical Low Frequency Stimulation of the Kindling Site Preserves the Electrophysiological Properties of the Rat Hippocampal CA1 Pyramidal Neurons From the Destructive Effects of Amygdala Kindling: The Basis for a Possible Promising Epilepsy Therapy. *Brain Stimul.* **2013**, *6*, 515–523. [CrossRef]
46. Minge, D.; Bähring, R. Acute Alterations of Somatodendritic Action Potential Dynamics in Hippocampal CA1 Pyramidal Cells after Kainate-Induced Status Epilepticus in Mice. *PLoS ONE* **2011**, *6*, e26664. [CrossRef]
47. Pelletier, M.R.; Carlen, P.L. Repeated tetanic stimulation in piriform cortex in vitro: Epileptogenesis and pharmacology. *J. Neurophysiol.* **1996**, *76*, 4069–4079. [CrossRef]
48. Niesen, C.E.; Ge, S. Chronic epilepsy in developing hippocampal neurons: Electrophysiologic and morphologic features. *Dev. Neurosci.* **1999**, *21*, 328–338. [CrossRef]
49. Shah, M.; Anderson, A.E.; Leung, V.; Lin, X.; Johnston, D. Seizure-Induced Plasticity of h Channels in Entorhinal Cortical Layer III Pyramidal Neurons. *Neuron* **2004**, *44*, 495–508. [CrossRef]
50. Marcelin, B.; Chauviere, L.; Becker, A.; Migliore, M.; Esclapez, M.; Bernard, C. h channel-dependent deficit of theta oscillation resonance and phase shift in temporal lobe epilepsy. *Neurobiol. Dis.* **2009**, *33*, 436–447. [CrossRef]
51. Sanabria, E.R.G.; Su, H.; Yaari, Y. Initiation of network bursts by Ca 2+ -dependent intrinsic bursting in the rat pilocarpine model of temporal lobe epilepsy. *J. Physiol.* **2001**, *532*, 205–216. [CrossRef] [PubMed]
52. Yaari, Y.; Yue, C.; Su, H. Recruitment of apical dendritic T-type Ca2+channels by backpropagating spikes underliesde novointrinsic bursting in hippocampal epileptogenesis. *J. Physiol.* **2007**, *580*, 435–450. [CrossRef] [PubMed]
53. Royeck, M.; Kelly, T.; Opitz, T.; Otte, D.-M.; Rennhack, A.; Woitecki, A.; Pitsch, J.; Becker, A.; Schoch, S.; Kaupp, U.B.; et al. Downregulation of Spermine Augments Dendritic Persistent Sodium Currents and Synaptic Integration after Status Epilepticus. *J. Neurosci.* **2015**, *35*, 15240–15253. [CrossRef] [PubMed]
54. Peña-Ortega, F.; Bargas, J.; Tapia, R. Paired pulse facilitation is turned into paired pulse depression in hippocampal slices after epilepsy induced by 4-aminopyridine in vivo. *Neuropharmacology* **2002**, *42*, 807–812. [CrossRef]
55. Smirnova, E.Y.; Chizhov, A.; Zaitsev, A.V. Presynaptic GABAB receptors underlie the antiepileptic effect of low-frequency electrical stimulation in the 4-aminopyridine model of epilepsy in brain slices of young rats. *Brain Stimul.* **2020**, *13*, 1387–1395. [CrossRef]
56. Abegg, M.H.; Savić, N.; Ehrengruber, M.U.; McKinney, R.A.; Gähwiler, B.H. Epileptiform activity in rat hippocampus strengthens excitatory synapses. *J. Physiol.* **2004**, *554*, 439–448. [CrossRef]
57. Liao, D.; Hessler, N.A.; Malinow, R. Activation of postsynaptically silent synapses during pairing-induced LTP in CA1 region of hippocampal slice. *Nat. Cell Biol.* **1995**, *375*, 400–404. [CrossRef]
58. Choquet, D.; Triller, A. The Dynamic Synapse. *Neuron* **2013**, *80*, 691–703. [CrossRef]
59. Newpher, T.M.; Ehlers, M.D. Glutamate Receptor Dynamics in Dendritic Microdomains. *Neuron* **2008**, *58*, 472–497. [CrossRef] [PubMed]
60. Opazo, P.; Sainlos, M.; Choquet, D. Regulation of AMPA receptor surface diffusion by PSD-95 slots. *Curr. Opin. Neurobiol.* **2012**, *22*, 453–460. [CrossRef]
61. Lisman, J.E.; Raghavachari, S.; Tsien, R.W. The sequence of events that underlie quantal transmission at central glutamatergic synapses. *Nat. Rev. Neurosci.* **2007**, *8*, 597–609. [CrossRef]
62. Tang, A.-H.; Chen, H.; Li, T.P.; Metzbower, S.R.; MacGillavry, H.; Blanpied, T.A. A trans-synaptic nanocolumn aligns neurotransmitter release to receptors. *Nature* **2016**, *536*, 210–214. [CrossRef]
63. Rajasekaran, K.; Todorovic, M.; Kapur, J. Calcium-permeable AMPA receptors are expressed in a rodent model of status epilepticus. *Ann. Neurol.* **2012**, *72*, 91–102. [CrossRef]
64. Rakhade, S.N.; Zhou, C.; Aujla, P.K.; Fishman, R.; Sucher, N.J.; Jensen, F.E. Early Alterations of AMPA Receptors Mediate Synaptic Potentiation Induced by Neonatal Seizures. *J. Neurosci.* **2008**, *28*, 7979–7990. [CrossRef]
65. Joshi, S.; Rajasekaran, K.; Sun, H.; Williamson, J.; Kapur, J. Enhanced AMPA receptor-mediated neurotransmission on CA1 pyramidal neurons during status epilepticus. *Neurobiol. Dis.* **2017**, *103*, 45–53. [CrossRef]
66. Russo, I.; Bonini, D.; La Via, L.; Barlati, S.; Barbon, A. AMPA Receptor Properties are Modulated in the Early Stages Following Pilocarpine-induced Status Epilepticus. *Neuromol. Med.* **2013**, *15*, 324–338. [CrossRef]
67. Peled, E.S.; Newman, Z.L.; Isacoff, E.Y. Evoked and Spontaneous Transmission Favored by Distinct Sets of Synapses. *Curr. Biol.* **2014**, *24*, 484–493. [CrossRef] [PubMed]
68. Kaeser, P.S.; Regehr, W.G. Molecular Mechanisms for Synchronous, Asynchronous, and Spontaneous Neurotransmitter Release. *Annu. Rev. Physiol.* **2014**, *76*, 333–363. [CrossRef] [PubMed]
69. Kavalali, E.T. The mechanisms and functions of spontaneous neurotransmitter release. *Nat. Rev. Neurosci.* **2015**, *16*, 5–16. [CrossRef] [PubMed]

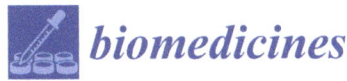

Article

Activation of Calcium-Activated Chloride Channels Suppresses Inherited Seizure Susceptibility in Genetically Epilepsy-Prone Rats

Miracle Thomas, Mark Simms and Prosper N'Gouemo *

Department of Physiology and Biophysics, Howard University College of Medicine, Washington, DC 20059, USA; miracle.thomas@bison.howard.edu (M.T.); mark.simms@bison.howard.edu (M.S.)
* Correspondence: prosper.ngouemo@howard.edu; Tel.: +1-202-806-9708

Abstract: Inherited seizure susceptibility in genetically epilepsy-prone rats (GEPR-3s) is associated with increased voltage-gated calcium channel currents suggesting a massive calcium influx resulting in increased levels of intraneuronal calcium. Cytosolic calcium, in turn, activates many processes, including chloride channels, to restore normal membrane excitability and limit repetitive firing of the neurons. Here we used EACT and T16Ainh-A01, potent activator and inhibitor of calcium-activated channels transmembrane protein 16A (TMEM16A), respectively, to probe the role of these channels in the pathophysiology of acoustically evoked seizures in the GEPR-3s. We used adult male and female GEPR-3s. Acoustically evoked seizures consisted of wild running seizures (WRSs) that evolved into generalized tonic-clonic seizures (GTCSs) and eventually culminated into forelimb extension (partial tonic seizures). We found that acute EACT treatment at relatively higher tested doses significantly reduced the incidences of WRSs and GTCSs, and the seizure severity in male GEPR-3s. Furthermore, these antiseizure effects were associated with delayed seizure onset and reduced seizure duration. Interestingly, the inhibition of TMEM16A channels reversed EACT's antiseizure effects on seizure latency and seizure duration. No notable antiseizure effects were observed in female GEPR-3s. Together, these findings suggest that activation of TMEM16A channels may represent a putative novel cellular mechanism for suppressing GTCSs.

Keywords: acoustically evoked seizures; EACT; generalized tonic-clonic seizures; inherited epilepsy; TMEM1A channels; wild running seizures

Citation: Thomas, M.; Simms, M.; N'Gouemo, P. Activation of Calcium-Activated Chloride Channels Suppresses Inherited Seizure Susceptibility in Genetically Epilepsy-Prone Rats. *Biomedicines* **2022**, *10*, 449. https://doi.org/10.3390/biomedicines10020449

Academic Editor: Joanna Pera

Received: 30 November 2021
Accepted: 9 February 2022
Published: 15 February 2022

Publisher's Note: MDPI stays neutral with regard to jurisdictional claims in published maps and institutional affiliations.

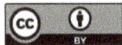

Copyright: © 2022 by the authors. Licensee MDPI, Basel, Switzerland. This article is an open access article distributed under the terms and conditions of the Creative Commons Attribution (CC BY) license (https://creativecommons.org/licenses/by/4.0/).

1. Introduction

Epilepsy is one of the most common chronic neurological disorders characterized by recurrent seizures, which result from hypersynchronous discharges of neurons in specific brain networks. This disorder is associated with increased morbidity and death, and generalized tonic-clonic seizures (GTCSs) are the most common risk factor of sudden unexpected death in epilepsy, the leading cause of death in patients with epilepsy [1,2]. Significant progress has enhanced our understanding of the pathogenesis and pathophysiology of seizures and epilepsy, resulting in numerous antiseizure medications. However, some seizures are still refractory to optimal treatment with two or more antiseizure medications in about one-third of patients with epilepsy [3–6]. Therefore, there is an urgent need to develop additional therapeutic approaches based on new mechanisms underlying neuronal hyperexcitability that leads to seizures. Elevated levels of intraneuronal Ca^{2+} contributed to the generation and propagation of seizure activity and activated multiple Ca^{2+}-dependent mechanisms, including Ca^{2+}-activated chloride channels (CaCCs) [7–10]. Hence, systemic administration of inhibitors of voltage-gated Ca^{2+} channels (VGCCs) and activator of small conductance Ca^{2+}-activated K^+ channels markedly suppressed acoustically evoked seizures in the genetically epilepsy-prone rats (GEPRs) and DBA/2 mice [11–15]. These findings suggested a functional and molecular remodeling of these channels, at least in the inferior colliculus (IC), the site for initiating acoustically evoked seizures in the GEPRs [11–15]. Accordingly, we found an upregulation of VGCCs and current density in the IC of the GEPR-3s, the moderated seizure severity strain of the GEPR [16,17]. Although a significant accumulation of intraneuronal chloride accompanies seizure activity, the role of CaCCs in the initiation and propagation of seizures has not been fully understood [18,19]. CaCCs are voltage-gated channels activated by rising intracellular Ca^{2+} concentration and play multiple physiological roles, including neuronal excitability regulation [20,21]. Anoctamin and bestrophin are the significant components of CaCCs; furthermore, anoctamins form a family of transmembrane (TMEM16) proteins, including TMEM16A, TMEM16B, and TMEM16C [22–26]. Interestingly, TMEM16A mRNA and proteins were expressed in auditory brainstem nuclei; such expression may also occur in the IC [27]. Here, we probe the role of TMEM16A channels in the mechanisms underlying seizures by evaluating the effects of EACT and T16Ainh-A01, potent activator and inhibitor of TMEM16A channels, respectively, on acoustically evoked seizure susceptibility in the GEPR-3, a model of inherited generalized tonic-clonic epilepsy.

2. Materials and Methods

2.1. Animals

The present study used 54 GEPR-3s (eight-week-old, male, and female) obtained from our animal colony maintained at Howard University College of Medicine. The GEPR-3s were housed in a temperature/humidity-controlled room on a 12 h/12 h light/dark cycle with free access to food and water. We made all possible efforts to minimize the number of animals used in experiments and their discomfort. Thus, the same animals were used as controls for each tested dosage of a given pharmacological agent. The Institutional Animal Care and Use Committee approved all experimental procedures (Protocol MED-20-04) following the National Institutes of Health Guide for the Care and Use of Laboratory Animals [28].

2.2. Acoustically Evoked Seizure Testing

Following administration of vehicle, EACT, and T16Ainh-A01, GEPR-3s were placed in an acoustic chamber (Med Associates, St. Albans, VT, USA) and tested for acoustically evoked susceptibility at 0.5 h, 1 h, and 2 h post-treatment. To evaluate the long-lasting effects of EACT and T16Ainh-A01, the GEPR-3s were again tested for acoustically evoked susceptibility 24 h later. To induce seizures, an acoustic stimulus that consisted of pure tones at a 100–105 decibels sound pressure level (Med Associated, St. Albans, VT, USA) was presented until either seizure was elicited, or 60 s passed with no seizure activity. The GEPR-3s were closely monitored following the administration of EACT and T16Ainh-A01. The phenotype of seizures was classified into seven stages [29]. stage 0, no seizures in response to an acoustic stimulus; stage 1, wild running seizures (WRSs); stage 2, two or more episodes of WRSs; stage 3, one episode of WRSs followed by generalized tonic-clonic seizures (GTCSs) characterized by tonic dorsiflexion of the neck, tonic flexion of shoulder and bouncing clonic seizures (or clonus, i.e., tonic-clonic seizures while the animal is lying on its belly); stage 4, two episodes of WRSs followed by GTCSs, stage 5, one episode of WRS followed by GTCSs and tonic forelimb extension (FLE, partial tonic seizures); and stage 6, two episodes of WRSs followed by GTCSs and FLE.

In another set of experiments, male and female GEPR-3s ($n = 6$/group) were used to assess the general behavior (up to 48 h) following administration of EACT at the dose of 2.5, 5, and 10 mg/kg body weight (p.o.) and T16Ainh-A01 at the dose of 10 mg/kg body weight (p.o.). We recorded the occurrence of lethargy, ataxia, tremor, Straub's tail, change in body temperature, and spontaneous seizures. We humanely euthanized all animals at the end of the experiments.

2.3. Pharmacological Treatments

To evaluate the role of CaCCs in inherited seizure susceptibility in the GEPR-3, we used EACT (3,4,5-Trimethoxy-*N*-(2-methoxyethyl)-*N*-(4-phenyl-2-thiazolyl)benzamide) (R&D systems, Minneapolis, MN, USA), and T16Ainh-A01 (2-[(5-Ethyl-1,6-dihydro-4-methyl-6-oxo-2-pyrimidinyl)thio]-*N*-[4-(4-methoxyphenyl)-2 thiazolyl]acetamide (R&D Systems, Minneapolis, MN, USA), potent activator and inhibitor of TMEM16A channels, respectively. For EACT and T16Ainh-A01 experiments, the GEPR-3s were randomly separated into groups of $n = 9$ and $n = 6$, respectively, and were used as their controls. The GEPR-3s were first tested for acoustically evoked seizures 30 min following vehicle administration. Those GEPR-3s exhibiting seizures were referred to as controls and subsequently used for pharmacological studies one hour later. Eact (2.5, 5 and 10 mg/kg body weight) and T16Ainh-A01 (10 mg/kg body weight) were dissolved in dimethyl sulfonic acid (1%) and sterile water using sonication (80 kHz, 100% power); the solutions were filtered and administered 30 min before seizure testing. The vehicle, Eact, and T16Ainh-A01 were given per os (p.o.) by gastric intubation with a volume of 0.2 mL/100 g body weight using an 18-gauge stainless steel feeding needle (round tip, ball diameter 3 mm). The tested dose range and the 30 min timeframe interval were chosen based on our previously published in vivo pharmacological studies and preliminary data. The order of seizure testing was randomized and counterbalanced by dose and sex. For EACT experiments, each seizure testing dosage was performed at a minimum of 72 h to allow its washout.

2.4. Data Analysis

The investigators were blinded to group allocation during experiments and data analysis. The Origin 2021 software (Origin Northampton, MA, USA) and Primer 6th edition software (Primer of Biostatistics, McGraw-Hill, NY, USA) were used for statistical analyses and to create graphs. Following EACT pretreatment and seizure testing, the GEPR-3s that did not display seizures within the 60 s observation period were considered protected from seizure activity. Therefore, only data obtained in control conditions and following administration of EACT and T16Ainh-A01 were included in the analysis. The incidences of WRSs, GTCSs, and FLE were recorded for each group. The time interval from the start of acoustic stimulus to the onset of the first episode of WRSs was recorded as the seizure latency (or seizure onset). The incidences of WRSs, GTCSs, and FLE were analyzed using Fisher Exact test. The seizure severity was analyzed using the Wilcoxon signed-rank test or Mann Whitney test. The seizure latency was analyzed using one-way ANOVA followed by Bonferroni correction; before performing ANOVA, data were subjected to the Kolmogorov Smirnov test for normality and Levene's test for homogeneity of variances. The cut-off for statistical significance was $p < 0.05$. Data are presented as percentages (%) for the incidences of WRSs and GTCSs, mean ± S.E.M. for seizure latency, and median score ± median average deviation score for the seizure severity.

3. Results

Twenty-four-hour monitoring revealed that administration of EACT at the tested doses did not alter the gross behavior of the GEPR-3s. No loss of righting reflex, Straub tail, sedation, lethargy, ataxia, and spontaneous seizures were observed following EACT and T16Ainh-A01 treatments. In addition, we did not observe an exacerbation of seizure severity (e.g., the occurrence of complete tonic seizures characterized by forelimb and hindlimb extension) in the GEPR-3s subjected to seizure testing. We also did not find notable changes in body temperature.

3.1. Effects on EACT at the Dose of 2.5 mg/kg on Acoustically Evoked Seizures in GEPR-3s

First, we evaluated the effects of acute EACT treatment at the dose of 2.5 mg/kg on acoustically evoked seizure susceptibility in the GEPR-3s. In the control testing conditions (pre-EACT treatment), all-male ($n = 9$) and all-female ($n = 9$) GEPR-3s experienced WRSs (Figure 1A,B), and GTCSs (Figure 1C,D); FLE was observed in one female but not in male

GEPR-3s. Fisher Exact test showed that EACT pretreatment did not considerably reduce the incidence of the occurrence of WRSs in male GERP-3s at 0.5, 1, 2, and 24 h post-treatment time points compared with the control testing conditions (Figure 1A). Similarly, EACT also did not considerably reduce the incidence of the occurrence of WRSs in female GEPR-3s at 0.5, 1, 2, and 24 h post-treatment time points compared with the control testing conditions (Figure 1B). The analysis showed that EACT significantly reduced the incidence of the occurrence of GTCSs in male GEPR-3s by 56% ($p < 0.029$) at 2 h but not 0.5, 1, and 24 h post-treatment time points compared with the control testing conditions (Figure 1C). In female GEPR-3s, EACT did not considerably reduce the incidence of the occurrence GTCSs at all tested post-treatment time points compared with the control testing conditions (Figure 1D).

In addition to the incidence of the occurrence of seizures, we also evaluated the effects of EACT's treatment on the seizure latency and duration (Figure 1E–H). In the control conditions, the seizure latency was 19.78 ± 3.79 s ($n = 9$) and 19.44 ± 2.54 s ($n = 9$) in male and female GEPR-3s, respectively (Figure 1E,F); the seizure duration was 24.44 ± 2.12 s ($n = 9$) and 26.67 ± 3.22 s ($n = 9$) in male and female GEPR-3s, respectively. ANOVA showed that, in male GEPR-3s, EACT did not considerably delay the seizure latency and decreased the seizure duration at all tested post-treatment time points compared with the control testing conditions (Figure 1E,G). Quantification also showed that, in female GEPR-3s, EACT did not considerably delay the seizure latency and decrease the seizure duration at all tested post-treatment time points compared with the control testing conditions (Figure 1F,G).

We also examined the effects of EACT on the severity of acoustically evoked seizures. Wilcoxon signed-rank test showed that EACT significantly reduced the seizure severity in male GEPR-3s at 2 h ($z = 2.16$, $p < 0.031$), but not at 0.5, 1, and 24 h post-treatment time points compared to the control testing conditions (Figure 2A). However, in female GEPR-3s, EACT did not alter the seizure severity at all tested post-treatment time points compared with the control testing conditions (Figure 2B).

3.2. Effects on EACT at the Dose of 5 mg/kg on Acoustically Evoked Seizures in GEPR-3s

Next, we evaluated the efficacy of EACT at 5 mg/kg (p.o.) to determine if this dose can either alter the seizure susceptibility in female GEPR-3s or completely suppress seizure susceptibility in male GEPR-3s. In the control testing conditions (pre-EACT treatment), all-male ($n = 9$) and all-female ($n = 9$) GEPR-3s experienced WRSs and GTCSs (Figure 3A–D); FLE was not observed in the GEPR-3s. The Fisher Exact test revealed that, in male GEPR-3s, EACT significantly reduced the incidence of the occurrence of WRSs by 56% ($p < 0.029$) and 67% ($p < 0.009$) at 2 and 24 h post-treatment time points, respectively, compared with control testing conditions (Figure 3A). Furthermore, EACT did not considerably reduce the incidence of the occurrence of WRS at 0.5 h and 2 h post-treatment time points, respectively, compared with control testing conditions (Figure 3A). However, in the females, EACT did not reduce the incidence of the occurrence of WRSs at all tested post-treatment time points compared with the control testing conditions (Figure 3B). Quantification also showed that pretreatment with 5 mg/kg EACT significantly reduced the incidence of the occurrence of GTCSs in male GEPR-3s by 56% ($p < 0.029$), and 56% ($p < 0.029$), and 67% ($p < 0.002$) at 1, 2 and 24 h post-treatment time points, respectively, compared with control testing conditions. However, EACT did not considerably reduce the incidence of the occurrence of WRSs at 0.5 h post-treatment compared to the control testing conditions (Figure 3C). Furthermore, in female GEPR-3s, EACT treatment did not considerably reduce the incidence of the occurrence of GTCSs at all tested post-treatment time points compared with the control testing conditions (Figure 3D).

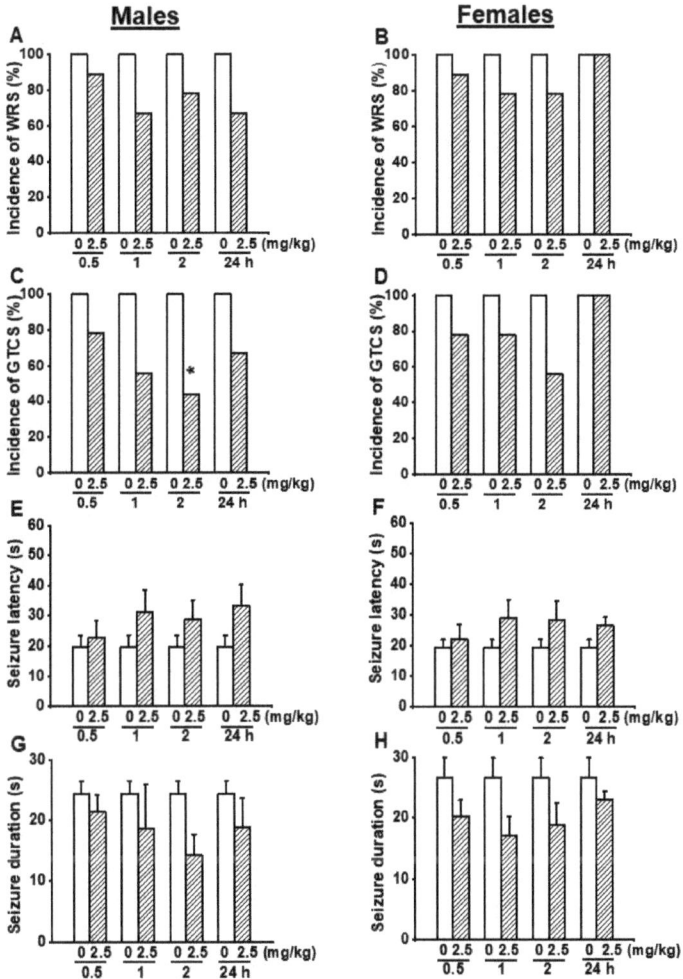

Figure 1. Effects of acute EACT treatment at the dose of 2.5 mg/kg on acoustically evoked seizures. The putative seizure suppressive effects EACT, a potent activator of TMEM16A, were evaluated at different post-treatment time points of 0.5, 1, 2, and 24 h in adult male ($n = 9$) and female ($n = 9$) GEPR-3s. (**A**) EACT treatment did not considerably reduce the incidence of the occurrence of WRSs in males. (**B**) Similarly, EACT treatment also did not considerably reduce the incidence of the occurrence of WRSs in females. (**C**) EACT treatment significantly reduced the incidence of the occurrence of GTCSs at the 2 h post-treatment time point in males. (**D**) However, EACT treatment did not considerably reduce the incidence of the occurrence of GTCSs in females. (**E**) EACT treatment did not considerably delay the seizure latency in males. (**F**) Similarly, EACT treatment also did not considerably delay the seizure onset in females. (**G**) EACT treatment did not considerably reduce the seizure duration in males. (**H**) Similarly, EACT treatment also did not considerably reduce the seizure duration in females. Data from the incidence of the occurrence of WRSs and GTCSs were represented as a mean percentage (%), and the Fisher Exact test was used for analysis. Data from the seizure latency and duration were presented as mean ± S.E.M., and one-way ANOVA followed by Bonferroni correction was used for analysis. Opened and filled bar graphs represent control-treated (pre-EACT) and EACT-treated GEPR-3s, respectively. * $p < 0.05$.

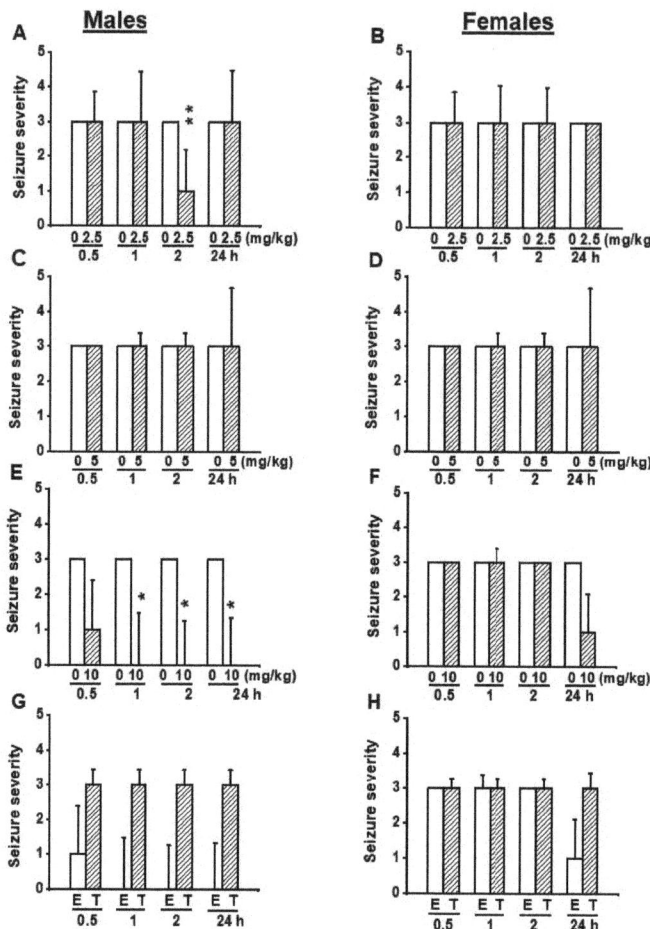

Figure 2. Effects of acute treatment with EACT (E) and T16Ainh-A01 (T), a potent blocker of TMEM16A channels, on the severity of acoustically evoked seizures. The effects of EACT, a potent activator of TMEM16A channels, on the seizure severity were evaluated at various doses (2.5, 5, and 10 mg/kg, p.o.), and at different post-treatment time points (0.5, 1 h, 2 h, and 24 h) in adult male and female GEPR-3s. T16Ainh-A01 was tested only at the dose of 10 mg/kg, p.o.) and the data were compared with EACT (10 mg/kg, p.o.) (**A**) EACT treatment significantly reduced the seizure severity at the 2 h post-treatment time point in males. (**B**) EACT treatment did not alter the seizure severity in females. (**C**) EACT treatment significantly suppressed the seizure severity at 2 and 2 h post-treatment time points in males. (**D**) EACT treatment did not considerably alter the seizure severity in females. (**E**) EACT treatment significantly suppressed the seizure severity at 1, 2, and 24 h post-treatment time points in males. (**F**) EACT treatment did not considerably alter the seizure severity in females. (**G**) In males, T16Ainh-A01 treatment (T) reversed the antiseizure effects following EACT administration (E), but no statistical significance was reached. (**H**) In females, T16Ainh-A01 did alter the effects of EACT. The seizure severity data were represented as median ± median average deviation, and the Wilcoxon signed-rank test was used to compare paired EACT data or T16Ainh-A01 data, and the Mann-Whitney test was used to compare the EACT and T16Ainh-A01 groups. Opened and filled bar graphs represent control-treated (pre-EACT) and EACT treated GEPR-3s ($n = 9$), respectively. * $p < 0.05$, ** $p < 0.01$.

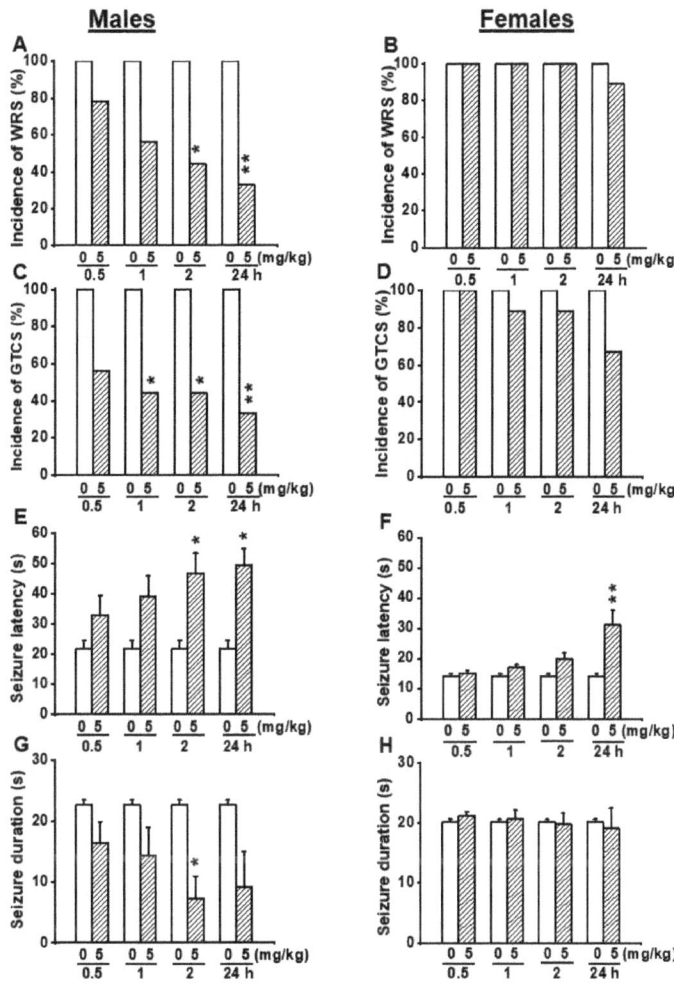

Figure 3. Effects of acute EACT treatment at the dose of 5 mg/kg on acoustically evoked seizures. The effects EACT, a potent activator of TMEM16A, were evaluated at different post-treatment time points of 0.5, 1, 2, and 24 h in adult male ($n = 9$) and female ($n = 9$) GEPR-3s. (**A**) EACT treatment significantly reduced the incidence of the occurrence of WRSs at 2 and 24 h post-treatment time points in males. (**B**) EACT treatment did not considerably reduce the incidence of the occurrence of WRSs in females. (**C**) EACT treatment significantly reduced the incidence of the occurrence of GTCSs at 1, 2, and 24 h post-treatment time points in males. (**D**) EACT treatment did not considerably reduce the incidence of the occurrence of GTCSs in females. (**E**) EACT treatment significantly delayed the seizure onset at 2 and 24 h post-treatment time points in males. (**F**) In females. EACT treatment also significantly delayed the seizure onset at the 24 h post-treatment time point. (**G**) EACT treatment significantly reduced the seizure duration at the 2 h post-treatment time point in males. (**H**) EACT treatment did not alter the seizure duration in females. Data from the incidence of the occurrence of WRSs and GTCSs were represented as a mean percentage (%), and Fisher Exact test was used for analysis. Data from the seizure latency and seizure duration were presented as mean ± S.E.M., and one-way ANOVA followed by Bonferroni correction was used for analysis. Opened and filled bar graphs represent control-treated (pre-EACT) and EACT treated GEPR-3s, respectively. * $p < 0.05$, ** $p < 0.01$.

We also evaluated the effects of EACT's treatment on seizure latency and duration (Figure 3E–H). In the control conditions, the seizure latency was 21.67 ± 2.93 s ($n = 9$) and 14.33 ± 0.79 s ($n = 9$) in male and female GEPR-3s, respectively (Figure 3E,F); seizure duration was 22.67 ± 0.79 s ($n = 9$) and 20.11 ± 0.48 s ($n = 9$) in male and female GEPR-3s, respectively (Figure 3G,H). ANOVA showed that EACT pretreatment significantly altered the seizure latency in male GEPR-3s ($F_{(4,40)} = 3.488$, $p < 0.015$). Multiple comparisons revealed that the seizure onset was delayed at 2 h ($t = 2.962$, $p < 0.005$) and 24 h ($t = 3.79$, $p < 0.002$) post-treatment time points compared to control testing conditions; the seizure latency was not considerably altered at 0.5 and 1 h post-treatment time points (Figure 3E). The analysis also showed that EACT pretreatment significantly altered the seizure duration. Multiple comparisons revealed that EACT significantly reduced the seizure duration at 2 h ($t = 3.075$, $p < 0.038$) post-treatment time point compared to control testing conditions; the seizure duration was not considerably reduced at 0.5, 1, and 24 h post-treatment time points (Figure 3G). In female GEPR-3s, ANOVA showed that EACT pretreatment significantly alters the seizure latency ($F_{(4,40)} = 7.846$, $p < 0.00009$). Multiple comparisons revealed that EACT significantly delayed the seizure onset at 24 h ($t = 4.895$, $p < 0.002$) post-treatment time points compared with control testing conditions; the seizure latency was not considerably increased at 0.5, 1, and 2 h post-treatment time points (Figure 3F). The analysis also showed that EACT treatment did not alter the seizure duration in females GEPR-3s (Figure 1H).

We also evaluated the effects of EACT pretreatment on the severity of acoustically evoked seizures. Wilcoxon signed-rank test showed that at a dose of 5mg/kg, EACT treatment significantly suppressed the seizure severity in male GEPR-3s at 2 h ($z = 2.22$, $p < 0.033$), and 24 h ($z = 2.33$, $p < 0.031$) post-treatment time points compared with the control testing conditions; the seizure severity was not considerably reduced or changed at 1 and 0.5 h post-treatment, respectively (Figure 2C). In female GEPR-3s, EACT did not alter the seizure severity compared with the control testing conditions (Figure 2D).

3.3. Effects on EACT at the Dose of 10 mg/kg on Acoustically Evoked Seizures in GEPR-3s

Since no anticonvulsant effects were seen in female GEPR-3s following administration of EACT at the doses of 2.5 and 5 mg/kg, we evaluated the effects of EACT pretreatment at the dose of 10 mg/kg on acoustically evoked seizure susceptibility in the GEPR-3s. In the control testing conditions (pre-EACT treatment), all-male ($n = 9$) and all-female ($n = 9$) GEPR-3s experienced WRSs and GTCSs (Figure 4A–D). FLE was not observed in both male and female GEPR-3s. The Fisher Exact test showed that the incidence of the occurrence of WRSs, in male GEPR-3s, was significantly reduced by 56% ($p < 0.029$) and 67% ($p < 0.009$) at 2 and 24 h post-treatment time points compared with control testing conditions; no considerable reduction of the incidence of the occurrence of WRSs was seen at 0.5 and 1 h post-treatment time points (Figure 4A). However, in females, EACT did not considerably alter the incidence of the occurrence of WRSs at all tested post-treatment time points compared with the control testing conditions (Figure 4B). We also evaluated the effects of EACT on the incidence of the occurrence of GTCSs. Analysis revealed that EACT significantly reduced the incidence of the occurrence of GTCSs, in male GEPR-3s, by 67% ($p < 0.009$) and 78% ($p < 0.002$) at 2 and 24 h post-treatment time points compared with control testing conditions; no considerable reduction of the incidence of the occurrence of GTCSs was seen at 0.5 h and 1 h post-treatment time points (Figure 4C). In female GEPR-3s, EACT significantly reduced the incidence of the occurrence of GTCSs by 56% ($p < 0.029$) at 24 h post-treatment time point compared with the control testing conditions; no considerable change was observed at other post-treatment time points (Figure 4D).

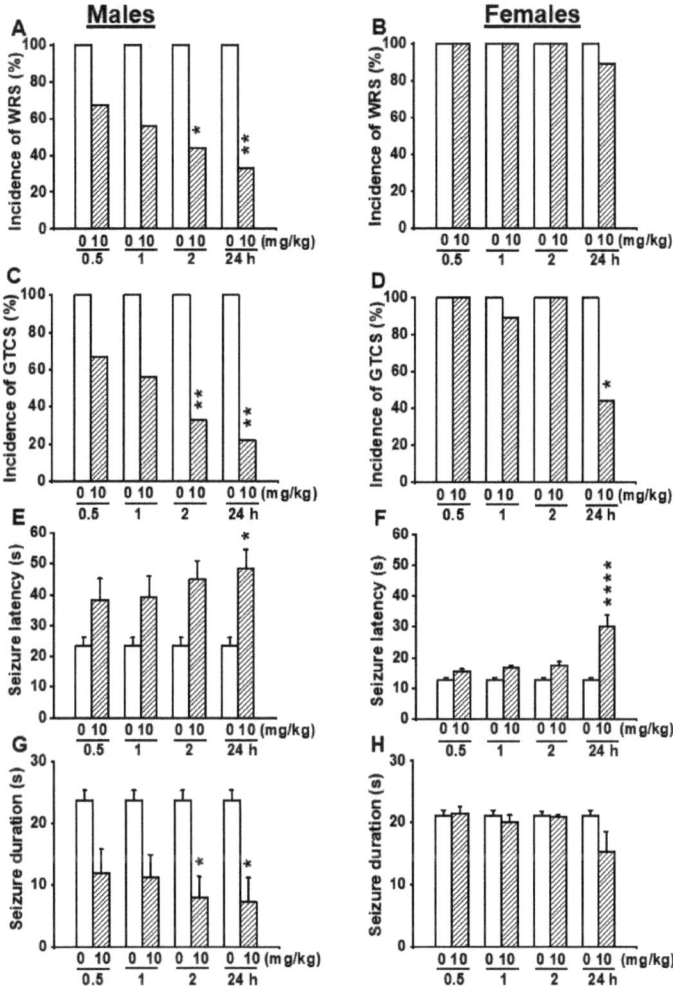

Figure 4. Effects of acute EACT treatment at the dose of 10 mg/kg on acoustically evoked seizures. The effects of EACT, a potent activator of TMEM16A, were evaluated at different post-treatment time points of 0.5, 1 h, 2 h, and 24 h in adult male and female GEPR-3s. (**A**) EACT treatment significantly reduced the incidence of the occurrence of WRSs at 2 and 24 h time points in males. (**B**) However, EACT treatment did not considerably alter the incidence of the occurrence of WRSs in females. (**C**) EACT treatment significantly reduced the incidence of the occurrence of GTCSs at 2 and 24 h post-treatment time points in males. (**D**) EACT treatment also significantly reduced the incidence of the occurrence of GTCSs at 24 h post-treatment time point in females. (**E**) EACT treatment significantly delayed the seizure onset at 24 h post-treatment time points in males. (**F**) Similarly, EACT treatment also significantly delayed the seizure onset at 24 h post-treatment time point in females. (**G**) EACT treatment significantly reduced the seizure duration at 2 and 24 h post-treatment time points in males. (**H**) However, in females, EACT did not considerably alter the seizure duration. Data from the incidence of WRSs and GTCSs were represented as a mean percentage (%), and Fisher Exact test was used for analysis. Data from the seizure latency and seizure duration were presented as mean ± S.E.M., and one-way ANOVA followed by Bonferroni correction was used for analysis. Opened and filled bar graphs represent control-treated (pre-EACT) and EACT treated GEPR-3s ($n = 9$), respectively. * $p < 0.05$, ** $p < 0.01$, **** $p < 0.0001$.

We also evaluated the effects of EACT pretreatment on the severity of acoustically evoked seizures. The Wilcoxon signed-rank test showed that EACT significantly reduced the seizure severity in male GEPR-3s at 1 h (z = 2.22, $p < 0.031$), 2 h (z = 2.22, $p < 0.031$), and 24 h (z = 2.33, $p < 0.019$) post-treatment time points compared with control testing conditions. However, the seizure severity was not considerably decreased at the 0.5 h post-treatment time point (Figure 2E). In females, EACT did not considerably alter the seizure severity up to 2 h post-treatment time points compared to the control conditions (Figure 2F).

We also quantified the effects of EACT pretreatment on seizure latency and seizure duration. In the control conditions, the seizure latency was 23.56 ± 2.49 s (n = 9) and 12.78 ± 0.68 s (n = 9) in male and female GEPR-3s, respectively (Figure 4E,F); the seizure duration was 23.67 ± 1.67 s (n = 9) and 21.11 ± 0.90 s (n = 9) in male and female GEPR-3s, respectively (Figure 4G,H). ANOVA showed that EACT pretreatment significantly alter the seizure latency in male GEPR-3s ($F_{(4,40)}$ = 2.786, $p < 0.0393$). Multiple comparisons revealed that EACT significantly delayed the seizure onset at the 24 h (t = 3.024, $p < 0.043$) post-treatment time point in male GEPR-3s compared with control testing conditions. No considerable delay of the seizure onset was seen at the other tested post-treatment time points (Figure 4E,F). In female GEPR-3s, the analysis showed that EACT pretreatment significantly alter the seizure latency ($F_{(4,40)}$ = 12.159, $p < 0.000001$). Multiple comparisons revealed that the seizure onset was only significantly delayed at the 24 h (t = 6.351, $p < 0.0001$) post-treatment time point compared with the control testing conditions. EACT did not considerably alter the seizure latency at the other tested post-treatment time points (Figure 4F). We also evaluated the effects of EACT pretreatment on the seizure duration. Analysis also showed that EACT pretreatment significantly alters the seizure duration in male GEPR-3s ($F_{(4,40)}$ = 3.776, $p < 0.0107$). Multiple comparisons revealed that, in male GEPR-3s, EACT significantly reduced the seizure duration at 2 h (t = 3.254, $p < 0.0232$) and 24 h (t = 3.417, $p < 0.0147$) post-treatment time points compared with control testing conditions. No considerable changes in the seizure duration were seen at other post-treatment time points (Figure 4G). However, EACT did not considerably alter the seizure duration in female GEPR-3s (Figure 4H).

In another set of experiments, we probed the extent to which inhibition of TMEM16A channels reversed the antiseizure effects seen following activation of these channels. Thus, we evaluated the effects of T16Ainh-A01 (10 mg/kg, body weight, p.o.), a potent inhibitor of TMEM16A channels on the acoustically evoked seizure susceptibility in both male (n = 6) and female (n = 6) GEPR-3s. Quantification showed that T16Ainh-A01 pretreatment did not alter the incidence of the occurrence of WRSs and GTCSs, the seizure latency, the seizure duration, and the seizure severity (compare Figures 4 and 5, and see Figure 2E–H). Comparison of the effects of EACT and T16Ainh-A01 on the seizure susceptibility revealed T16Ainh-A01 significantly rescued EACT-induced delay of the seizure latency (Figure 5E) and EACT-induced decreases in the seizure duration (Figure 5H) in male GEPR-3s. In female GEPR-3s, T16Ainh-A01 significantly rescued EACT-induced increases in the seizure latency 24-h post-treatment (Figure 5F). T16Ainh-A01 also increased the seizure duration compared to EACT pretreatment in female GEPR-3s at all tested post-treatment time points (Figure 5H). However, both EACT and T16Ainh-A01 did not alter the incidence of the occurrence of WRSs in both male and female GEPR-3s (Figure 5A,B). T16Ainh-A01 also did not considerably rescue the suppressive effects of EACT on the incidence of the occurrence GTCSs (Figure 5C,D) and the seizure severity (Figure 2G,H) in both male and female GEPR-3s.

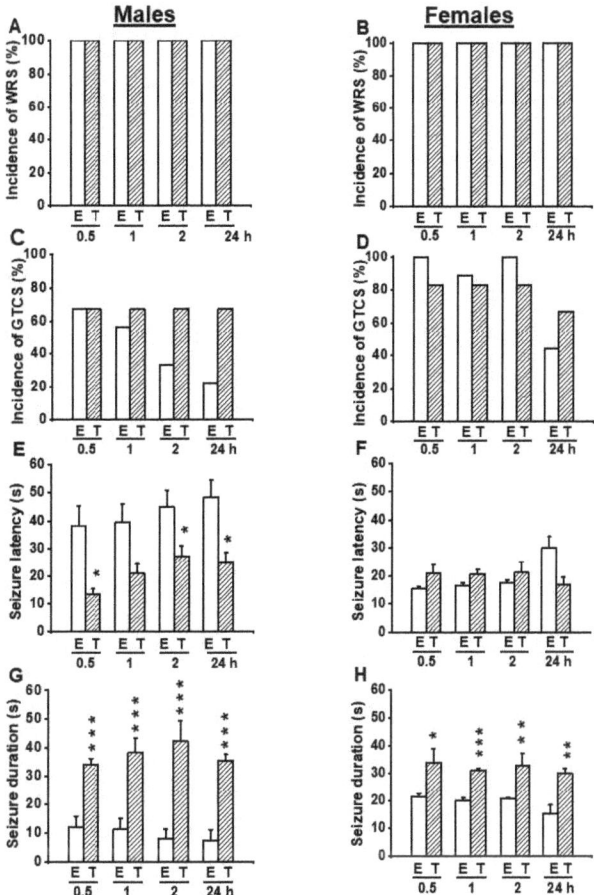

Figure 5. Effects of acute treatment with EACT (E) and T16Ainh-A01 (T), a potent activator and blocker of TMEM16A channels, respectively. The effects of EACT ($n = 9$) and T16Ainh-A01 ($n = 6$) on acoustically evoked seizures were evaluated at the dose of 10 mg/kg and at various posttreatment time points (0.5, 1 h, 2 h, and 24 h) in adult male and female GEPR-3s. Data were compared to determine the extent to which T16Ain-A01 treatment reverses the antiseizure effects seen in the EACT-treated group. (**A**) The incidence of the occurrence of WRSs was similar in both the EACT-treated and the T16Ainh-A01-treated groups in males. (**B**) Likewise, the incidence of the occurrence of WRSs was similar in both the EACT-treated group and T16Ainh-A01-treated group in females. (**C**) T16Ainh-A01 treatment reversed the reduced incidence of GTCSs seen in the EACT-treated group in males, but this effect did not reach statistical significance. (**D**) Similarly, T16Ainh-A01 treatment did alter the effects of EACT on the incidence of the occurrence of WRSs in female GEPR-3s. (**E**) T16Ainh-A01 treatment significantly reversed the effect of EACT treatment on the seizure latency in males. (**F**) In females, T16Ainh-01 also significantly reversed the effect of EACT on the seizure latency. (**G**) T16Ainh-A01 treatment significantly reversed the effect of EACT treatment on the seizure duration in males. (**H**) In females, T16Ainh-01 also significantly reversed the effect of EACT on the seizure duration. Data from the incidence of the occurrence of WRSs and GTCSs were represented as a mean percentage (%), and Fisher Exact test was used for analysis. Data from the seizure latency and duration were presented as mean ± S.E.M., and one-way ANOVA followed by Bonferroni correction was used for analysis. Opened and filled bar graphs represent EACT-treated GEPR-3s (E) and T16Ainh-A01-treated GEPR-3s (T). * $p < 0.05$, ** $p < 0.01$, *** $p < 0.001$.

Finally, we evaluated the effects of seizure susceptibility between male and female GEPR-3s used in this study. Analysis revealed no considerable changes in the seizure latency, seizure severity, incidence of the occurrence of WRSs and GTCSs, and seizure severity between male and female GEPR-3s (data not shown).

4. Discussion

In this study, we evaluated the role of activating TMEM16A channels as a putative novel mechanism for seizure suppression in the GEPR-3s. We found that activation of TMEM16A channels reduced the occurrence of both WRSs and GTCSs, and the seizure severity. We also found that activation of TMEM16A channels delayed the seizure onset and reduced the seizure duration. These antiseizure effects were primarily seen in male GEPR-3s. The effects on the seizure latency and duration (and seizure severity to a lesser extent) were markedly reversed by inhibiting TMEM16A channels. Together, these findings suggest that TMEM1A channels may play essential roles in the pathophysiology of inherited seizure susceptibility in the GEPR-3s. The prolonged seizure onset following activation of TMEM16A channels suggests that these channels may play a role in the propagation of seizure activity from the initiation site to networks responsible for the expression of seizure phenotypes. The reduced seizure duration following activation of TMEM16A channels indicates that these channels may play a role in the mechanisms underlying seizure termination. Finally, the suppression of the seizure severity suggests a role of TMEM16A channels on the seizure threshold and seizure initiation.

Acoustically evoked seizure susceptibility is associated with increased VGCC currents in IC neurons, suggestive of massive Ca^{2+} influx resulting in abnormal levels of intracellular Ca^{2+} that can activate chloride channels among other Ca^{2+}-dependent mechanisms. Therefore, CaCCs may play a role in the mechanisms underlying neuronal hyperexcitability that leads to seizures. Accordingly, selective deletion of TMEM16C channels in the brain exhibited enhanced susceptibility to hyperthermia-induced tonic-clonic seizures and decreased the seizure latency in rodent pups [30]. Furthermore, knockdown of TMEM16B channels in thalamocortical neurons reduced spike frequency adaptation and significantly decreased the afterhyperpolarization conductance, consistent with the enhanced neuronal excitability that can lead to seizures [31]. Interestingly, reduced spike frequency adaptation and slow afterhyperpolarization conductance were found in CA1 and CA3 neurons of the hippocampus in the GEPR-9, the most severe seizure severity strain of the GEPRs [32,33]. Such altered spike frequency adaptation and slow afterhyperpolarization may also occur in the GEPR-3s and contribute to enhancing the seizure susceptibility [14,34]. The mechanisms of how activation of CaCCs suppresses seizures are complex. Nevertheless, we posit that activation of CaCCs allows chloride influx that contributes to hyperpolarization of the neurons and modulates the spike-frequency adaptation via the shunting effect, leading to seizure suppression in the GEPR-3s [35–38]. Activation of CaCCs also contributes to elevated intraneuronal chloride levels, which have been reported to accompany seizure activity [18,19,39]. However, elevated intraneuronal chloride loading by itself does not trigger a complete ictal activity [39].

Other molecular targets can mediate the antiseizure effects of EACT. Evidence indicates that EACT also activates the transient receptor potential vanilloid 1 (TRPV1) channel in addition to CaCCs, suggesting a potential role of these channels in EACT's antiseizure effects [40]. However, we previously reported that capsazepine, a potent inhibitor of TRPV1 channels, completely suppressed the seizure susceptibility in female (but not male, as seen in the present study with EACT) GEPR-3s [41]. These findings ruled out the possible role of TRPV1 channels in EACT's antiseizure effects in male GEPR-3s. In the present study, we also found that EACT's antiseizure effects were mainly seen in male but not female GEPR-3s, suggesting that male GEPR-3s are more sensitive to the activation of CaCCs. The underlying biological mechanisms for the differential sex effect of EACT's antiseizure effects are unknown in GEPR-3s. Nevertheless, sex-related EACT's antiseizure effects may be due to sex differences in inherited seizure susceptibility in GEPR-3s. However, this study found no notable differences in the parameters and phenotypes of acoustically evoked seizures between male and female GEPR-3s. Steroid hormones and endogenous neuro-steroids have been implicated as factors contributing to sex differences in epilepsy and may play a role in the lack of EACT's antiseizure effects in female GEPR-3s [42]. However, female GEPR-3s consistently exhibited seizures over 30 days of repetitive acoustic stimulations, ruling out the possible role of steroids and neuro-steroids in EACT's antiseizure effects [43]. A potential sex-related mechanism of the EACT's antiseizure effects may include altered function and expression of TMEM16A channels, at least in the IC, the initiation site of acoustically evoked seizures in the GEPR.

Despite the novelty of our findings, this study has a limitation of its translational value because no mutations of the genes encoding for CaCCs are yet associated with seizure phenotypes and epilepsy syndromes in humans [2,44].

In conclusion, activation of TMEM16A channels is sufficient to suppress seizure susceptibility in the male GEPR-3s, providing a putative novel cellular mechanism for controlling tonic-clonic seizures and epilepsy.

Author Contributions: Conceptualization, P.N.; methodology, P.N.; analysis, M.T., M.S., P.N.; investigation, M.T., M.S., P.N.; writing—original draft preparation: P.N.; writing—review and editing M.T., M.S., P.N.; supervision, P.N.; funding acquisition, P.N. All authors have read and agreed to the published version of the manuscript.

Funding: This work was partially funded by the National Institute of Alcoholism and Alcohol Abuse (R01 AA027660 grant to P.N.) at the National Institutes of Health.

Institutional Review Board Statement: The study was conducted according to the National Institutes of Health Guide for the Care and Use of Laboratory Animals and approved by the Institutional Animal and Use Committee of Howard University (protocol number MED-20-04; approved on 12 July 2021).

Data Availability Statement: Data are available upon request from the corresponding author.

Conflicts of Interest: The authors declare no conflict of interest.

References

1. Devinsky, O.; Bundock, E.; Hesdorffer, D.; Donner, E.; Moseley, B.; Cihan, E.; Hussain, F.; Friedman, D. Resolving ambiguities in SUDEP classification. *Epilepsia* **2018**, *59*, 1220–1233. [CrossRef] [PubMed]
2. Coll, M.; Oliva, A.; Grassi, S.; Brigada, R.; Campuzano, O. Update on the genetic basis of sudden unexpected death in Epilepsy. *Int. J. Mol. Sci.* **2019**, *20*, 1979. [CrossRef] [PubMed]
3. Zack, M.M.; Kobau, R. National and State Estimates of the Numbers of Adults and Children with Active Epilepsy—United States, 2015. *Morb. Mortal. Wkly. Rep.* **2017**, *66*, 821–825. [CrossRef] [PubMed]
4. WHO. *World Health Organization: Epilepsy: Epidemiology, Aetiology, and Prognosis*; WHO Factsheet; WHO: Geneva, Switzerland, 2001.
5. French, J.A. Refractory epilepsy: Clinical overview. *Epilepsia* **2007**, *48* (Suppl. S1), 3–7. [CrossRef]
6. Kwan, P.; Arzimanoglou, A.; Berg, A.T.; Brodie, M.J.; Allen Hauser, W.; Mathern, G.; Moshé, S.L.; Perucca, E.; Wiebe, S.; French, J. Definition of drug resistant epilepsy: Consensus proposal by the ad hoc Task Force of the ILAE Commission on Therapeutic Strategies. *Epilepsia* **2010**, *51*, 1069–1107. [CrossRef]
7. Lux, H.D.; Heinemann, U. Ionic changes during experimentally induced seizure activity. *Electrencephalogr. Clin. Neurophysiol.* **1978**, *34*, 289–297.
8. Heinemann, U.; Konnerth, A.; Pumain, R.; Wadman, W.J. Extracellular calcium and potassium concentration changes in chronic epileptic brain tissue. *Adv. Neurol.* **1986**, *44*, 641–661.
9. Albowitz, B.; König, P.; Kuhnt, U. Spatiotemporal distribution of intracellular calcium transients during epileptiform activity in guinea pig hippocampal slices. *J. Neurophysiol.* **1997**, *77*, 491–501. [CrossRef]
10. Delorenzo, R.J.; Sun, D.A.; Deshpande, L.S. Cellular mechanisms underlying acquired epilepsy: The calcium hypothesis of the induction and maintenance of epilepsy. *Pharmacol. Ther.* **2005**, *105*, 229–266. [CrossRef]
11. De Sarro, G.; De Sarro, A.; Federico, F.; Meldrum, B.S. Anticonvulsant properties of some calcium antagonists on sound-induced seizures in genetically epilepsy prone rats. *Gen. Pharmacol.* **1990**, *21*, 768–778. [CrossRef]
12. De Sarro, G.; Ascioti, C.; Di Paola, E.D.; Vidal, M.J.; De Sarro, A. Effects of antiepileptic drugs, calcium channel blockers and other compounds on seizures induced by activation of voltage-dependent L calcium channel in DBA/2 mice. *Gen. Pharmacol.* **1992**, *23*, 1205–1216. [CrossRef]

13. De Sarro, G.; Russo, E.; Citraro, R.; Meldrum, B.S. Genetically epilepsy-prone rats (GEPRs) and DBA/2 mice: Two animal models of audiogenic reflex epilepsy for the evaluation of new generation AEDs. *Epilepsy Behav.* **2017**, *71*, 165–173. [CrossRef] [PubMed]
14. Khandai, P.; Forcelli, P.A.; N'Gouemo, P. Activation of small conductance calcium-activated potassium channels suppresses seizure susceptibility in the genetically epilepsy-prone rats. *Neuropharmacology* **2020**, *163*, 107865. [CrossRef] [PubMed]
15. Faingold, C.L. Neuronal networks in the genetically epilepsy-prone rat. *Adv. Neurol.* **1999**, *79*, 311–321.
16. N'Gouemo, P.; Faingold, C.L.; Morad, M. Calcium channel dysfunction in inferior colliculus neurons of the genetically epilepsy-prone rat. *Neuropharmacology* **2009**, *56*, 665–675. [CrossRef]
17. N'Gouemo, P.; Yasuda, R.P.; Faingold, C. Seizure susceptibility is associated with altered protein expression of voltage-gated calcium channel subunits in inferior colliculus neurons of the genetically epilepsy-prone rats. *Brain Res.* **2010**, *1308*, 153–157. [CrossRef]
18. Raimondo, J.V.; Burman, R.J.; Katz, A.A.; Akerman, C.J. Ion dynamics during seizures. *Front. Cell. Neurosci.* **2015**, *9*, 419. [CrossRef]
19. Raimondo, J.V.; Joyce, B.; Kay, L.; Schlagheck, T.; Newey, S.E.; Srinivas, S.; Akerman, C.J. A genetically encoded chloride and pH sensor for dissociating ion dynamics in the nervous system. *Front. Cell. Neurosci.* **2013**, *7*, 202. [CrossRef]
20. Mayer, M. A calcium-activated chloride current generates the after-hyperpolarization of rat sensory neurons in culture. *J. Physiol. Lond.* **1985**, *364*, 217–239. [CrossRef]
21. Hartzell, C.; Putzier, I.; Arreola, J. Calcium-activated chloride channels. *Annu. Rev. Physiol.* **2005**, *67*, 719–758. [CrossRef]
22. Shroeder, B.C.; Cheng, T.; Jan, Y.N.; Jan, L.Y. Expression cloning of TMEM16A as a calcium-activated chloride channel subunit. *Cell* **2008**, *134*, 1019–1029. [CrossRef] [PubMed]
23. Caputo, A.; Caci, E.; Ferrera, L.; Pedemonte, N.; Sondo, E.; Pfeffer, U.; Ravazzolo, R.; Zegarra-Moran, O.; Galietta, L.J. TMEM16A, a membrane protein associated with calcium-dependent chloride channel activity. *Science* **2008**, *322*, 590–594. [CrossRef] [PubMed]
24. Yang, Y.D.; Cho, H.; Koo, J.Y.; Tak, M.H.; Cho, Y.; Shim, W.S.; Park, S.P.; Lee, J.; Lee, B.; Kim, B.M.; et al. TMEM16A confers receptor-activated calcium dependent chloride conductance. *Nature* **2008**, *455*, 1210–1215. [CrossRef] [PubMed]
25. Kunzelmann, K.; Kongsuphol, P.; Aldehni, F.; Tian, Y.; Ousingsawat, J.; Warth, R.; Schreiber, R. Bestrophin and TMEM16-Ca^{2+} activated Cl$^-$ channels with different functions. *Cell Calcium* **2009**, *46*, 233–241. [CrossRef]
26. Kunzelmann, K.; Kongsuphol, P.; Chootip, K.; Toledo, C.; Martins, J.R.; Almaca, J.; Tian, Y.; Witzgall, R.; Ousingsawat, J.; Schreiber, R. Role of Ca^{2+}-activated Cl$^-$ channels bestrophin and anoctamin in epithelial cells. *Biol. Chem.* **2009**, *392*, 125–134. [CrossRef]
27. Cho, S.J.; Jeon, J.H.; Chun, D.I.; Yeo, S.W.; Kim, I.-B. Anoctamin 1 expression in the mouse auditory brainstem. *Cell Tissue Res.* **2014**, *357*, 563–569. [CrossRef]
28. National Research Council (U.S.); Institute for Laboratory Animal Research (U.S.); National Academies Press (U.S.). *Guide for the Care and Use of Laboratory Animals*; National Academies Press: Washington, DC, USA, 2011.
29. Mishra, P.K.; Dailey, J.W.; Reigel, C.E.; Jobe, P.C. Audiogenic convulsions in moderate seizure genetically epilepsy-prone rats (GEPR-3s). *Epilepsy Res.* **1989**, *3*, 191–198. [CrossRef]
30. Wang, T.A.; Chen, C.; Huang, F.; Feng, S.; Tien, J.; Braz, J.M.; Basbaum, A.I.; Jan, Y.N.; Jan, L.Y. TMEM16C is involved in thermoregulation and protects rodent pups from febrile seizures. *Proc. Natl. Acad. Sci. USA* **2021**, *118*, e2023342118. [CrossRef]
31. Ha, G.E.; Cheon, G. Calcium-activated chloride channels: New target to control the spiking pattern of neurons. *BMR Rep.* **2017**, *50*, 109–110. [CrossRef]
32. Verma-Ahuja, S.; Pencek, T.L. Hippocampal CA1 neurons properties in the genetically epilepsy-prone rats. *Epilepsy Res.* **1994**, *18*, 205–215. [CrossRef]
33. Verma-Ahuja, S.; Evans, M.S.; Pencek, T.L. Evidence for decreased calcium dependent potassium conductance in hippocampal CA3 neurons of the genetically epilepsy-prone rats. *Epilepsy Res.* **1995**, *22*, 137–144. [CrossRef]
34. N'Gouemo, P.; Yasuda, R.P.; Faingold, C.L. Protein expression of small conductance calcium-activated potassium channels is altered in inferior colliculus neurons of the genetically epilepsy-prone rat. *Brain Res.* **2009**, *1270*, 107–111. [CrossRef]
35. Huang, W.C.; Xiao, S.; Huang, F.; Harfe, B.D.; Jan, Y.N.; Jan, L.Y. Calcium-activated chloride channels (CaCCs) regulate action potential and synaptic response in hippocampal neurons. *Neuron* **2012**, *74*, 179–192. [CrossRef] [PubMed]
36. Zhan, W.; Schmelzeisen, S.; Parthier, D.; Möhrlen, F. Anoctamin and calcium-activated chloride channels may modulate inhibitory transmission in the cerebellar cortex. *PLoS ONE* **2015**, *10*, e0142160.
37. Ha, G.E.; Lee, J.; Kwak, H.; Song, K.; Kwon, J.; Jung, S.-Y.; Hong, J.; Chang, G.-E.; Hwang, E.M.; Shin, H.-S.; et al. The Ca^{2+}-activated chloride channel anoctamin-2 mediates spike-frequency adaptation and regulates sensory transmission in thalamocortical neurons. *Nat. Commun.* **2016**, *7*, 13791–13803. [CrossRef] [PubMed]
38. Wang, L.; Simms, J.; Peters, C.J.; Tynan-La Fontaine, M.; Li, K.; Gill, M.; Jan, Y.N.; Jan, L.Y. TMEM16B calcium activated chloride channels regulate action potential firing in lateral septum and aggression in male mice. *J. Neurosci.* **2019**, *39*, 7102–7117. [CrossRef]
39. Alfonsa, H.; Merricks, E.M.; Codadu, N.K.; Cunningham, M.O.; Deisseroth, K.; Racca, C.; Trevelyan, A.J. The contribution of raised intraneuronal chloride to epileptic network activity. *J. Neurosci.* **2015**, *35*, 7715–7726. [CrossRef]
40. Liu, S.; Feng, J.; Luo, J.; Yang, P.; Brett, T.J.; Hu, H. Eact, a small molecule activator of TMEM16A, activates TRPV1 and elicits pain- and itch-related behaviours. *Br. J. Pharmacol.* **2016**, *173*, 1208–1218. [CrossRef]
41. Akita, T.; Fukuda, A. Intracellular Cl$^-$ dysregulation causing and caused by pathological neuronal activity. *Pflügers Arch.-Eur. J. Physiol.* **2020**, *472*, 977–987. [CrossRef]

42. Cho, S.J.; Vaca, M.A.; Miranda, C.J.; N'Gouemo, P. Inhibition of transient potential receptor vanilloid type 1 suppresses seizure susceptibility in the genetically epilepsy-prone rat. *CNS Neurosci. Ther.* **2018**, *24*, 18–28. [CrossRef]
43. Naritoku, D.K.; Mecozzi, L.B.; Aiello, M.T.; Faingold, C.L. Repetition of audiogenic seizures in genetically epilepsy-prone rats induces cortical epileptiform activity and additional seizure behaviors. *Exp. Neurol.* **1992**, *115*, 317–324. [CrossRef]
44. Martinez, L.A.; Lai, Y.-C.; Holder, J.L.; Anderson, A.E. Genetics in epilepsy. *Neurol. Clin.* **2021**, *39*, 743–777. [CrossRef] [PubMed]

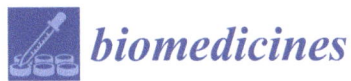

Article

Increased TRPV1 Channels and FosB Protein Expression Are Associated with Chronic Epileptic Seizures and Anxiogenic-like Behaviors in a Preclinical Model of Temporal Lobe Epilepsy

Willian Lazarini-Lopes [1], Gleice Kelli Silva-Cardoso [2], Christie Ramos Andrade Leite-Panissi [2] and Norberto Garcia-Cairasco [1,3,*]

[1] Neuroscience and Behavioral Sciences Department, Ribeirão Preto School of Medicine, University of São Paulo, Ribeirão Preto 14049-900, Brazil; willian.lopes@usp.br
[2] Psychology Department, Faculty of Philosophy, Science, and Letters, University of São Paulo, Ribeirão Preto 14040-901, Brazil; cardoso.gkrs@usp.br (G.K.S.-C.); christie@usp.br (C.R.A.L.-P.)
[3] Physiology Department, Ribeirão Preto School of Medicine and Neuroscience and Behavioral Sciences Department, University of São Paulo, Ribeirão Preto 14049-900, Brazil
* Correspondence: ngcairas@usp.br

Abstract: Epilepsies are neurological disorders characterized by chronic seizures and their related neuropsychiatric comorbidities, such as anxiety. The Transient Receptor Potential Vanilloid type-1 (TRPV1) channel has been implicated in the modulation of seizures and anxiety-like behaviors in preclinical models. Here, we investigated the impact of chronic epileptic seizures in anxiety-like behavior and TRPV1 channels expression in a genetic model of epilepsy, the Wistar Audiogenic Rat (WAR) strain. WARs were submitted to audiogenic kindling (AK), a preclinical model of temporal lobe epilepsy (TLE) and behavioral tests were performed in the open-field (OF), and light-dark box (LDB) tests 24 h after AK. WARs displayed increased anxiety-like behavior and TRPV1R expression in the hippocampal CA1 area and basolateral amygdala nucleus (BLA) when compared to control Wistar rats. Chronic seizures increased anxiety-like behaviors and TRPV1 and FosB expression in limbic and brainstem structures involved with epilepsy and anxiety comorbidity, such as the hippocampus, superior colliculus, and periaqueductal gray matter. Therefore, these results highlight previously unrecognized alterations in TRPV1 expression in brain structures involved with TLE and anxiogenic-like behaviors in a genetic model of epilepsy, the WAR strain, supporting an important role of TRPV1 in the modulation of neurological disorders and associated neuropsychiatric comorbidities.

Keywords: epilepsy; anxiety; TRPV1 channels; neuronal activity; neuropsychiatric comorbidity; immunofluorescence; temporal lobe epilepsy; audiogenic kindling

Citation: Lazarini-Lopes, W.; Silva-Cardoso, G.K.; Leite-Panissi, C.R.A.; Garcia-Cairasco, N. Increased TRPV1 Channels and FosB Protein Expression Are Associated with Chronic Epileptic Seizures and Anxiogenic-like Behaviors in a Preclinical Model of Temporal Lobe Epilepsy. *Biomedicines* **2022**, *10*, 416. https://doi.org/10.3390/biomedicines10020416

Academic Editor: Joanna Pera

Received: 18 December 2021
Accepted: 20 January 2022
Published: 10 February 2022

Publisher's Note: MDPI stays neutral with regard to jurisdictional claims in published maps and institutional affiliations.

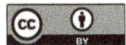

Copyright: © 2022 by the authors. Licensee MDPI, Basel, Switzerland. This article is an open access article distributed under the terms and conditions of the Creative Commons Attribution (CC BY) license (https://creativecommons.org/licenses/by/4.0/).

1. Introduction

Epilepsies are neurological disorders characterized by chronic epileptic seizures and their consequent neuropsychiatric comorbidities [1,2]. Among them, we can highlight anxiety, which is one of the most common comorbidities associated with epilepsies, not only because of the epileptogenic processes but also as a cause of its exacerbation, which indicates a bidirectional relationship between epilepsies and anxiety [3–5]. Therefore, anxiety symptoms, or anxiogenic-like behaviors, may be present either as intrinsic aspects of epileptic seizures or as events related to inter-ictal alterations [6–8]. Additionally, anxiety management can overlap epilepsy, and some antiseizure drugs may modulate anxiety in patients with epilepsies, while classical anxiolytic drugs also display antiseizure effects [2,3,9].

The phenomenon of the bidirectionality between neurological disorders and neuropsychiatric comorbidities has been frequently discussed in the literature [10,11]. Studies demonstrated that seizure severity is highly correlated with anxiety and other neuropsychiatric comorbidities, such as depression, in patients with epilepsies, supporting a direct relationship between seizures and affective disorders. Consequently, the diagnosis of epilepsies increases the chances of suicide and further diagnosis of anxiety, but the opposite is also true once patients with anxiety and depressive disorders have a higher risk of developing epilepsies in comparison to those who do not suffer from mood or anxiety disorders [3,5,6,12,13]. Additionally, it is worth noticing that brainstem and limbic structures, such as the periaqueductal gray matter (PAG), superior colliculus, basolateral amygdala nucleus (BLA), and hippocampus, are intrinsically involved with epileptic seizures manifestations [14–17], as well as with anxiogenic, emotional and defensive behaviors [18–21], indicating that neuroplastic and functional alterations in these neuronal networks can impact epilepsy and anxiety comorbidity.

Psychiatric and neurological disorders are commonly associated with changes in neural calcium ion signaling pathways. The transient receptor potential vanilloid (TRPV) channel family is composed of seven different subfamilies, and most of their members are closely related to the modulation of calcium influx. The TRPV type-1 (TRPV1) is a non-selective calcium-permeable cation channel with high Ca^{2+} permeability that has been associated with a wide range of biological functions, such as synaptic plasticity, anxiety, fear, stress, thermoregulation, and pain [22–26]. TRPV1 channels are widely expressed in the brain, but cortical and limbic structures present the highest levels of TRPV1 protein and mRNA [27,28]. Moreover, TRPV1 signaling is associated with other neurotransmitter systems related with neuropsychiatric disorders, especially the endocannabinoid [29–31], which makes its neurobiological function even more complex to understand.

Since TRPV1 receptors are involved with calcium mobilization, these channels have been shown to be intrinsically involved with synaptic excitability and, consequently, with epileptic seizure susceptibility and manifestation [32–34]. Increased mRNA and protein levels of TRPV1 channels were observed in the hippocampus and cortex of patients with temporal lobe epilepsy (TLE) [35] and preclinical models suggest an important role for TRPV1 in seizure susceptibility, especially because its pharmacological activation facilitates seizure manifestation [33,36,37]. Additionally, evidence supports the role of TRPV1 channels located in the brainstem and limbic structures in the modulation of emotional and anxiety-like behaviors [22,38,39].

The Wistar Audiogenic Rat (WAR) strain is a genetic model of epilepsy with animals susceptible to audiogenic seizures (AGS)—for a comprehensive review see [40]. Acute AGS mimics generalized tonic-clonic seizures associated with brainstem hyperactivity, where the inferior colliculus (IC), deep layers of the superior colliculus (DLSC), and dorsal PAG (dPAG) play an important role in seizure susceptibility and manifestation [15,41]. However, during the chronic protocol of AGS, the audiogenic kindling (AK), firstly demonstrated by Marescaux et al. [42], limbic seizures, modulated by cortical and limbic brains sites, coexist with brainstem seizures. Thus, AK in genetically susceptible rodents is considered a model of TLE with limbic recruitment characterized by electrographic and behavioral seizures [43–48], similar to those described by Racine in the amygdala kindling protocol [49]. It is worth noting that genetic selection for seizure susceptibility in the WAR strain also selected physiological and behavioral alterations associated with epilepsy related comorbidities [40,50]. Additionally, chronic seizures in WARs induce spatial memory deficits [51] and increase the expression of glutamate receptor subunits [52] and CB1 receptors [53] in limbic structures. Therefore, genetic susceptibility and chronic epileptic seizures are both involved with manifestations of neuropsychiatric comorbidities underlying epilepsy in the WAR strain.

However, the impact of both genetic background and chronic epileptic seizures on anxiety-like behaviors still needs to be appropriately investigated in WARs. Similarly, despite TRPV1 channels being closely related with epilepsies and their comorbidities, possible neuroplastic alterations in their expression have never been analyzed, either in WARs or in other genetic models of audiogenic seizures. Therefore, the present study aimed to investigate endogenous alterations in TRPV1 channels expression in the brainstem and limbic structures involved with seizure susceptibility and anxiogenic-like behaviors in the WAR strain. We also characterized the impact of AK, a model of TLE, on anxiety-like behaviors and TRPV1 and FosB expression in the brainstem and limbic structures involved with the comorbidity epilepsy and anxiety in animals of the WAR strain.

2. Materials and Methods

2.1. Animals

Adult male Wistar (n = 16) and WAR (n = 16) rats (2–4 months old) were provided by the Central Vivarium of the University of São Paulo, Ribeirão Preto, and by the Special Rat Strains' Vivarium of the Ribeirão Preto School of Medicine, respectively. Animals were kept at the Animal Housing Facility of the Physiology Department of the Ribeirão Preto School of Medicine, University of São Paulo, housed in groups of 3–4 animals per cage in a controlled temperature (23 ± 2 °C) under light/dark cycle of 12/12 h. (lights on at 6:00 a.m.), with access to food and water ad libitum. The experimental protocol was approved by the Ethics Committee in Animal Research of the Ribeirão Preto School of Medicine, University of São Paulo (Protocol number: 057/2017; approval date: 2 August 2017).

2.2. Chronic Audiogenic Seizure (AGS) Protocol: Audiogenic Kindling (AK)

Chronic AGS were induced as previously described [43,53]. Briefly, animals were placed into an acrylic cylindrical chamber located at a soundproof wood chamber. A small speaker connected to a computer was placed on the top of the acrylic chamber. In every test session, animals were placed into the chamber and after 1 min the sound (110–120 dB; 5–20 kHz) was manually triggered by the researcher and applied until the onset of a tonic seizure, or for a maximum of 60 s if no seizure was observed. Animal behavior was recorded for 1 min before sound, maximum of 1 min during sound exposure, and 1 min after sound. During the AK, WARs (n = 8) were submitted to 20 acoustic stimulations for 10 days (2 per day), every morning (8:00–9:00 a.m.) and afternoon (5:00–6:00 p.m.). The apparatus was cleaned with 5% ethanol solution after each test session.

Wistar rats (n = 8) were submitted to the same protocol, for two reasons: as a control of the specificity of the AK protocol to induce seizures only in genetically susceptible rats and to investigate if changes induced by the AK in WARs were, in fact, due to the epileptogenic process and not merely due to the chronic sound exposure. Additionally, to investigate possible endogenous alterations in anxiety-like behaviors, chronic neuronal hyperactivity, and TRPV1 expression in the WAR strain, control (non-stimulated) WARs (n = 8) and Wistars (n = 8) were submitted to a false AK (Sham) protocol, exactly as described for chronic stimulated animals, but the sound was never applied in these groups.

Brainstem seizure severity was analyzed according to the Brainstem index [54], where: 0 = no seizure; 1 = one running; 2 = one wild running (running with jumps and atonic falls); 3 = two wild runnings; 4 = tonic convulsion; 5 = tonic seizure followed by generalized clonic convulsion; 6 = index 5 plus head ventral flexion; 7 = index 6 plus forelimb hyperextension; 8 = index 7 plus hindlimb hyperextension. Limbic seizures were measured according to the Racine scale [49], where: 0 = no seizure; 1 = facial and years myoclonus; 2 = head myoclonus; 3 = forelimb myoclonus; 4 = forelimb myoclonus, followed by elevation; 5 = forelimb myoclonus, followed by elevation and fall.

2.3. Behavioral Tests for Anxiety

In the morning (8:00–11:00 a.m.) after the last AGS or sham exposure to the cylinder, animals were submitted to the open-field (OF) test followed by the light/dark box (LDB) test to investigate possible alterations in anxiety-like behaviors (see Figure 1).

The OF consists of an acrylic circular arena (90 cm diameter) with a 40 cm wall, and a floor divided into 12 equal areas. Animals were placed in the center of the apparatus (50 lux) and behaviors were recorded for 5 min by a camera located above the apparatus. The time spent in the central area of the apparatus was calculated and the locomotory activity was measured according to the number of crossings. Duration and frequency of vertical exploratory behaviors (rearings) and grooming were also measured.

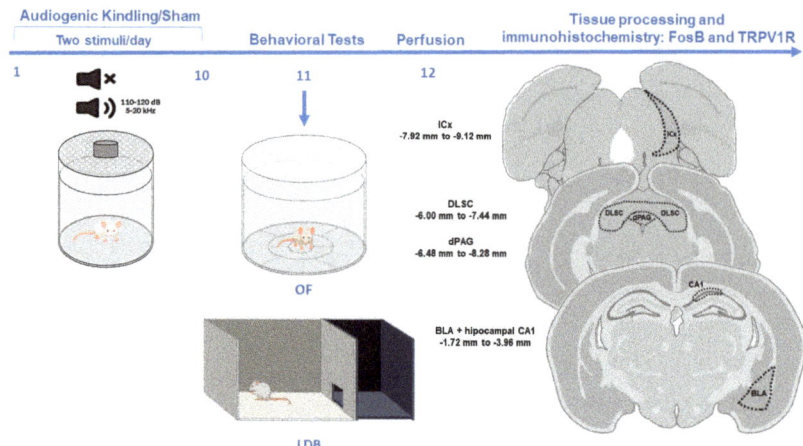

Figure 1. Experimental design. Animals were submitted to the audiogenic kindling (AK) protocol with 20 acoustic simulations. After that, animals were submitted to behavioral tests, and tissue was collected for immunohistochemistry. Abbreviations: OF—open field test, LDB—light/dark box test, ICx—inferior colliculus cortical area, dPAG—dorsal periaqueductal gray matter, DLSC—deep layers of superior colliculus, BLA—basolateral amygdala nucleus, CA1—dorsal hippocampus sub-region.

The light/dark box (LDB) test was performed 5 min after the OF in a different room. The apparatus consists of an acrylic box with overall dimensions of 100 × 50 × 40 cm (length, width, height) divided into a light and a dark compartment with a doorway (10 × 10 cm) communicating both sides. The lit side (65 lux) has floor and walls painted white, a transparent roof, and corresponds to 2/3 of the size of the apparatus. The dark compartment (0 lux) has floor, walls, and roof all painted black and corresponds to 1/3 of the size of the apparatus. Animals were individually placed in the center of the lit compartment turned back to the doorway separating both compartments. Behavior was recorded for 5 min by a camera located above the apparatus and the following parameters were measured: number of entries and time spent into the lit compartment, latency to the first transition to the dark compartment, latency to the first return to the lit compartment, and frequency and duration of rearings. The number of risk assessment behaviors, such as stretched attempt postures and pokes, were also measured. After each session, the OF and LDB were cleaned with 5% ethanol.

2.4. Tissue Processing and Immunohistochemistry

Animals were anesthetized with sodium thiopental (50 mg/kg; i.p.; Abbott, São Paulo, Brazil) and perfused with phosphate-buffered saline (PBS 0.1M, pH 7.4) followed by paraformaldehyde (PFA 4%, pH 7.4) 24 h after behavioral tests. Brains were post-fixed in PFA for 4 h and then cryoprotected in sucrose solution 30% at 4 °C and, after that, they were frozen in isopentane and dry ice. Using a cryostat (Microm HM-505-E, Microm International, Walldorf, Germany), serial coronal sections (40 μm) from the dorsal hippocampus, BLA, DLSC, dPAG, and the cortical area of the IC (ICx) were cut following the coordinates from Paxinos and Watson [55]. Slices were stored in a cryoprotection solution (50% PBS, 30% ethylene glycol, 20% glycerol) until immunohistochemical experiments. Representative images of each structure are illustrated in Figure 1.

Immunofluorescence for TRPV1 channels was performed in the DLSC, dPAG, BLA, and in the CA1 region of the dorsal hippocampus, as we have previously described [56]. Briefly, after washing in PBS, free-floating sections were incubated overnight in a mouse polyclonal antibody that recognizes the C-terminal of the TRPV1 receptor (Abcam, ab203103, Cambridge, UK) diluted in normal goat serum (1:1000). Tissues were washed in PBS and then incubated for 2 h in an anti-mouse IgG Rhodamine B (AP192R) diluted in normal goat serum (1:1000). The slides were mounted in Vectashield mounting medium (Vector Laboratories, Burlingame, CA, USA) and stored at 4 °C. Immunostaining for FosB+ neurons were performed in the ICx, DLSC, dPAG, and BLA as previously described [57]. Briefly, free-floating sections were washed in PBS and incubated overnight in a rabbit polyclonal primary antibody (1:1000; sc-48, Santa Cruz Biotechnology, Dallas, TX, USA) diluted in a 2% solution of bovine serum albumin solution (BSA, Amresco, Solon, OH, USA). On the next day, slices were washed in PSB and incubated for 2 h in a biotinylated secondary antibody anti-rabbit IgG (1:1.000; BA-1000, lot. Zb0318, Vector) diluted in BSA solution. Immunoreactive sites were visualized using the 3,3'-diaminobenzidine (DAB) peroxidase substrate with nickel (SK-4100, Vector). Slices were mounted on glass slides and coverslipped with Permount (Sigma-Aldrich, Inc., St. Louis, MO, USA).

For FosB and TRPV1R immunohistochemical protocols, negative control sections were incubated as described, but without the primary antibody, and immunoreactivity was absent in these sections.

2.5. Image Processing and Analysis

Immunoreactive sites were visualized and photographed in a scanning microscope (Olympus BX61VS). Tissues processed for TRPV1R immunofluorescence and FosB+ neurons were analyzed in 400× magnification and the software ImageJ (National Institute of Mental Health, Bethesda, MD, USA) was used for image processing analysis as we previously described [56,57].

To analyze the TRPV1 immunofluorescence images, we used the Integrated Optical Density (IOD) method. Six slices per animal were analyzed for each structure of interest, with a sample of six animals randomly selected per group. The intensity was analyzed using the software ImageJ (https://imagej.nih.gov/ij/ version 1.8.0; accessed on 20 November 2021) and the mean value of the integrated density (the product of the area and the mean gray value) was calculated using the mean value of the three regions of interest (ROI), randomly selected within each structure of each animal. In smaller areas, such as CA1 and dPAG, we used 3 ROIs with 2.500 μm^2, while in the BLA, DLSC, and IC, 3 ROI with 10.000 μm^2 were used. For FosB immunostaining, three slices per animal were analyzed for each region of interest, with a sample of five animals randomly selected per group. To analyze the number of FosB+ neurons, we opted for the manual counting method (blind researcher). For each animal, we used the arithmetic mean of the total number of FosB+ cells detected in 3 ROIs (10.000 mm^2 each one) randomly selected within each structure.

2.6. Statistical Analysis

Data were tested for normality using the Shapiro–Wilk test. Statistical analysis was performed using Two-Way ANOVA (variables: STRAIN and AK) followed by post hoc Tukey's test. Data were expressed as mean ± standard error of the mean, and the software GraphPad Prism 9.0 (GraphPad Software, Inc., La Jolla, CA, USA) was used to perform statistical analysis and to create the graphics. Significant differences: $p < 0.05$.

3. Results

3.1. Audiogenic Kindling (AK) Progression

In the beginning of the protocol, WARs developed brainstem AGS in response to intense sound stimulation; seizures were characterized by wild running with jumps and atonic falls followed by generalized tonic-clonic seizure behaviors, such as forelimb hyperextension, partial or generalized clonic seizures. During AK, limbic seizures coexist with those that originated from brainstem structures; this phenomenon is illustrated by the appearance of novel clonic seizure behaviors such as those described by Racine [49], similar to facial and forelimb myoclonus, followed by body elevation and fall (Figure 2). All WARs developed AGS during the AK protocol and 4/8 rats from the WAR-AK group developed severe limbic seizures (Racine ≥ 4) during the AK and were classified as forebrain-recruited; the remaining four WARs from this group developed consistent generalized tonic-clonic seizures, but limbic seizures were not detected. Wistar rats submitted to chronic auditory stimulation did not develop AGS.

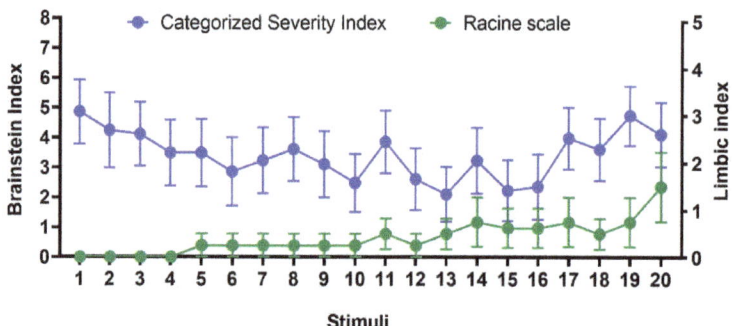

Figure 2. Evolution of audiogenic kindling (AK) in WARs. Mean of brainstem (blue circles) and limbic (green circles) seizure severity during AK. Only brainstem generalized tonic-clonic seizures were detected at the beginning of the protocol; however, during the AK, limbic seizures coexist with those that originated from the brainstem. Data are represented by mean ± standard error mean (n = 8/group).

3.2. Open-Field (OF) Test

Results from the OF test are presented in Figure 3. Firstly, regarding the time in the center of the OF, two-way ANOVA showed a significant effect of strain with WARs spending less time in the center ($F_{1, 28}$ = 5.626; p = 0.0248), but no AK effect ($F_{1, 28}$ = 0.9779; p = 0.3312) was detected, neither in WARs nor in Wistars.

Regarding the locomotor activity during the OF test, two-way ANOVA showed a powerful strain effect, with WAR presenting less crossings than Wistars ($F_{1, 28}$ = 73.23; p < 0.0001), but AK showed no significant effects ($F_{1, 28}$ = 0.04102; p = 0.8410).

Vertical exploratory activity was impaired in WARs in comparison with Wistars in both parameters, frequency ($F_{1, 28}$ = 23.44; p < 0.0001) and percentage of time ($F_{1, 28}$ = 21.52; p < 0.0001). However, neither AK (WARs) nor the chronic exposure to intense sound stimulation (Wistars) had any effect on frequency ($F_{1, 28}$ = 1.113; p = 0.3004) or percentage of time ($F_{1, 28}$ = 8.439 × 10^{-21}; p > 0.9999) of the vertical exploratory behaviors in WARs and Wistar, respectively.

Two-Way ANOVA showed a significant strain effect regarding grooming behavior, with WARs expressing increased number ($F_{1, 28}$ = 35.13; p < 0.0001) and duration ($F_{1, 28}$ = 4.756; p = 0.0377) of grooming patterns in comparison to Wistars. However, as for the previous parameters, neither AK (WARs) nor the chronic exposure to intense sound stimulation (Wistar) changed the frequency ($F_{1, 28}$ = 0.9138; p = 0.3473) or the percentage of time of grooming behaviors ($F_{1, 28}$ = 2.324; p = 0.1386).

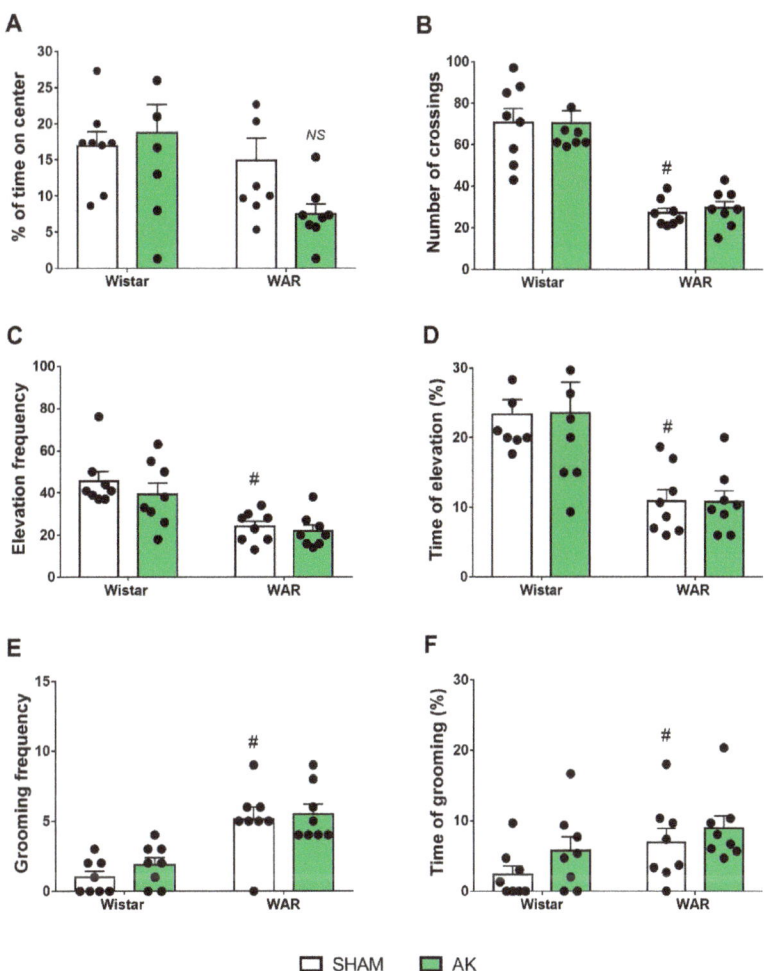

Figure 3. Assessment of anxiety-like behavior in the open-field (OF) test. The measures analyzed were (**A**) percentage of time in the center, (**B**) the number of crossings, (**C**) frequency of elevation, (**D**) time of elevation, (**E**) frequency of grooming, and (**F**) time of grooming. The behavioral tests in the OF were performed during 5 min on the 11th experimental day. $^{\#}$ $p < 0.05$ Tukey test comparing WAR-Sham and Wistar-Sham groups. NS = non-significant difference. Data are expressed as means ± standard error mean. N = 8/group.

3.3. Light Dark Box (LDB) Test

Results from the LDB test are illustrated in Figure 4. Firstly, regarding the percentage of time spent in the lit side of the LDB, Two-Way ANOVA revealed significant effects of both, strain (F1, 28 = 35.9; $p < 0.0001$) and AK (F1, 28 = 7.895; $p = 0.0089$). Tukey's post-test revealed that WARs spent less time spent in the lit side than Wistars ($p = 0.0262$). Additionally, the time in the lit side was reduced even more in WARs after AK ($p = 0.0184$), but the AK protocol did not change the time spent in the lit side of the LDB in Wistar rats ($p = 0.8502$).

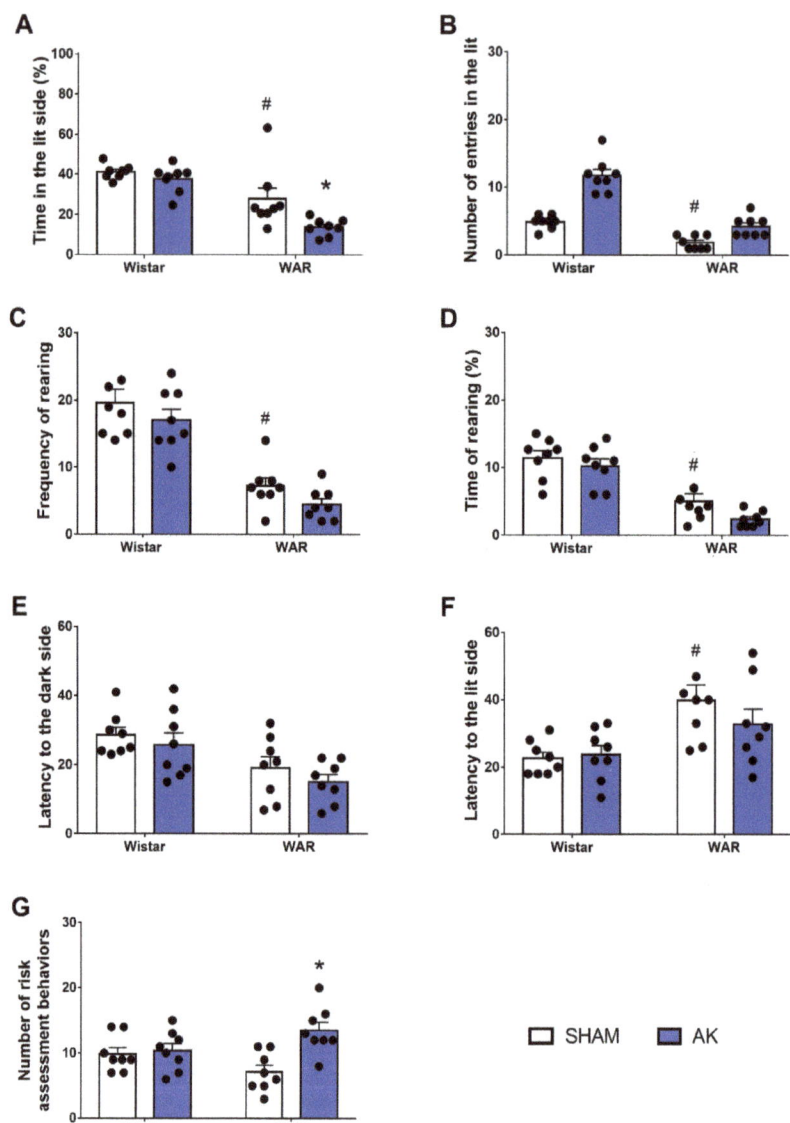

Figure 4. Assessment of anxiety-like behavior in the light/dark box (LDB) test. The measures analyzed were (**A**) percentage of time in the lit side of the box, (**B**) the number of crossings, (**C**) frequency rearing, (**D**) time of rearing, (**E**) latency to the dark side, (**F**) latency to the lit side, and (**G**) risk assessment behaviors. The LBD test was performed during 5 min on the 11th experimental day. * $p < 0.05$ Tukey test comparing WAR-AK and WAR-Sham. # $p < 0.05$ Tukey test compared to WAR-Sham and Wistar-Sham. Data are expressed as mean ± standard error mean. N = 8/group.

Two-Way ANOVA showed a significant strain effect in the number of entries in the lit side of the LDB, with WARs presenting a reduced number of entries in the lit side in comparison to Wistars ($F_{1, 28} = 70.10$; $p < 0.0001$). Again, the AK protocol showed no effects on the number of entries in the lit side, neither in WARs nor in Wistars ($F_{1, 28} = 0.9333$; $p = 0.3423$).

Similar to that observed in the OF test, vertical exploratory activity was impaired in WARs when compared to Wistars in both, frequency (F1, 28 = 70.23; $p < 0.0001$) and duration (F1, 28 = 54.96; $p < 0.0001$). However, AK showed no significant impact, either in frequency (F1, 28 = 3.279; $p = 0.0809$) or in duration (F1, 28 = 4.088; $p = 0.528$) of vertical exploratory behaviors.

Regarding the first latency to the dark compartment, two-Way ANOVA showed a significant strain effect with WARs presenting a shorter latency than Wistars (F1, 28 = 12.86; $p = 0.0013$). The AK protocol did not modify the latency to the dark compartment (F1, 28 = 1.501; $p = 0.2317$). The latency to the first return to the lit compartment was significantly increased in WARs in comparison to Wistars (F1, 28 = 13.75; $p = 0.0009$), Multiple comparisons test showed that animals from the WAR-Sham group had a higher latency to their first return to the lit compartment in comparison to Wistar-Sham ($p = 0.1$).

Risk assessment behaviors were measured based on the number of stretched attempt postures and pokes displayed by animals. Despite no significant strain effect (F1, 28 = 0.02965; $p = 0.8645$), there is an effect of the AK protocol (F1, 28 = 9.965; $p = 0.0038$), as well as an interaction between both factors (F1, 28 = 7.277; $p = 0.0117$). Multiple comparisons analysis showed an increased number of risk assessment behaviors in WARs submitted to AK in comparison to the WAR-Sham group ($p = 0.0016$).

3.4. Immunohistochemistry for FosB+ Neurons

Results from FosB immunostaining are illustrated in Figure 5. In the ICx, two-way ANOVA showed strain (F1, 16 = 26.93; $p < 0.0001$) and AK effects (F1, 16 = 19.67; $p = 0.0004$), besides an interaction between both factors (F1, 16 = 19.21; $p = 0.0005$). Post hoc analysis revealed that the WAR-AK group presented an increased number of FosB+ neurons in comparison to all the other experimental groups ($p < 0.0001$).

In the DLSC significant strain (F1, 14 = 7.539; $p = 0.0158$) and AK effects (F1, 14 = 8.540; $p = 0.0111$) were detected, as well as a significant interaction between both factors (F1, 14 = 6.360; $p = 0.0244$). Additionally, post hoc analysis showed that the WAR-AK group presented an increased number of FosB+ neurons in the DLSC when compared to all the other groups ($p \leq 0.0108$).

FosB expression in the dPAG was significantly affected by strain (F1, 15 = 50.33; $p < 0.0001$) and AK effects (F1, 15 = 53.37; $p < 0.0001$). Two-way ANOVA also detected an interaction between both factors (F1, 15 = 43.54; $p < 0.0001$). Post hoc analysis showed significant differences only when comparing the WAR-AK group with the other experimental groups ($p < 0.0001$).

Finally, regarding the FosB expression in the BLA, significant strain (F1, 16 = 28.09; $p < 0.0001$) and AK effects (F1, 16 = 34.97; $p < 0.0001$) were detected. Additionally, two-way ANOVA showed significant interaction between strain and AK (F1, 16 = 27.17; $p < 0.0001$). As observed in the other structures, post hoc analysis showed that the WAR-AK group presented an increased number of FosB+ neurons in comparison to all the other groups ($p < 0.0001$).

3.5. Immunofluorescence for TRPV1 Channels

Results from immunofluorescence for TRPV1 channels are presented in Figure 6. Two-way ANOVA revealed significant strain (F 1, 20 = 70.05; $p < 0.0001$) and AK (F1, 20 = 70.17; $p < 0.0001$) effects of TRPV1R immunofluorescence in the DLSC. Additionally, a significant interaction between strain and AK (F1, 20 = 70.40; $p < 0.0001$) was detected. Post hoc analysis showed no difference between WAR-Sham and Wistar-Sham groups ($p > 0.9999$), however, chronic seizures increased TRPV1 expression in the DLSC in the WAR-AK group in comparison to all experimental groups ($p < 0.0001$). Chronic exposure to intense sound stimulation did not change TRPV1 expression in the DLSC of Wistar rats ($p > 0.9999$).

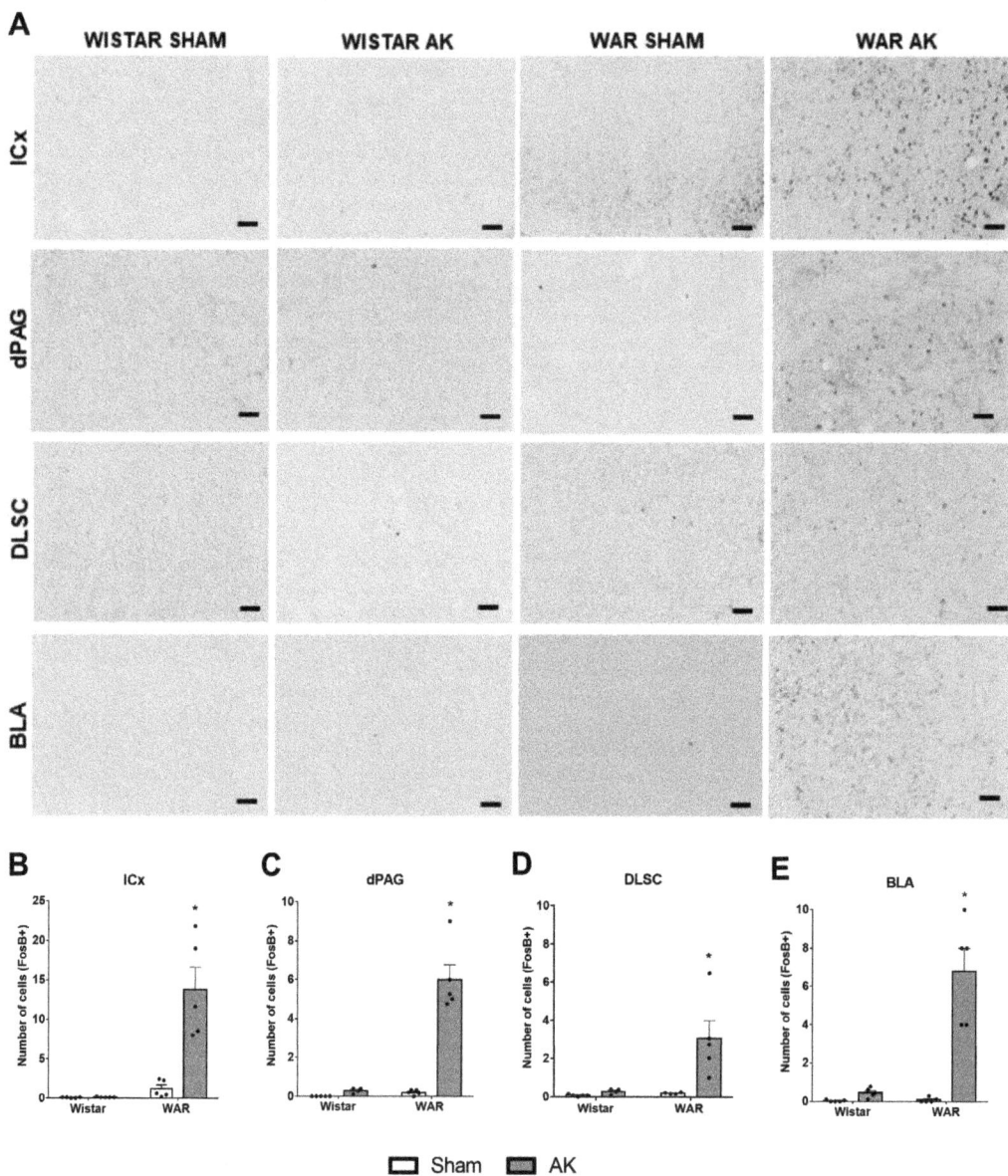

Figure 5. FosB immunostaining after the audiogenic kindling (AK) protocol. (A) Representative images of every analyzed area in each experimental group. FosB+ neurons are characterized by black dots, which indicate the nucleus of each immunopositive neuron. (B) inferior colliculus cortical area—ICx. (C) dorsal periaqueductal gray matter—dPAG. (D) deep layers of superior colliculus—DLSC. (E) basolateral amygdala nucleus—BLA. * $p < 0.05$ Tukey test compared to WAR-Sham. Data are expressed as mean ± standard error mean. N = 4–5/group. Scale bars = 200 μm.

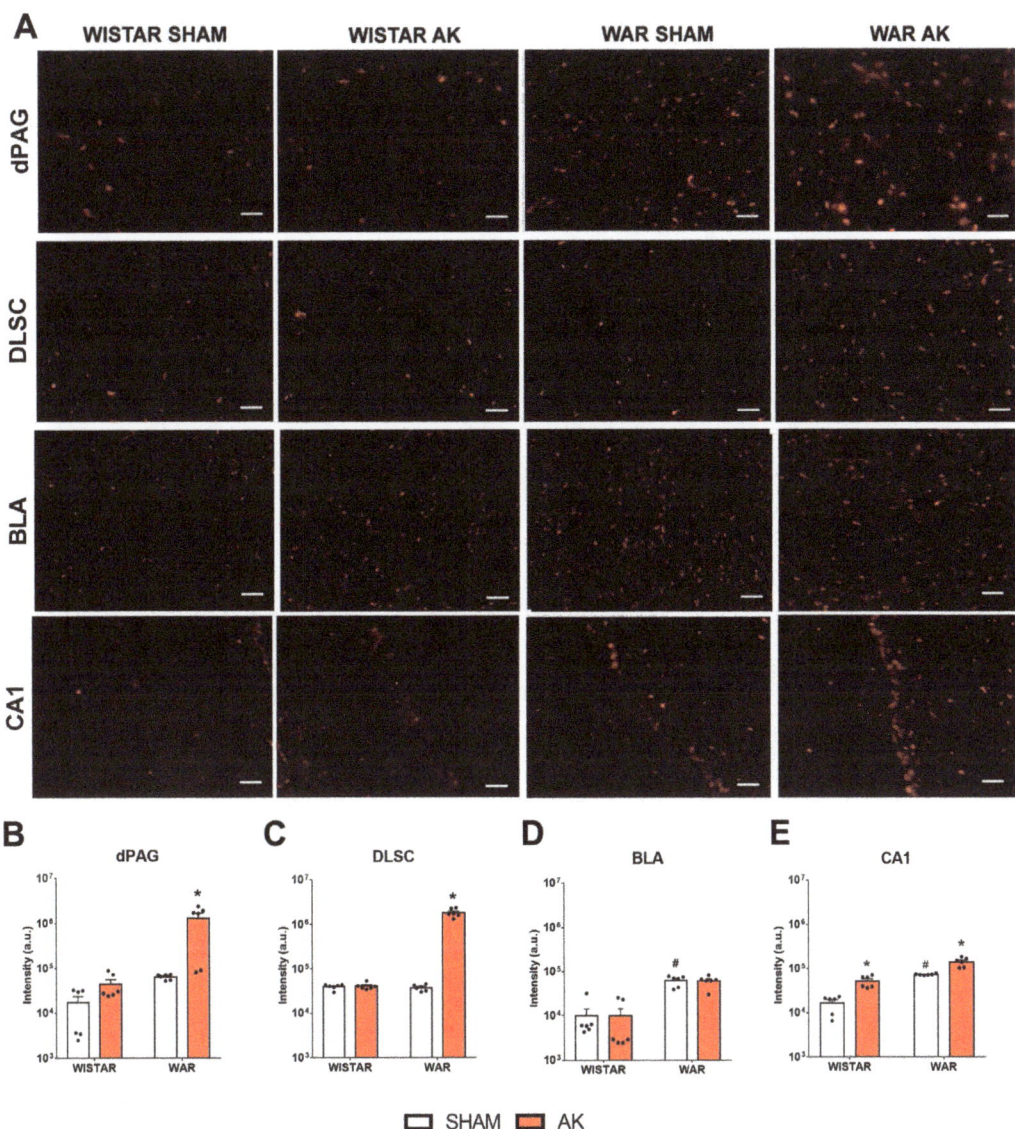

Figure 6. Immunofluorescence for TRPV1 channels after the audiogenic kindling (AK) protocol. (**A**) Representative images of every analyzed area in each experimental group. (**B**) dorsal periaqueductal gray matter—dPAG. (**C**) deep layers of superior colliculus—DLSC. (**D**) basolateral amygdala nucleus—BLA. (**E**) CA1 area of the dorsal hippocampus. # $p < 0.05$ Tukey test compared to Wistar-Sham. * $p < 0.05$ Tukey test compared to WAR-Sham. N = 6 animals/group. Scale bars = 200 μm.

In the dPAG, significant strain ($F_{1, 20} = 10.71$; $p = 0.0038$) and AK ($F_{1, 20} = 10.07$; $p = 0.0048$) effects were observed in TRPV1R expression. Significant interaction between both factors was detected ($F_{1, 20} = 9.21$; $p = 0.0065$). Post hoc analysis showed no difference between Wistar and WAR Sham groups ($p = 0.9983$), but chronic seizures increased TRPV1R expression in the WAR-AK group in comparison to all experimental groups ($p < 0.0015$).

Chronic exposure to intense sound stimulation did not affect TRPV1R expression in Wistars ($p = 0.9997$).

In the BLA, significant strain (F1, 20 = 79.01; $p < 0.0001$), but no AK (F1, 20 = 0.0071; $p = 0.9337$) effects were detected. No significant interaction was detected by two-way ANOVA (F1, 20 = 0.0064; $p = 0.9370$). Post hoc analysis revealed that WARs present increased TRPV1R expression than Wistars, regardless of the experimental condition ($p < 0.0001$). However, neither the chronic seizures in WARs ($p = 0.9994$), nor the chronic exposure to intense sound stimulation in Wistars ($p > 0.9999$) changed TRPV1R expression in the BLA.

In the CA1 of the dorsal hippocampus, two-way ANOVA revealed significant strain (F1, 20 = 87.47; $p < 0.0001$) and AK (F1, 20 = 44.74; $p < 0.0001$) effects. Significant interaction between factors were detected (F1, 20 = 4,862; $p = 0.0393$). Post hoc analysis demonstrated endogenous differences between non-stimulated Wistar and WARs, with WARs presenting increased TRPV1R expression ($p = 0.0003$). Additionally, AK increased TRPV1R expression in CA1 of WARs ($p < 0.0001$), as well as the chronic exposure to intensity sound stimulation increased TRPV1R immunofluorescence in CA1 of Wistars ($p = 0.0229$).

4. Discussion

In the present study, we demonstrated that increased TRPV1 immunoreactivity in limbic brain structures, such as the hippocampus and BLA, is associated with genetic susceptibility to epileptic seizures and increased anxiety-like behavior in a genetic model of epilepsy, the WAR strain. Additionally, the AK protocol, a preclinical model of TLE, increased anxiety-like behaviors and TRPV1 immunoreactivity in the dPAG, DLSC, and CA1 in the WAR-AK group compared to control animals. Supporting these alterations, WARs submitted to chronic seizures also displayed an increased number of FosB+ neurons in brainstem and limbic regions related to seizure and anxiety-like behavior manifestation, such as the ICx, dPAG, DLSC, and BLA, indicating increased chronic hyperactivity in these areas.

AK progression in WARs developed similarly as previously described [43,44,58]. Initially, acoustic stimulation induced generalized tonic-clonic seizures, but during the AK, a preclinical model of TLE [43], epileptogenic events modify seizures patterns, which leads to the expression of limbic seizures typical of forebrain recruitment [44,46,58]. It is worth noting that Wistars (non-epileptic control rats) submitted to the AK protocol did not develop AGS, and the chronic high intense sound stimulation had no impact on anxiety or chronic neuronal hyperactivity and only a minor effect on TRPV1 expression. The increased TRPV1 expression in the CA1 of Wistars chronically stimulated was, initially, an unexpected result, especially because it was not associated with any FosB or anxiogenic-like alterations. However, previous data showed that hippocampal TRPV1 signaling is an important mechanism of stress adaptation, once stress effects on hippocampal synaptic activity and spatial memory were prevented by focal and systemic capsaicin administration [59]. Therefore, the increased TRPV1 expression in the CA1 of Wistar rats submitted to chronic intense sound stimulation could be a reflex of adaptive neuroplastic changes in response to chronic stressful situations, such as intense sound exposure.

To our knowledge, the present study is the first to investigate neuroplastic alterations in TRPV1 channels associated with seizure susceptibility in a genetic model of epilepsy, but similar neuroplastic changes have already been reported in other preclinical models. TRPV1 knock-out mice were less susceptible to febrile seizures than control mice; however, seizure development increased TRPV1 mRNA and protein levels in the cortex and hippocampal formation of control mice [60]. Increased TRPV1 protein levels were detected in the dentate gyrus of mice during the acute and chronic phase of the pilocarpine-induced *Status Epilepticus* (SE) model [34,36]. Additionally, bath application of capsaicin increased synaptic transmission in hippocampal slices from epileptic rats but showed no effect on basal synaptic transmission in tissue from control animals [34]. Thus, our results of increased TRPV1 expression in the BLA and dorsal hippocampus agree with previous studies that used febrile and chemical models of epileptic seizures. Furthermore, we also measured TRPV1 immunofluorescence in brainstem structures involved with generalized tonic-clonic seizures and, similar as observed in the BLA, increased TRPV1 expression was detected in the dPAG and DLSC. Therefore, our results suggest an important role of TRPV1 channels in brainstem generalized tonic-clonic and limbic seizures, and these neuroplastic alterations in the BLA, when associated with increased FosB+ neurons, might be related to the intensification of anxiogenic behavior and chronic seizures manifestation.

Previous studies reported anxiogenic-like behaviors in several genetic models of epilepsies. Similar to the results from the present study, animals from the Genetically Epilepsy Prone Rats (GEPR) and Krushinsky-Molodkina (KM), which are also strains genetically susceptible to AGS, display increased anxiety- and depressive-like behaviors [61,62], supporting the presence of emotional behavioral alterations that mimic neuropsychiatric comorbidities in those models. Here, it is crucial to mention that although it is still unclear if alterations in TRPV1 expression and functionality are involved with emotional behavioral alterations found in GEPRs [61], its antagonism with capsazepine have already been shown to attenuate AGS in male and female GEPRs [63]. Furthermore, genetic models of childhood absence epilepsy, such as the Wistar Albino Glaxo from Rijswijk (WAG/Rij) and the Genetic Absence Epilepsy Rats from Strasbourg (GAERS) strains, display increased anxiety- and depressive-like behaviors [64,65]. Similarly, increased anxiogenic-like behaviors and cognitive impairments were detected in the Scn1a +/− mouse model of Dravet syndrome [66], as well as in chemical models of limbic seizures induced by chronic and sub-chronic pentylenetetrazole (PTZ) administration [67,68]. Anxiogenic-like behaviors were also observed in rodents submitted to the pilocarpine-induced SE during the acute (6–10 days after SE) and chronic (3 and 10 months after SE) phase of the model, suggesting that increased anxiogenic-like behavior may underlie epileptogenic events that lead to further seizure manifestation [69–71]. Therefore, the present results are in line with previous data and support the presence of the neuroplastic changes in TRPV1 expression underlying the comorbidity of epilepsy and anxiety in genetic and chemical models of epilepsies.

Strikingly, in a previous study, authors performed several behavioral analyses in Wistar and WAR rats, including sucrose preference, forced swimming test, social preference, aversive memory tests, OF, and EPM [72]. WARs displayed several behavioral alterations in these tests, but no difference was detected in the exploration of the open and enclosed arms of the EPM. Briefly, a study conducted with the original WAR strain [50] detected decreased exploration of the open arms in the EPM. However, results from Castro et al. [72] are from a branch of the original WARs, maintained in a different location (Federal University of Minas Gerais, Belo Horizonte, Brazil). Powell et al. [73], compared seizures, behavior, and brain morphology between four different GAERs colonies and they detected variations in seizure severity, anxiety- and depressive-like behaviors. Such behavioral divergences could be associated, therefore, with epigenetic signatures (e.g.,: DNA methylation, histone modifications, and noncoding RNAs). We speculate that several of these factors are also involved in the variations observed between WARs from different colonies.

Neuronal networks involved with generalized tonic-clonic and limbic seizures manifestations are closely related to emotional and anxiogenic-like behaviors [15,18,19]. This relationship can be particularly observed in the WAR strain. Once the IC is the main brainstem structure involved with auditory processing associated with seizures, it plays a key role in AGS susceptibility and manifestation [74], especially the ICx area, which presents increased epileptogenic activity and sends glutamatergic projections to the dPAG and DLSC [75–77]. Thus, the hypersynchronism and hyperactivity in these structures mediate the motor manifestation of generalized tonic-clonic seizures [15,78]. During AK, chronic brainstem hyperactivity, especially in excitatory projections from the ICx to the medial geniculate body and then to the BLA, hippocampal formation, and several cortical areas, lead to the phenomenon called limbic recruitment. Once recruited, forebrain regions such as cortical and limbic areas display epileptogenic activities associated with the expression of electrographic and behavioral limbic seizures [42–46,48,58].

Differently from other models of TLE, such as the pilocarpine-induced SE [79], in the AK, the hippocampus does not present neuronal loss, and it is extremely resistant to recruitment; however, c-Fos immunostaining becomes evident in the BLA after 5–10 AGS, when limbic seizures start to coexist with brainstem seizures [76]. Nevertheless, the hippocampus of WARs does present neuroplastic alterations associated with epilepsy susceptibility and neuropsychiatric alterations, such as reduced GABAergic currents in hippocampal neurons [80,81], increased CB1 expression [53], hippocampal hyperplasia [82], and increased calcium concentration in hippocampal synaptosomes [83]. The amygdaloid complex, especially the BLA, is probably the limbic structure most susceptible to AK epileptogenic events, presenting neuronal loss and increased neo-Timm+ staining (Zn^+ sprouting) [58], as well as increased neuronal hyperactivity and CB1 expression [53,57].

Additionally, fully kindled GEPR-9s have their post-tonic clonic seizure abolished after administration of a selective adenylyl cyclase inhibitor directly into the lateral amygdala nucleus [84]. Similar results were also observed in kindled GEPR-3s who had limbic seizures prevented by administering the NMDA receptor antagonist AP7 into the same structure [85]. Thus, the increased TRPV1 expression endogenously detected in the hippocampus and BLA of WARs is in line with previous neuroplastic alterations and add new information regarding epilepsy susceptibility and calcium mobilization in these limbic brain sites.

Although the dPAG and DLSC are involved with AGS expression [16,17,41,86], they are also intrinsically associated with anxiety-like, defensive, and panic-like behaviors [87–89]. Pharmacological manipulations of TRPV1 channels in these structures have also been shown to modulate anxiety. Capsaicin administration into the dPAG increased anxiogenic-like behaviors in rodents [90,91], while TRPV1 antagonism with capsazepine induced the opposite effects [91]. Although TRPV1 channels from neurons located in the superior colliculus have been shown to play an important role in long-term synaptic plasticity [92], there is still a lack of studies investigating their role on either epilepsy or anxiety. Therefore, our results indicate that increased TRPV1 expression and signaling in the dPAG and DLSC of chronically stimulated WARs may be involved with the increased number of FosB+ neurons in the same area. Together these neuroplastic alterations might play an important role on seizure susceptibility and anxiogenic-like behaviors displayed by epileptic rats.

In forebrain sites, activation of TRPV1 located at the dorsal hippocampus induced anxiogenic-like behaviors [29], while its antagonism in the ventral hippocampus induced anxiolytic-like behaviors [39]. Furthermore, anxiolytic-like effects induced microinjection of anandamide within the BLA were shown to be dependent on previous antagonism of TRPV1 located in the same structure, suggesting that anxiolytic effects were associated with CB1 activation [93]. While the local activation of CB1 inhibits calcium channels and excitatory neuronal activity [94], TRPV1 activation promotes calcium influx and glutamate release [95,96]. Thus, once TRPV1R are activated by the endogenous cannabinoid anandamide and its signaling leads to intracellular calcium mobilization and increasing neuronal excitability [31], its increased expression in the analyzed brain structures may explain, at least in part, the genetic susceptibility to epilepsy and the anxiogenic-like behaviors displayed by WARs. Therefore, given the dual role of these receptors in the modulation of emotional behaviors [97], the results from the present study may be associated with the increased CB1 expression previously detected in limbic brain sites of WARs [53], where CB1 receptors could be up-regulated in response to the increased excitability related to increased TRPV1 expression and signaling.

Although we did not perform a co-localization immunohistochemical study to verify if increased TRPV1R immunoreactivity was present in FosB+ neurons, our results from both immunohistochemical protocols, coupled with behavioral analysis, suggest that the increased neuronal hyperexcitability detected in chronically stimulated WARs is due to the increased TRPV1 expression and activity in these neurons, increasing calcium signaling and neuronal firing. This explanation is supported by the increased number of FosB+ neurons in the ICx, DLSC, dPAG, and BLA, and the increased TRPV1R expression in the dPAG, DLSC, BLA, and hippocampal CA1 region. Furthermore, using a genetic model coupled with a chronic protocol of epileptic seizures (AK) and histological analyses are important tools for translational neuroscience, especially in the context of neuropsychiatric comorbidities commonly observed in patients with epilepsies. Intriguingly, several of the mentioned neural substrates or neuronal networks are extensively overlapped when we study either defense systems associated with panic or flight behaviors [19,87,88,98] or those involved in the behavioral and electrographic expression of epileptic seizures [15–17,57]. The actual meaning of these overlayed substrates in the context of behavioral and evolutive neuroscience, although not the main goal of the current study, deserves further examination. Indeed, that challenge has been taken brightly in a recent comprehensive literature review by Inga Poletaeva´s research group [99].

In conclusion, increased TRPV1 channels expression in the hippocampus and BLA are associated with seizure susceptibility and anxiogenic-like behaviors in the WAR strain. Additionally, epileptogenic events underlying the limbic recruitment intensified anxiogenic-like behaviors and increased TRPV1 expression in the brainstem and limbic regions involved with the modulation of seizures and emotional behavior. Therefore, the present study added new neuropathological information about the epileptogenic process underlying the limbic recruitment associated with AK, a TLE model, and the consequent development of neuropsychiatric comorbidities. These data shade light on an important role for TRPV1 channels and calcium mobilization in the regulation of endogenous mechanisms related to seizure susceptibility in animals genetically susceptible to epilepsies, supporting a key role for this receptor in epilepsy and anxiety as comorbidities.

Author Contributions: W.L.-L., G.K.S.-C. and N.G.-C. designed the study. W.L.-L. conducted and analyzed behavioral experiments. W.L.-L. and G.K.S.-C. conducted immunohistochemical experiments, imaging protocols, and analysis. W.L.-L. and G.K.S.-C. wrote the manuscript and prepared figures. C.R.A.L.-P. and N.G.-C. provided critical reviews of the manuscript and obtained funding. All authors have read and agreed to the published version of the manuscript.

Funding: Coordenação de Aperfeiçoamento de Pessoal de Nível Superior (CAPES—Brazil—Finance Code 001). Fundação de Amparo à Pesquisa do Estado de São Paulo, Brazil (FAPESP): Ph.D. Scholarship (2018/06877-5); Regular Research Funding (2019/05957-8). Conselho Nacional de Desenvolvimento Científico e Tecnológico—CNPq—Brazil—305883/2014-3 (NGC). CLP and NGC hold CNPq Research Fellowships.

Institutional Review Board Statement: The experimental protocol was approved by the Ethics Committee in Animal Research of Ribeirão Preto School of Medicine, University of São Paulo (Protocol number: 057/2017).

Informed Consent Statement: Not applicable.

Data Availability Statement: The data presented in this study are available on request from the corresponding author.

Conflicts of Interest: The authors declare no conflict of interest.

References

1. Fisher, R.S.; Acevedo, C.; Arzimanoglou, A.; Bogacz, A.; Cross, J.H.; Elger, C.E.; Engel, J., Jr.; Forsgren, L.; French, J.A.; Glynn, M.; et al. ILAE Official Report: A practical clinical definition of epilepsy. *Epilepsia* **2014**, *55*, 475–482. [CrossRef] [PubMed]
2. Kanner, A.M. Psychiatric comorbidities in new onset epilepsy: Should they be always investigated? *Seizure* **2017**, *49*, 79–82. [CrossRef] [PubMed]
3. Beyenburg, S.; Mitchell, A.J.; Schmidt, D.; Elger, C.E.; Reuber, M. Anxiety in patients with epilepsy: Systematic review and suggestions for clinical management. *Epilepsy Behav.* **2005**, *7*, 161–171. [CrossRef] [PubMed]
4. Verrotti, A.; Carrozzino, D.; Milioni, M.; Minna, M.; Fulcheri, M. Epilepsy and its main psychiatric comorbidities in adults and children. *J. Neurol. Sci.* **2014**, *343*, 23–29. [CrossRef]
5. Kanner, A.M. Anxiety Disorders in Epilepsy: The Forgotten Psychiatric Comorbidity. *Epilepsy Curr.* **2011**, *11*, 90–91. [CrossRef] [PubMed]
6. Salpekar, J.A.; Salpekar, J.A.; Basu, T.; Basu, T.; Thangaraj, S.; Thangaraj, S.; Maguire, J.; Maguire, J. The intersections of stress, anxiety and epilepsy. *Int. Rev. Neurobiol.* **2020**, *152*, 195–219. [CrossRef] [PubMed]

7. Scott, A.; Sharpe, L.; Loomes, M.; Gandy, M. Systematic Review and Meta-Analysis of Anxiety and Depression in Youth with Epilepsy. *J. Pediatr. Psychol.* **2020**, *45*, 133–144. [CrossRef] [PubMed]
8. Scott, A.; Sharpe, L.; Hunt, C.; Gandy, M. Anxiety and depressive disorders in people with epilepsy: A meta-analysis. *Epilepsia* **2017**, *58*, 973–982. [CrossRef]
9. Davydov, O.S. Antiepileptic Drugs Beyond Epilepsy (Use of Anticonvulsants in the Treatment of Pain Syndromes). *Neurosci. Behav. Physiol.* **2014**, *44*, 772–778. [CrossRef]
10. Hesdorffer, D.C.; Ishihara, L.; Mynepalli, L.; Webb, D.J.; Weil, J.; Hauser, W.A. Epilepsy, suicidality, and psychiatric disorders: A bidirectional association. *Ann. Neurol.* **2012**, *72*, 184–191. [CrossRef]
11. Mula, M. Bidirectional link between epilepsy and psychiatric disorders. *Nat. Rev. Neurol.* **2012**, *8*, 252–253. [CrossRef]
12. Johnson, E.K.; Jones, J.E.; Seidenberg, M.; Hermann, B.P. The Relative Impact of Anxiety, Depression, and Clinical Seizure Features on Health-related Quality of Life in Epilepsy. *Epilepsia* **2004**, *45*, 544–550. [CrossRef] [PubMed]
13. Kanner, A.M. Management of psychiatric and neurological comorbidities in epilepsy. *Nat. Rev. Neurol.* **2016**, *12*, 106–116. [CrossRef] [PubMed]
14. Lazarini-Lopes, W.; Silva, R.A.D.V.-D.; da Silva-Júnior, R.M.P.; Cunha, A.O.S.; Garcia-Cairasco, N. Cannabinoids in Audiogenic Seizures: From Neuronal Networks to Future Perspectives for Epilepsy Treatment. *Front. Behav. Neurosci.* **2021**, *15*, 2. [CrossRef]
15. Faingold, C.L.; Raisinghani, M.; N'Gouemo, P. Chapter 26-Neuronal Networks in Epilepsy: Comparative Audiogenic Seizure Networks. In *Neuronal Networks in Brain Function, CNS Disorders, and Therapeutics*; Faingold, C.L., Blumenfeld, H., Eds.; Academic Press: San Diego, CA, USA, 2014; pp. 349–373. [CrossRef]
16. N'Gouemo, P.; Faingold, C. Periaqueductal gray neurons exhibit increased responsiveness associated with audiogenic seizures in the genetically epilepsy-prone rat. *Neuroscience* **1998**, *84*, 619–625. [CrossRef]
17. Soper, C.; Wicker, E.; Kulick, C.V.; N'Gouemo, P.; Forcelli, P.A. Optogenetic activation of superior colliculus neurons suppresses seizures originating in diverse brain networks. *Neurobiol. Dis.* **2015**, *87*, 102–115. [CrossRef]
18. Baas, J.M.; Milstein, J.; Donlevy, M.; Grillon, C. Brainstem Correlates of Defensive States in Humans. *Biol. Psychiatry* **2006**, *59*, 588–593. [CrossRef]
19. Brandão, M.L.; Troncoso, A.C.; de Souza Silva, M.A.; Huston, J.P. The relevance of neuronal substrates of defense in the midbrain tectum to anxiety and stress: Empirical and conceptual considerations. *Eur. J. Pharmacol.* **2003**, *463*, 225–233. [CrossRef]
20. Gu, Y.; Piper, W.; Branigan, L.A.; Vazey, E.M.; Aston-Jones, G.; Lin, L.; LeDoux, J.E.; Sears, R.M. A brainstem-central amygdala circuit underlies defensive responses to learned threats. *Mol. Psychiatry* **2019**, *25*, 640–654. [CrossRef]
21. Tye, K.M.; Prakash, R.; Kim, S.-Y.; Fenno, L.E.; Grosenick, L.; Zarabi, H.; Thompson, K.R.; Gradinaru, V.; Ramakrishnan, C.; Deisseroth, K. Amygdala circuitry mediating reversible and bidirectional control of anxiety. *Nature* **2011**, *471*, 358–362. [CrossRef]
22. Aguiar, D.; Moreira, F.; Terzian, A.; Fogaça, M.; Lisboa, S.; Wotjak, C.; Guimaraes, F. Modulation of defensive behavior by Transient Receptor Potential Vanilloid Type-1 (TRPV1) Channels. *Neurosci. Biobehav. Rev.* **2014**, *46*, 418–428. [CrossRef] [PubMed]
23. Benítez-Angeles, M.; Morales-Lázaro, S.L.; Juárez-González, E.; Rosenbaum, T. TRPV1: Structure, Endogenous Agonists, and Mechanisms. *Int. J. Mol. Sci.* **2020**, *21*, 3421. [CrossRef] [PubMed]
24. Du, Q.; Liao, Q.; Chen, C.; Yang, X.; Xie, R.; Xu, J. The Role of Transient Receptor Potential Vanilloid 1 in Common Diseases of the Digestive Tract and the Cardiovascular and Respiratory System. *Front. Physiol.* **2019**, *10*, 1064. [CrossRef] [PubMed]
25. Edwards, J.G. TRPV1 in the Central Nervous System: Synaptic Plasticity, Function, and Pharmacological Implications. In *Capsaicin as a Therapeutic Molecule, Progress in Drug Research*; Abdel-Salam, O.M.E., Ed.; Springer: Basel, Switzerland, 2014; pp. 77–104. [CrossRef]
26. Zhang, M.; Ruwe, D.; Saffari, R.; Kravchenko, M.; Zhang, W. Effects of TRPV1 Activation by Capsaicin and Endogenous N-Arachidonoyl Taurine on Synaptic Transmission in the Prefrontal Cortex. *Front. Neurosci.* **2020**, *14*, 91. [CrossRef] [PubMed]
27. Tóth, A.; Boczán, J.; Kedei, N.; Lizanecz, E.; Bagi, Z.; Papp, Z.; Édes, I.; Csiba, L.; Blumberg, P.M. Expression and distribution of vanilloid receptor 1 (TRPV1) in the adult rat brain. *Mol. Brain Res.* **2005**, *135*, 162–168. [CrossRef]
28. Zschenderlein, C.; Gebhardt, C.; Halbach, O.V.B.U.; Kulisch, C.; Albrecht, D. Capsaicin-Induced Changes in LTP in the Lateral Amygdala Are Mediated by TRPV1. *PLoS ONE* **2011**, *6*, e16116. [CrossRef]
29. Hakimizadeh, E.; Oryan, S.; Hajizadeh moghaddam, A.; Shamsizadeh, A.; Roohbakhsh, A. Endocannabinoid System and TRPV1 Receptors in the Dorsal Hippocampus of the Rats Modulate Anxiety-like Behaviors. *Iran. J. Basic Med. Sci.* **2012**, *15*, 795–802.
30. Lee, S.-H.; Ledri, M.; Tóth, B.; Marchionni, I.; Henstridge, C.M.; Dudok, B.; Kenesei, K.; Barna, L.; Szabo, S.I.; Renkecz, T.; et al. Multiple Forms of Endocannabinoid and Endovanilloid Signaling Regulate the Tonic Control of GABA Release. *J. Neurosci.* **2015**, *35*, 10039–10057. [CrossRef]
31. Van Der Stelt, M.; Trevisani, M.; Vellani, V.; De Petrocellis, L.; Moriello, A.S.; Campi, B.; McNaughton, P.; Geppetti, P.; Di Marzo, V. Anandamide acts as an intracellular messenger amplifying Ca2+ influx via TRPV1 channels. *EMBO J.* **2005**, *24*, 3026–3037. [CrossRef] [PubMed]
32. Fu, M.; Xie, Z.; Zuo, H. TRPV1: A potential target for antiepileptogenesis. *Med. Hypotheses* **2009**, *73*, 100–102. [CrossRef]
33. Nazıroglu, M. TRPV1 Channel: A Potential Drug Target for Treating Epilepsy. *Curr. Neuropharmacol.* **2015**, *13*, 239–247. [CrossRef] [PubMed]
34. Saffarzadeh, F.; Eslamizade, M.; Mousavi, S.; Abraki, S.; Hadjighassem, M.; Gorji, A. TRPV1 receptors augment basal synaptic transmission in CA1 and CA3 pyramidal neurons in epilepsy. *Neuroscience* **2016**, *314*, 170–178. [CrossRef] [PubMed]

35. Sun, F.-J.; Guo, W.; Zheng, D.-H.; Zhang, C.-Q.; Li, S.; Liu, S.-Y.; Yin, Q.; Yang, H.; Shu, H.-F. Increased Expression of TRPV1 in the Cortex and Hippocampus from Patients with Mesial Temporal Lobe Epilepsy. *J. Mol. Neurosci.* **2012**, *49*, 182–193. [CrossRef] [PubMed]
36. Bhaskaran, M.D.; Smith, B.N. Cannabinoid-Mediated Inhibition of Recurrent Excitatory Circuitry in the Dentate Gyrus in a Mouse Model of Temporal Lobe Epilepsy. *PLoS ONE* **2010**, *5*, e10683. [CrossRef] [PubMed]
37. Shirazi, M.; Izadi, M.; Amin, M.; Rezvani, M.E.; Roohbakhsh, A.; Shamsizadeh, A. Involvement of central TRPV1 receptors in pentylenetetrazole and amygdala-induced kindling in male rats. *Neurol. Sci.* **2014**, *35*, 1235–1241. [CrossRef] [PubMed]
38. Campos, A.C.; Guimarães, F.S. Evidence for a potential role for TRPV1 receptors in the dorsolateral periaqueductal gray in the attenuation of the anxiolytic effects of cannabinoids. *Prog. Neuro-Psychopharmacol. Biol. Psychiatry* **2009**, *33*, 1517–1521. [CrossRef]
39. Santos, C.J.; Stern, C.A.; Bertoglio, L.J. Attenuation of anxiety-related behaviour after the antagonism of transient receptor potential vanilloid type 1 channels in the rat ventral hippocampus. *Behav. Pharmacol.* **2008**, *19*, 357–360. [CrossRef]
40. Garcia-Cairasco, N.; Umeoka, E.; de Oliveira, J.A.C. The Wistar Audiogenic Rat (WAR) strain and its contributions to epileptology and related comorbidities: History and perspectives. *Epilepsy Behav.* **2017**, *71*, 250–273. [CrossRef]
41. Garcia-Cairasco, N.; Terra, V.; Doretto, M. Midbrain substrates of audiogenic seizures in rats. *Behav. Brain Res.* **1993**, *58*, 57–67. [CrossRef]
42. Marescaux, C.; Vergnes, M.; Kiesmann, M.; Depaulis, A.; Micheletti, G.; Warter, J. Kindling of audiogenic seizures in Wistar rats: An EEG study. *Exp. Neurol.* **1987**, *97*, 160–168. [CrossRef]
43. Moraes, M.F.D.; Galvis-Alonso, O.Y.; Garcia-Cairasco, N. Audiogenic kindling in the Wistar rat: A potential model for recruitment of limbic structures. *Epilepsy Res.* **2000**, *39*, 251–259. [CrossRef]
44. Garcia-Cairasco, N.; Wakamatsu, H.; Oliveira, J.; Gomes, E.; Del Bel, E.; Mello, L. Neuroethological and morphological (Neo-Timm staining) correlates of limbic recruitment during the development of audiogenic kindling in seizure susceptible Wistar rats. *Epilepsy Res.* **1996**, *26*, 177–192. [CrossRef]
45. Naritoku, D.K.; Mecozzi, L.B.; Aiello, M.T.; Faingold, C.L. Repetition of audiogenic seizures in genetically epilepsy-prone rats induces cortical epileptiform activity and additional seizure behaviors. *Exp. Neurol.* **1992**, *115*, 317–324. [CrossRef]
46. Romcy-Pereira, R.; Garcia-Cairasco, N. Hippocampal cell proliferation and epileptogenesis after audiogenic kindling are not accompanied by mossy fiber sprouting or fluoro-jade staining. *Neuroscience* **2003**, *119*, 533–546. [CrossRef]
47. Moraes, M.; Chavali, M.; Mishra, P.; Jobe, P.; Garcia-Cairasco, N. A comprehensive electrographic and behavioral analysis of generalized tonic-clonic seizures of GEPR-9s. *Brain Res.* **2005**, *1033*, 1–12. [CrossRef]
48. Vinogradova, L.V. Audiogenic kindling and secondary subcortico-cortical epileptogenesis: Behavioral correlates and electrographic features. *Epilepsy Behav.* **2017**, *71*, 142–153. [CrossRef]
49. Racine, R.J. Modification of seizure activity by electrical stimulation: II. Motor seizure. *Electroencephalogr. Clin. Neurophysiol.* **1972**, *32*, 281–294. [CrossRef]
50. Garcia-Cairasco, N.; Oliveira, J.; Wakamatsu, H.; Bueno, S.; Guimarães, F. Reduced exploratory activity of audiogenic seizures suceptible Wistar rats. *Physiol. Behav.* **1998**, *64*, 671–674. [CrossRef]
51. Cunha, A.; de Oliveira, J.; Almeida, S.; Garcia-Cairasco, N.; Leão, R. Inhibition of long-term potentiation in the schaffer-CA1 pathway by repetitive high-intensity sound stimulation. *Neuroscience* **2015**, *310*, 114–127. [CrossRef]
52. Gitaí, D.L.G.; Martinelli, H.N.; Valente, V.; Pereira, M.G.A.G.; Oliveira, J.A.C.; Elias, C.F.; Bittencourt, J.C.; Leite, J.P.; Costa-Neto, C.M.; Garcia-Cairasco, N.; et al. Increased expression of GluR2-flip in the hippocampus of the Wistar audiogenic rat strain after acute and kindled seizures. *Hippocampus* **2009**, *20*, 125–133. [CrossRef]
53. Lazarini-Lopes, W.; Da Silva-Júnior, R.M.P.; Servilha-Menezes, G.; Silva, R.A.D.V.-D.; Garcia-Cairasco, N. Cannabinoid Receptor Type 1 (CB1R) Expression in Limbic Brain Structures After Acute and Chronic Seizures in a Genetic Model of Epilepsy. *Front. Behav. Neurosci.* **2020**, *14*, 602258. [CrossRef]
54. Rossetti, F.; Rodrigues, M.C.A.; de Oliveira, J.A.C.; Garcia-Cairasco, N. EEG wavelet analyses of the striatum–substantia nigra pars reticulata–superior colliculus circuitry: Audiogenic seizures and anticonvulsant drug administration in Wistar audiogenic rats (War strain). *Epilepsy Res.* **2006**, *72*, 192–208. [CrossRef]
55. Paxinos, G.; Watson, C. *The Rat Brain in Stereotaxic Coordinates: Hard Cover Edition*; Elsevier: Amsterdam, The Netherlands, 2006.
56. Silva-Cardoso, G.K.; Lazarini-Lopes, W.; Hallak, J.E.; Crippa, J.A.; Zuardi, A.W.; Garcia-Cairasco, N.; Leite-Panissi, C.R. Cannabidiol effectively reverses mechanical and thermal allodynia, hyperalgesia, and anxious behaviors in a neuropathic pain model: Possible role of CB1 and TRPV1 receptors. *Neuropharmacology* **2021**, *197*, 108712. [CrossRef]
57. Lazarini-Lopes, W.; Do Val-Da Silva, R.A.; da Silva-Júnior, R.M.P.; Silva-Cardoso, G.K.; Leite-Panissi, C.R.A.; Leite, J.P.; Garcia-Cairasco, N. Chronic cannabidiol (CBD) administration induces anticonvulsant and antiepileptogenic effects in a genetic model of epilepsy. *Epilepsy Behav.* **2021**, *119*, 107962. [CrossRef]
58. Galvis-Alonso, O.Y.; De Oliveira, J.C.; Garcia-Cairasco, N. Limbic epileptogenicity, cell loss and axonal reorganization induced by audiogenic and amygdala kindling in wistar audiogenic rats (WAR strain). *Neuroscience* **2004**, *125*, 787–802. [CrossRef]
59. Li, H.-B.; Mao, R.-R.; Zhang, J.-C.; Yang, Y.; Cao, J.; Xu, L. Antistress Effect of TRPV1 Channel on Synaptic Plasticity and Spatial Memory. *Biol. Psychiatry* **2008**, *64*, 286–292. [CrossRef]
60. Huang, W.-X.; Yu, F.; Sanchez, R.M.; Liu, Y.-Q.; Min, J.-W.; Hu, J.-J.; Bsoul, N.B.; Han, S.; Yin, J.; Liu, W.-H.; et al. TRPV1 promotes repetitive febrile seizures by pro-inflammatory cytokines in immature brain. *Brain Behav. Immun.* **2015**, *48*, 68–77. [CrossRef]

61. Aguilar, B.; Malkova, L.; N'Gouemo, P.; Forcelli, P. Genetically Epilepsy-Prone Rats Display Anxiety-Like Behaviors and Neuropsychiatric Comorbidities of Epilepsy. *Front. Neurol.* 2018, 9, 476. [CrossRef]
62. Sarkisova, K.Y.; Fedotova, I.B.; Surina, N.M.; Nikolaev, G.M.; Perepelkina, O.V.; Kostina, Z.A.; Poletaeva, I.I. Genetic background contributes to the co-morbidity of anxiety and depression with audiogenic seizure propensity and responses to fluoxetine treatment. *Epilepsy Behav.* 2017, 68, 95–102. [CrossRef]
63. Cho, S.J.; Vaca, M.A.; Miranda, C.J.; N'Gouemo, P. Inhibition of transient potential receptor vanilloid type 1 suppresses seizure susceptibility in the genetically epilepsy-prone rat. *CNS Neurosci. Ther.* 2017, 24, 18–28. [CrossRef]
64. Jones, N.C.; Salzberg, M.R.; Kumar, G.; Couper, A.; Morris, M.; O'Brien, T. Elevated anxiety and depressive-like behavior in a rat model of genetic generalized epilepsy suggesting common causation. *Exp. Neurol.* 2008, 209, 254–260. [CrossRef] [PubMed]
65. Sarkisova, K.; van Luijtelaar, G. The WAG/Rij strain: A genetic animal model of absence epilepsy with comorbidity of depressiony. *Prog. Neuro-Psychopharmacol. Biol. Psychiatry* 2010, 35, 854–876. [CrossRef]
66. Ricobaraza, A.; Mora-Jimenez, L.; Puerta, E.; Sanchez-Carpintero, R.; Mingorance, A.; Artieda, J.; Nicolas, M.J.; Besne, G.; Bunuales, M.; Gonzalez-Aparicio, M.; et al. Epilepsy and neuropsychiatric comorbidities in mice carrying a recurrent Dravet syndrome SCN1A missense mutation. *Sci. Rep.* 2019, 9, 14172. [CrossRef]
67. Anesti, M.; Stavropoulou, N.; Atsopardi, K.; Lamari, F.N.; Panagopoulos, N.T.; Margarity, M. Effect of rutin on anxiety-like behavior and activity of acetylcholinesterase isoforms in specific brain regions of pentylenetetrazol-treated mice. *Epilepsy Behav.* 2019, 102, 106632. [CrossRef]
68. Wang, S.; Mao, S.; Yao, B.; Xiang, D.; Fang, C. Effects of low-frequency repetitive transcranial magnetic stimulation on depression- and anxiety-like behaviors in epileptic rats. *J. Integr. Neurosci.* 2019, 18, 237–243. [CrossRef]
69. Gröticke, I.; Hoffmann, K.; Löscher, W. Behavioral alterations in the pilocarpine model of temporal lobe epilepsy in mice. *Exp. Neurol.* 2007, 207, 329–349. [CrossRef]
70. Lopes, M.W.; Lopes, S.C.; Santos, D.B.; Costa, A.P.; Gonçalves, F.M.; de Mello, N.; Prediger, R.D.; Farina, M.; Walz, R.; Leal, R.B. Time course evaluation of behavioral impairments in the pilocarpine model of epilepsy. *Epilepsy Behav.* 2016, 55, 92–100. [CrossRef]
71. Otsuka, S.; Ohkido, T.; Itakura, M.; Watanabe, S.; Yamamori, S.; Iida, Y.; Saito, M.; Miyaoka, H.; Takahashi, M. Dual mechanisms of rapid expression of anxiety-related behavior in pilocarpine-treated epileptic mice. *Epilepsy Res.* 2016, 123, 55–67. [CrossRef]
72. Castro, G.P.; Medeiros, D.; Guarnieri, L.D.O.; Mourão, F.; Pinto, H.P.P.; Pereira, G.; Moraes, M.F.D. Wistar audiogenic rats display abnormal behavioral traits associated with artificial selection for seizure susceptibility. *Epilepsy Behav.* 2015, 71, 243–249. [CrossRef]
73. Powell, K.; Tang, H.; Ng, C.; Guillemain, I.; Dieuset, G.; Dezsi, G.; Çarçak, N.; Onat, F.; Martin, B.; O'Brien, T.; et al. Seizure expression, behavior, and brain morphology differences in colonies of Genetic Absence Epilepsy Rats from Strasbourg. *Epilepsia* 2014, 55, 1959–1968. [CrossRef]
74. Garcia-Cairasco, N. A critical review on the participation of inferior colliculus in acoustic-motor and acoustic-limbic networks involved in the expression of acute and kindled audiogenic seizures. *Hear. Res.* 2002, 168, 208–222. [CrossRef]
75. Coleman, J.R.; Clerici, W.J. Sources of projections to subdivisions of the inferior colliculus in the rat. *J. Comp. Neurol.* 1987, 262, 215–226. [CrossRef] [PubMed]
76. Simler, S.; Vergnes, M.; Marescaux, C. Spatial and Temporal Relationships between C-Fos Expression and Kindling of Audiogenic Seizures in Wistar Rats. *Exp. Neurol.* 1999, 157, 106–119. [CrossRef]
77. Snyder-Keller, A.M.; Pierson, M.G. Audiogenic seizures induce c-fos in a model of developmental epilepsy. *Neurosci. Lett.* 1992, 135, 108–112. [CrossRef]
78. Ross, K.; Coleman, J. Developmental and genetic audiogenic seizure models: Behavior and biological substrates. *Neurosci. Biobehav. Rev.* 2000, 24, 639–653. [CrossRef]
79. Cavalheiro, E.A.; Leite, J.P.; Bortolotto, Z.A.; Turski, W.A.; Ikonomidou, C.; Turski, L. Long-Term Effects of Pilocarpine in Rats: Structural Damage of the Brain Triggers Kindling and Spontaneous I Recurrent Seizures. *Epilepsia* 1991, 32, 778–782. [CrossRef]
80. Cunha, A.O.S.; Ceballos, C.; De Deus, J.L.; Pena, R.F.D.O.; De Oliveira, J.A.C.; Roque, A.C.; Garcia-Cairasco, N.; Leão, R.M. Intrinsic and synaptic properties of hippocampal CA1 pyramidal neurons of the Wistar Audiogenic Rat (WAR) strain, a genetic model of epilepsy. *Sci. Rep.* 2018, 8, 10412. [CrossRef]
81. Mesquita, F.; Aguiar, J.F.; Oliveira, J.A.; Garcia-Cairasco, N.; Varanda, W.A. Electrophysiological properties of cultured hippocampal neurons from Wistar Audiogenic Rats. *Brain Res. Bull.* 2005, 65, 177–183. [CrossRef]
82. Lee, Y.; Rodriguez, O.C.; Albanese, C.; Santos, V.R.; de Oliveira, J.A.C.; Donatti, A.L.F.; Fernandes, A.; Garcia-Cairasco, N.; N'Gouemo, P.; Forcelli, P.A. Divergent brain changes in two audiogenic rat strains: A voxel-based morphometry and diffusion tensor imaging comparison of the genetically epilepsy prone rat (GEPR-3) and the Wistar Audiogenic Rat (WAR). *Neurobiol. Dis.* 2017, 111, 80–90. [CrossRef]
83. dos Santos, R.R.; Bernardino, T.C.; da Silva, M.C.M.; de Oliveira, A.C.; Drumond, L.E.; Rosa, D.V.; Massensini, A.R.; Moraes, M.F.; Doretto, M.C.; Romano-Silva, M.A.; et al. Neurochemical abnormalities in the hippocampus of male rats displaying audiogenic seizures, a genetic model of epilepsy. *Neurosci. Lett.* 2021, 761, 136123. [CrossRef]
84. Tupal, S.; Faingold, C. Inhibition of adenylyl cyclase in amygdala blocks the effect of audiogenic seizure kindling in genetically epilepsy-prone rats. *Neuropharmacology* 2010, 59, 107–111. [CrossRef] [PubMed]

85. Raisinghani, M.; Faingold, C.L. Neurons in the amygdala play an important role in the neuronal network mediating a clonic form of audiogenic seizures both before and after audiogenic kindling. *Brain Res.* **2005**, *1032*, 131–140. [CrossRef] [PubMed]
86. Doretto, M.C.; Cortes-De-Oliveira, J.A.; Rossetti, F.; Garcia-Cairasco, N.; Cortes-De-Oliveira, J.A. Role of the superior colliculus in the expression of acute and kindled audiogenic seizures in Wistar audiogenic rats. *Epilepsia* **2009**, *50*, 2563–2574. [CrossRef] [PubMed]
87. Almada, R.; Genewsky, A.J.; Heinz, D.E.; Kaplick, P.M.; Coimbra, N.C.; Wotjak, C.T. Stimulation of the Nigrotectal Pathway at the Level of the Superior Colliculus Reduces Threat Recognition and Causes a Shift From Avoidance to Approach Behavior. *Front. Neural Circuits* **2018**, *12*, 36. [CrossRef]
88. Brandão, M.L.; Zanoveli, J.; Ruiz-Martinez, R.C.; Oliveira, L.C.; Landeira-Fernandez, J. Different patterns of freezing behavior organized in the periaqueductal gray of rats: Association with different types of anxiety. *Behav. Brain Res.* **2008**, *188*, 1–13. [CrossRef]
89. Vargas, L.C.; Marques, T.D.A.; Schenberg, L.C. Micturition and defensive behaviors are controlled by distinct neural networks within the dorsal periaqueductal gray and deep gray layer of the superior colliculus of the rat. *Neurosci. Lett.* **2000**, *280*, 45–48. [CrossRef]
90. Mascarenhas, D.C.; Gomes, K.S.; Nunes-De-Souza, R.L. Anxiogenic-like effect induced by TRPV1 receptor activation within the dorsal periaqueductal gray matter in mice. *Behav. Brain Res.* **2013**, *250*, 308–315. [CrossRef]
91. Terzian, A.L.B.; De Aguiar, D.C.; Guimarães, F.S.; Moreira, F.A. Modulation of anxiety-like behaviour by Transient Receptor Potential Vanilloid Type 1 (TRPV1) channels located in the dorsolateral periaqueductal gray. *Eur. Neuropsychopharmacol.* **2008**, *19*, 188–195. [CrossRef]
92. Maione, S.; Cristino, L.; Migliozzi, A.L.; Georgiou, A.L.; Starowicz, K.; Salt, T.E.; Di Marzo, V. TRPV1 channels control synaptic plasticity in the developing superior colliculus. *J. Physiol.* **2009**, *587*, 2521–2535. [CrossRef]
93. John, C.S.; Currie, P.J. N-Arachidonoyl-serotonin in the basolateral amygdala increases anxiolytic behavior in the elevated plus maze. *Behav. Brain Res.* **2012**, *233*, 382–388. [CrossRef]
94. Vaughan, C.W.; Connor, M.; Bagley, E.; Christie, M. Actions of cannabinoids on membrane properties and synaptic transmission in rat periaqueductal gray neurons in vitro. *Mol. Pharmacol.* **2000**, *57*, 288–295. [PubMed]
95. Starowicz, K.; Maione, S.; Cristino, L.; Palazzo, E.; Marabese, I.; Rossi, F.; De Novellis, V.; Di Marzo, V. Tonic Endovanilloid Facilitation of Glutamate Release in Brainstem Descending Antinociceptive Pathways. *J. Neurosci.* **2007**, *27*, 13739–13749. [CrossRef] [PubMed]
96. Xing, J.; Li, J. TRPV1 Receptor Mediates Glutamatergic Synaptic Input to Dorsolateral Periaqueductal Gray (dl-PAG) Neurons. *J. Neurophysiol.* **2007**, *97*, 503–511. [CrossRef] [PubMed]
97. Casarotto, P.; Terzian, A.L.B.; De Aguiar, D.C.; Zangrossi, H.; Guimaraes, F.S.; Wotjak, C.T.; Moreira, F.A. Opposing Roles for Cannabinoid Receptor Type-1 (CB1) and Transient Receptor Potential Vanilloid Type-1 Channel (TRPV1) on the Modulation of Panic-Like Responses in Rats. *Neuropsychopharmacology* **2011**, *37*, 478–486. [CrossRef]
98. Graeff, F.G.; Silveira, M.C.L.; Nogueira, R.L.; Audi, E.A.; Oliveira, R.M.W. Role of the amygdala and periaqueductal gray in anxiety and panic. *Behav. Brain Res.* **1993**, *58*, 123–131. [CrossRef]
99. Fedotova, I.B.; Surina, N.M.; Nikolaev, G.M.; Revishchin, A.V.; Poletaeva, I.I. Rodent Brain Pathology, Audiogenic Epilepsy. *Biomedicines* **2021**, *9*, 1641. [CrossRef]

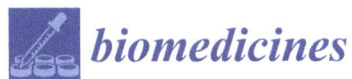

Review

Rodent Brain Pathology, Audiogenic Epilepsy

Irina B. Fedotova [1], Natalia M. Surina [1], Georgy M. Nikolaev [1], Alexandre V. Revishchin [2] and Inga I. Poletaeva [1,*]

[1] Department of Biology, Lomonosov Moscow State University, 119234 Moscow, Russia; lzglzg@yandex.ru (I.B.F.); Opera_ghost@Inbox.Ru (N.M.S.); humanoid15@yandex.ru (G.M.N.)
[2] Institute for Higher Nervous Activity, RAS, 119234 Moscow, Russia; revishchin@mail.ru
* Correspondence: ingapoletaeva@mail.ru

Abstract: The review presents data which provides evidence for the internal relationship between the stages of rodent audiogenic seizures and post-ictal catalepsy with the general pattern of animal reaction to the dangerous stimuli and/or situation. The wild run stage of audiogenic seizure fit could be regarded as an intense panic reaction, and this view found support in numerous experimental data. The phenomenon of audiogenic epilepsy probably attracted the attention of physiologists as rodents are extremely sensitive to dangerous sound stimuli. The seizure proneness in this group shares common physiological characteristics and depends on animal genotype. This concept could be the new platform for the study of epileptogenesis mechanisms.

Keywords: audiogenic epilepsy; rodents; fear reaction; behavior genetics

1. Introduction

It is widely known that the survival of animals (and of rodents in particular) in the wild depends on their acoustic sensitivity (and on their prompt reaction following danger stimulus). This obvious statement usually escapes the attention of investigators who analyze the rather well-known phenomenon of rodent audiogenic epilepsy (AE). At the onset of loud sound rats, mice, and hamsters of several strains develop typical audiogenic seizures. Such seizure fits develop according to the similar pattern in animals of different species and genotypes [1–6] and Figure 1. These fits start as violent running and jumpings, the stage named "wild run" or "clonic run" [7]. There were experimental evidences [8] that this stage of the audiogenic fit is "ambiguous" by its mechanisms; animal reaction reveals the traits of the violent flight reaction (defense behavior in order to escape aversive stimulation), but contains some type of forced movements as well, which are regarded as the signs of seizure process initiation. If the experiment is designed in such a way that during "wild run" an animal is able to escape from the sound source (into a safe place), some animals (but not all) will choose to escape [9]. Antipanic treatment ameliorates the wild run intensity [8]. It is likely that the "polygonal arena" for studying the escape reaction in rats could be of use as the device for further analysis of this ambiguity [10]. The further development of the audiogenic seizure in time is well described elsewhere [11–14]. Of course, the "wild run" stage in animal with audiogenic-epilepsy is different from that of a normal animal experiencing a panic state. But this difference is determined by differences in the CNS function in such animals. The panic state is induced usually by more complicated stimulus or stimulus situation (i.e., frightening environment, predators, etc.) and the prompt panic reaction help animal to find the safer place. Most animals usually don't develop "wild-run" in response to a loud sound. Non-AE-prone animals in their majority respond to sound onset by more or less intense startle-reaction. This could signify that sound sensitivity in AE-prone animals is abnormally enhanced. Nevertheless it has some features which resemble panic. The phenotypic similarity in movement patterns and the involvement of the similar brain regions (see below) could be the indications of their "relatedness".

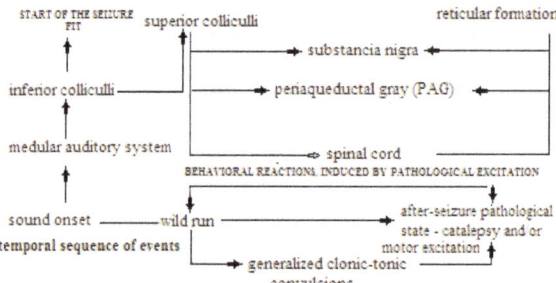

Figure 1. The schematic representation of both-brain structures, involved in the audiogenic seizure progress and the respective animal reactions, which unfold in parallel with certain structure involvement.

The same conclusions could be drawn concerning the "similarity" between post-ictal catalepsy in AE-prone animals and the freezing reaction of the normal rodent in response to a threatening situation in which presumably there is no way to escape. The common feature of these two states is the suppression of body movements, although significant differences between these two states do exist as well. For example, specific cataleptic muscle tone had been investigated rather extensively. This state models the important aspects of Parkinson's symptoms. It is widely known that haloperidol catalepsy develops due to abnormalities in striatal DA-receptors. At the same time the detailed research of this peculiar body muscles state (namely the body postural flexibility/rigidity) are not well known. Freezing is the component of the fear-anxiety reaction and it had been analyzed as a component of this state without special attention to muscle tone state *per se*.

This paper represents the attempt to demonstrate that rodent wild run, clonic, and tonic seizures in response to sound as well as the following catalepsy are the animal's exaggerated reactions to danger, which adopts the real pathological pattern due to the "constellation" of certain genetic elements. Such genetic anomalies could occur in rodent populations and discovered during laboratory breeding. The respective selection in laboratories increased the penetrance of these traits, so that the AE-prone lines could be created.

In other words, the successful selection of rats, mice and hamsters for high AE seizure intensity means that natural rodent populations harbor their respective genetic variants, although no data on AE seizures in wild populations could be found.

2. The General Pattern of AE Seizure Development

At the start of EEG era of neurology (around 1940s) Penfield and Jasper proposed that seizures became generalized as the pathological excitation spreads into the brain stem nuclei (i.e., medulla, pons and midbrain), including reticular formation (which had been described around this time). The brain stem structures are extensively connected to many brain regions and their excitation is the basis for epileptic discharge to become widespread.

The participation of brain stem structures in the genesis of audiogenic clonic-tonic seizures had been demonstrated independently in rats of audiogenic seizure prone strains such as the Krushinsky-Molodkina strain [14], which originated from Wistar population and GEPR (genetically epilepsy prone rats) from the Sprague-Dawley outbred strain. Later, the same pattern of AE seizure had been confirmed in the new strain, Wistar Audiogenic Rats (WAR) [6].

According to an explicit review of C. Faingold [12], based on GEPR data, the extensive firing in inferior colliculi (IC) increases before the seizure develops, which is the indication that this structure is the initial point of AE seizure fit development. The "wild running" expression depends on the activation of superior colliculi (SC) deep layers. The development of AE clonic-tonic seizures depends on the pontine reticular nucleus and periaqueductal gray (PAG), with further spread of excitation to the spinal cord [15]. During post-ictal depression, all areas except the pontine reticular nucleus are quiescent. This hierarchical neuronal network of AE, which determines this pathology, does not involve structures rostral to the midbrain.

The electrophysiological and neurochemical investigations made the serious impact concerning the participation of inferior-superior colliculi and other brain stem structures. The participation of PAG, ventral tegmental area (VTA) and *substantia nigra* as well as of other brain stem nuclei in the development of AE seizure [6,12,16,17] was established. Figure 2 (one of the first EEG records of AE seizure in KM rats) shows the neural excitation in the brain stem with typical lack of epileptic activity in the neocortex. However, it is worth noting that the reactivity of the visual cortex decreased after the seizure (less intense responses to light flashes) in comparison to pre-seizure recording.

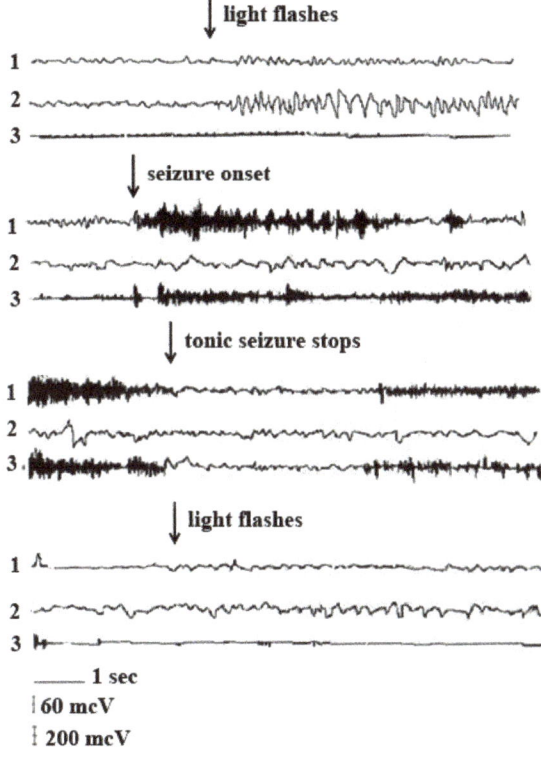

Figure 2. The electroencephalogram (EEG) and electromyogram (EMG) patterns, recorded from chronic electrodes in KM rat during experiment before seizure onset (upper part), during seizure (two middle parts) and after the seizure (the lower part of the figure). Electrodes positions: 1, brain stem; 2, visual cortex; 3, electromyogram (EMG). Calibration: horizontal bar-time scale, vertical bars, 60 mcV for EEG; 200 mcV for EMG (see also [18]).

3. The Neuroanatomical Correlates between AE Seizure Attack and Defense Reactions
3.1. Corpora Quardigemina

Inferior and superior colliculi had been recognized as the site of AE fit initiation rather long ago [19]. Among other experimental evidences is the fact that bilateral lesions of

IC abolished AE-fit development (see [16]). The onset of acoustic stimulus evokes the typical mammalian "startle" reaction, with IC and PAG mediating this reaction [20]. The review of IC role in this respect was performed by N. Garcia-Cairasco [6]. The initiation and propagation of AE activity relies upon hyperexcitability in the auditory system (and IC in particular) [16,21–23]. Thus, as it was mentioned above, the IC is considered to be the crucial structure for the AE-fit "ignition", and it was shown in mouse and rat AE models and in normal animals as well [24,25]. The activation pattern of different nuclei of IC as the process, which is causally connected with IC initiation, was proved using c-Fos immunoreactivity [13,26–30].

The genetic volumetric differences in IC of GEPR and WAR rat strains in comparison to controls were also demonstrated (with differences between these strains as well) [31].

At the same time, the IC is the structure responsible for the development of the innate defense reaction, at least in rodent brains, which could be expressed either as flight or as freezing [25,32–34]. The details were reported; ventral and dorsal IC regions are involved in the expression of the defensive reaction and audiogenic seizures, respectively [33], and aberrant neuronal reactions in the IC-SC system were described [22]. Ferreira-Netto et al. [33] demonstrated that in normal rats, freezing inducing chemical stimulation of these two brain regions activates different brain circuits, and apart from IC they include the forebrain structures.

The experimental data demonstrate that wild run could be the expression (or the -homologous) of the fear-induced flight reaction [2], which is the result of neuronal excitation spreading into lower-level brain stem structures [35] and the spinal cord. The special experiments and respective argumentation made it obvious that panic behavior is a phenomenon which is not similar to the anxiety traits [31,36]. Thus, the flight-like stage (wild run) of the AE fit could be regarded as the pathologically increased panic attack. The naturally occurring panic attacks (provoked in rats by ultrasonic stimulation) are the valid model of the respective human disorder [37]. Of course, panic behavior is the phenomenon which is not homogenous, and this was demonstrated by the effects of experimental interventions into the function of GABAergic and opioid systems in *corpora quarigemina, substantia nigra*, and other structures ([31,38–41], as the examples). The data obtained also demonstrated that forebrain excitation exert the plausible impact in panic-like behavior of different origin [42]. Thus, the AE-proneness is, presumably, the cause of IC auditory function disorder [43,44].

3.2. Brain Stem Structures (PAG in Particular)

The ventrolateral part of PAG (vlPAG) is responsible for mediating the excitation from IC [45] and for generation of the tonic AE stage [3,11,18,45,46]. It was demonstrated in GEPR-9 (in electrophysiological experiments) and confirmed in other AE models. It is worth noting that in cases of human partial epilepsy, these attacks sometimes resemble panic attacks as the patients experience the intense fear.

4. The Neurochemical Parallels between the AE Fit and Defense Reactions

Wild run (panic reaction). Some considerations in this respect were made above. Thus, the "wild run" stage of AE-seizure fit has the traits which permit to make the parallels with the panic-like animal behavior (namely in non-seizure prone animals). The panic-like behavior, realized as the successive neuronal excitation of IC, SC, PAG and other brain stem nuclei, share the neurochemical "sensitivity" with seizure fits induced by sound and demonstrate the participation of forebrain structures [47].

Freezing reaction. In rodents (and not only in rodents, but in other mammals as well) the encounter of fear-inducing situation evokes a freezing reaction (i.e., a normal response) which helps to avoid direct contact with danger. Freezing is expressed as the still posture (i.e., complete absence of body movements). The detailed analysis of this brain state in case of electrical stimulation of different PAG regions convinced authors [48] that there exist "at least four different kinds of freezing with specific neural substrates".

However, the brain stem stimulation creates the excitation pattern, which is different from the "natural" one when animal faces the natural danger. This means that direct comparisons are difficult to perform. As different intensities of IC electrical stimulation induced either freezing or escape reactions, the local infusions of semicarbazide or bicuculline (modulating GABAergic system) also induce these two types of reactions, respectively, demonstrating some type of similarity with AE neurochemical traits [49].

Catalepsy. The freezing reactions which are induced either in nature, or as the result of direct brain stimulations could be related to abnormal brain state-catalepsy. The cataleptic state induced by haloperidol (modulating dopamine transmission) was shown to be sensitive to aversive stimulations [50], and this type of cataleptic reactions could be modulated by changes in glutamatergic transmission in IC [51]. This could be regarded as the indication that cataleptic muscle tone pattern has probably some common links with the brain stem defense circuits. The special analysis of post-ictal catalepsy and/or of post sound cataleptic-like states in several rat strains indicated the relationship of AE seizures and this type of catalepsy [52]. The parallels of freezing-catalepsy expression could be partially confirmed by neurochemical and genetic data on pinch-induced catalepsy [53–56], which was shown to depend on brain tryptophan hydroxylase activity. Pinch-induced catalepsy (demonstrated in rats and mice) is regarded as a change in muscle tone, which resembles and probably is related to the non-responsiveness, developed in young pups when the mother transports them by holding the pup by the nape. The pinch-induced catalepsy in AE-prone rats of KM strain correlated with the intensity of their post-ictal catalepsy [55]. The special selection program for the spontaneous catalepsy from the Wistar population demonstrated several peculiarities in this strain such asthe appearance of "nervous" animals in the population of rats, selected for catalepsy as well as the certain percentage of animals which were AE-prone [54].

The schematic description of neurochemical substrate of AE seizure. It was shown rather long ago [24] that injecting metal ions and pyridoxal-5′-phosphate to normal mice made them prone to AE, and this change was accompanied by the elevation of glutamate and aspartate levels and the decrease of gamma-amino butyrate in IC. Thus, this chemical mimicking of AE seizure proved that the excitability level of this structure is connected with AS. The neuronal excitation (in norm and pathology) depends to a large extent on the glutamatergic brain system, which was demonstrated by induction of seizures by Glu-receptors agonists. The normal brain function depends on the balance between glutamate and GABA systems, which is deteriorated in cases of epilepsy. In AE, the misbalance of these neuronal circuits had been demonstrated in IC, SC and PAG [29,57–59].

Numerous studies demonstrated the involvement of glutamatergic, GABAergic, opioid, serotonin, and dopamine neurotransmitter systems in expression of reactions which belong to the "defense" domain. They are panic-like run, freezing, startle and AE [28,33,35,60–65]. Panicolytic-like effect of BDNF in the rat brain stem was also reported [66]. The hamster AE-prone strain demonstrated behavioral and molecular effects as the reaction to cannabidiol and valproate administration [67].

5. Genetics of AE

The expression of genetic acoustic peculiarities in rat and mouse AE strains. It is natural to ask question, whether the acoustic sensitivity in AE-prone animals is to blame for the audiogenic epilepsy in rodents. There were no data on KM rats, but other models are more or less investigated in this respect [12,68–70] (for details see the review in [71]).

Acoustic "equipment" in AE animals, single mutations. The finding that acoustic thresholds in AE-prone rodents were elevated, was common for AE data. Cochlea morphological anomalies, differing in details, were present in almost all studies. It is worthwhile to note the following. The defect in acoustic sensitivity was found in Black Swiss mouse strain, carrying the *jams1* gene, which is responsible for AE. However, this acoustic defect and AE-proneness were shown to be independent traits in these mice [69]. The detailed analysis of cochlear functions in albino Frings mice, namely in their inbred descendants, was also performed [72]. The thresholds of cochlear action potentials of the AE-susceptible RB/1 bg mice were abnormally high, while the AE resistant inbred RB/3 bg mice had normal audiograms of evoked potentials. The F1 hybrid mice were heterotic for cochlear function. This RB/1 bg line showed little age-related cochlear loss, which probably accounts for its robust sensitivity to audiogenic seizures over most of its lifespan. Earlier studies demonstrated that in the susceptible RB line, they demonstrated robust evoked potentials with little or no cochlear microphonic events. The susceptible RB/1 bg mice had well-defined potentials and cochlear microphonic [72]. Thus, we see that of course the acoustic anomalies accompany AE traits. However, they probably develop in parallel (i.e., they are not the cause of this pathology).

Frings mice are also the reliable genetic model of AE susceptibility with the gene mass1 (*monogenic audiogenic seizure-susceptible*, now referred to as Mgr1) being identified as responsible for this pathology. This gene codes for the membrane protein, which does not belong to ion channels "family". Frings mice display a robust AE, demonstrating sound-induced c-Fos immunoreactivity including the external and dorsal nuclei of the inferior colliculi. The subthreshold acoustic stimulation activates c-Fos immunoreactivity in the central nucleus of the IC [27]. Recently the genetic variant of this gene was found in AE prone WAR strain which is thought to be responsible for AE-proneness of these animals [73]. Homozygous carriers of Scn8a gene mutation in mouse, which affects generalized seizure susceptibility, demonstrated also the typical audiogenic epilepsy with high amplitude EEG signals and c-fos immunohistochemistry labelling in the IC [26,30,59].

Polygenic inheritance. The successful selection of rat strains for elevated incidences of AE seizures was the first indication that the AE is the genetically determined trait.

The diallel cross and F2 hybrids analysis [14,71,74,75] of AE-proneness in KM strain demonstrated the recessive polygenic nature inheritance, the data on genetic basis of GEPR and WAR strains is rather sparse [17,76–78]. Ribak and Morin [26] and Ribak [59] demonstrated that the IC GABA levels in GEPR were increased in comparison to controls and the number of GABAergic neurons was also atypical with the significantly large number of small GABAergic cells. The anomalies in GABAergic cells in IC and SC were found in KM rats, although the histological pattern of differences between AE-prone and resistant animals was different [73,79]. The IC ERK1/2 kinases activity was shown to be different between KM rats and Wistars [80]. The possible animal model for anticonvulsant mechanism was suggested by Arida et al. [81], namely the spiny rat *Proechimys guyannensis*, in which the decreased seizure proneness to forebrain convulsions was found. Although no data on AE in this species could be found.

Acoustic startle reaction. The genetic basis of differences in startle reaction in strains, which differ in AE-proneness and/or in defense reactions, was also shown [25,82,83]. The precise location of the chromosome fragment in mice was indicated, which is responsible for pinch-induced catalepsy [56]. These data are of importance as they signify the plausible ways for further investigation of AE-proneness mechanisms and thus for the origin of epilepsy phenomenon.

More information on genetic differences in neurochemical indices. The features which could be interpreted as common within pairs "wild run-panic", and "catalepsy-freezing" are perceived as distant ones in normal "non-epileptic brain". Although in cases of KM, GEPR and WAR strains numerous neurochemical anomalies were described which could be due to pathological transition from panic flight into wild run stage and from freezing as a defense reaction into catalepsy. The neurochemical deviations from non-AE normal state which are presumably of genetic origin were found in all three best investigated AE-prone rat strains (KM, GEPR and WAR). The brain monoamine system was analyzed as the first one [84–93], but deviations in other brain systems, which plausibly could affect behavioral reactions, were also noted (e.g., oxidative stress reactivity and histaminergic brain system) [94,95], as well as early gene expression patterns [96]. These neurochemical deviations were described not only in AE-prone animals; it seems that they are inherent to the "epileptic brain" in general [97,98]. It should be noted that these neurochemical peculiarities lay apart from already described glutamate-GABA misbalance in epilepsy.

The genetic basis of these deviations could be searched in the early stages of CNS development. It looks more or less plausible that the disturbances in gene expression patterns, which occur rather early in development, could be responsible for the expression of AE. Such disturbances (mutations) nevertheless permit the embryo to develop into the phenotype, which is still compatible with the embryo survival and future viability of an organism (which, probably, is reduced, as these mutation effects were found in laboratory only). The respective mutations are not yet identified, although several examples which probably fit this line of considerations, are now available. It was found that simultaneous genetic inactivation of three transcriptional factors (*PAR bZip* proteins, connected with circadian rhythms-albumin D-site-binding protein proline, hepatic leukemia factor, and thyrotrophic embryonic factor) induce the audiogenic epilepsy in young mice [99]. The target gene of this transcription factors family is the pyridoxal kinase (*Pdxk*), which catalyzes the conversion of vitamin B12 derivatives into pyridoxal-phosphate. The latter is the coenzyme of many enzymes participating in the neurotransmitter metabolism. It was demonstrated that in the triple mouse KOs the levels of brain pyridoxal-phosphate, serotonin and dopamine were decreased [99].

Mutations of other genes, which are identified as being involved in the early stages of CNS development, could also be possible candidates for AE-type dysfunction. These could be also the *disheveled* genes, as proteins, coded by this gene family, which are the important signaling components of *beta-catenin/Wnt pathway*, are important for developmental processes (cell proliferation and patterning etc.). $Dvl3 (-/-)$ mice died prenatally with several developmental defects, the detected stereocilia orientation anomaly in the organ of Corti being the example, which attracts attention [100].

The hypothesized abnormal "developmental" genes could induce the CNS anomalies, AE symptoms being among them. Such anomalies could cause the channelopathies in the certain brain regions (or in the brain as a whole), which are crucial for AE expression. As channelopathies (the full list not yet described) are the regular findings in many human epilepsy cases, AE models for respective investigations being of certain clinical value. One should not forget that the rodent brain is especially vulnerable for extreme acoustic stimulation for animals that avoid danger in natural habitats.

The general outline presented in this paper does not consider the mechanisms of so-called audiogenic kindling (i.e., the development of specific myoclonic seizures (type of "jerks")), which have the forebrain localization and appear after systemic repetitive daily sound exposures [1]. This phenomenon is the result of ascending influences from the (abnormally functioning) brain-stem structures of AE-prone animals. At the same time there are two clear indications that the reverse influences (i.e., from the forebrain to brain stem) also exist, as strong olfactory stimulation resulted in the decrease of AE-seizure intensity [101,102].

6. The Experimental Evidences Which Are Not Compatible with the Hypothesis Presented

Of course, the parallels which could be derived between wild run AE stage and panic reaction and between cataleptic traits and behavioral freezing are not "complete" as biological variability exists in physiological processes determining the AE. This "similarity" could not be "ideal", and the respective evidences presented above are not totally convincing. Some arguments against these parallels could be found, as they concern the metabolic correlates of seizure state. The seizure intensity in human patients and in experimental animals depends on the blood pH values and on the NMDA-receptors' excitability [103,104]. The acidosis (low pH) was described as occurring during seizure process as well [105,106]. The analysis of the brain stem area "responsible" for respiration function was found to be different in WAR in comparison to controls [107]. Schimitel et al. [108] presented the results of complicated study of CO_2 and PAG stimulation effects on panic-like behavior in rats with the detailed description of animals' autonomic reactions. Panic expression increased as the result of sodium lactate and inhalation of 5% CO_2 in panic-predisposed patients [108]. This inspired authors to analyze this issue in animal model. Exposure to CO_2 induced some kind of behavioral arousal, but also attenuated PAG-evoked immobility (i.e., the homologue of freezing reaction). This data as well as those, cited above, are in contrast with the CO_2 seizure attenuating effects demonstrated in KM strain, which were found by L.V. Krushinsky as early as the begin of 1950s, this being one of the first experimental data obtained in this model.

7. The General Comparison of Normal and Pathological Reactions in AE Models

The general outline of rodent abnormal reaction as the response to loud sound ("audiogenic seizures") is presented, which could probably be instructive as the comparison was made with the patterns of normal animal behavioral reactions. One may find that the wild run stage resembles the species-typical (although pathologically exaggerated) flight, wherein an animal aims to avoid imminent danger. Similarly, the drastic change in the muscle tone (catalepsy), occurring after the tonic AE-seizure stage could be regarded as pathologically exaggerated biologically normal freezing reaction. As described above, this resemblance could probably be determined by the close brain stem topographical locations of brain substrates of these two types of behavioral reactions. It could be that this parallelism is a mere coincidence. However, the question of the AE origin stays unanswered. Another hypothesis could be tested as well, namely that such region-specific channelopathies arise in rats and mice as the result of the abnormal pattern of CNS development *per se*, the rodent brain being especially vulnerable for loud sound as these animals rely on sound sensitivity in avoiding danger in natural habitats.

The dysfunction of ion-channels (channelopathy) is known not only for AE [109,110], but for epilepsy and neuromuscular pathology in general [111–114]. Thus the membrane-potential disturbances look like the most crucial proximate cause of AE and other seizure states.

The complex interconnections between genetic elements and behavior are different in different AE strains. Although one may conclude the existence of hypothetical "common pathway", namely the mechanism which underlie the seizure state (and AE) and defense behavior. One may also hypothesize the *endophenotype* for audiogenic epilepsy—the specific seizure provoking constellation of genetic and (further) neurochemical events (distortions), which function, probably, at both levels—in peripheral hearing organ and in brain structures. The development of regional specific channelopathies and/or of the misbalance in GABA and glutamate systems (both central and cochlear) could be the possible links which would help to delineate the AE endophenotype. The key components of any identified endophenotype are heritability and stability (state independence). Endophenotype approach is useful as, according to I.I. Gottesman and T.D. Gould [115], "it reduces the complexity of symptoms and multifaceted behaviors", successful identifying of "units" for analysis being the positive result.

The data presented above in a short way demonstrated that apart from phenotypical similarity of AE seizures there are not many traits common for all AE models explored (non- identical hearing system defects and the pattern of brain neurotransmitter systems misbalance). The data of modern volumetric estimation of brains from WAR and GEPR is also the illustration [31]. The dysfunction patterns of brain neurotransmitter systems in cases of AE not always coincide in different AE genotypes.

One more moment should be mentioned in this respect, namely the attempt of Traub et al. [116] to transfer the notion of "central pattern generator", CPG (which is used in invertebrate neurobiology and neuroethology) to the domain of circuits, generating vertebrate motor patterns. Authors suggest that the concept of CPG could be useful for analyzing not only normal cortical oscillations, but also the transition of normal activity pattern to epileptiform pathology. The generality of CPG notion could be the helpful theoretical framework for further studies of seizure development.

The final summarizing Tables 1 and 2 are presented (containing the facts and literature references) which could help to acknowledge the new aspect on AE data presented in this review.

Table 1. The data evidencing the neurobiological parallels between defense behavior and AE phenomena.

The Phenomenon Described	The Connection to AE Phenotype	References
Flight behavior and panic reaction	The involvement of colliculi inferior in both states (AE and defense behavior)	[2,25,31–34,36]
Behavioral freezing	Cataleptic states	[48–52]
The specific neurochemical state in brain stem nuclei	The common misbalance in glutamate-GABA signaling	[28,33,35,60–65]

Table 2. The genetic data on AE susceptibility origins.

The Type of Inheritance	The Neurobiological "Unit" Affected	References
Monogenic	Cochlea	[43,68–70]
	Non-"channel" coding gene *mass1 (Mgr1)*	[27]
	Different channellopathies	[30,109,110]
	Several genes, expressed in early development, coding *for PAR bZip* proteins, e.g., *Pdxk*. Participant of *wnt* cascade *Dvl3* gene	[114,115]
Polygenic	Dominant-recessive inheritance, diallel cross	[14,17,72,74–78]

8. Conclusions

The literature analysis, presented above, represents an attempt to find the "biological roots" of the peculiar trait, inherent to the series of rodent species, namely the production of intense seizure reaction in response to sound. As these seizures typically start as the wild run and jumps, the first parallel, which crosses the observers mind, is that an animal is eager to run away from the source of the unpleasant sensation. This excitation, being enhanced in certain genotypes, could be followed by motor seizures as this abnormal excitation spreads into the brain stem and further downstream to the motor centers. The parallelism between audiogenic epilepsy and abnormally enhanced escape reaction could be perceived as exotic. However, a range human epilepsy cases (first) and the necessity (second) for the search of epileptogenesis roots (taking the whole brain) is not sufficient to reject this point of view.

Author Contributions: Conceptualization, I.I.P., I.B.F., G.M.N.; software, I.I.P.; validation, I.I.P., I.B.F., A.V.R.; resources, N.M.S.; data curation, G.M.N.; writing—original draft preparation, I.I.P.; writing—review and editing, I.I.P.; supervision, I.B.F.; funding acquisition, I.I.P., I.B.F. All authors have read and agreed to the published version of the manuscript.

Funding: The work was partly supported State Scientific Assignment No.121032500080-8 for Moscow State University and by Interdisciplinary Scientific and Educational School of Moscow University Brain, cognitive systems, artificial intellect.

Institutional Review Board Statement: Not applicable.

Informed Consent Statement: Not applicable.

Data Availability Statement: Not applicable.

Conflicts of Interest: The authors declare no conflict of interest.

References

1. Moraes, D.M.F.; Galvis-Alonso, O.Y.; Garcia-Cairasco, N. Audiogenic kindling in the Wistar rat: A potential model for recruitment of limbic structures. *Epil. Res.* **2000**, *39*, 251–259. [CrossRef]
2. Moraes, M.F.; Chavali, M.; Mishra, P.K.; Jobe, P.C.; Garcia-Cairasco, N. A comprehensive electrographic and behavioral analysis of generalized tonic-clonic seizures of GEPR-9s. *Brain Res.* **2005**, *1033*, 1–12. [CrossRef]
3. N'Gouemo, P.; Faingold, C.L. Periaqueductal gray neurons exhibit increased responsiveness associated with audiogenic seizures in the genetically epilepsy-prone rat. *Neuroscience* **1998**, *84*, 619–625. [CrossRef]
4. Midzyanovskaya, I.S.; Galina, D.; Kuznetsova, G.D.; Liudmila, V.; Vinogradova, L.V.; Shatskova, A.B.; Coenen, A.M.L.; van Luijtelaar, G. Mixed forms of epilepsy in a subpopulation of WAG/Rij rats. *Epilepsy Behav.* **2004**, *5*, 655–661. [CrossRef] [PubMed]
5. Francois, J.; Boehrer, A.; Nehlig, A. Effects of carisbamate (RWJ-333369) in two models of genetically determined generalized epilepsy, the GAERS and the audiogenic Wistar AS. *Epilepsia* **2008**, *49*, 393–399. [CrossRef] [PubMed]
6. Garcia-Cairasco, N. A critical review on the participation of inferior colliculus in acoustic-motor and acoustic-limbic networks involved in the expression of acute and kindled audiogenic seizures. *Hear. Res.* **2002**, *168*, 208–222. [CrossRef]
7. Fehr, C.; Shirley, R.L.; Metten, P.; Kosobud, A.E.K.; Belknap, J.K.; Crabbe, J.C.; Buck, K.J. Potential pleiotropic effects of Mpdz on vulnerability to seizures. *Genes Brain Behav.* **2004**, *3*, 8–19. [CrossRef] [PubMed]
8. de Paula, H.M.; Hoshino, K. Antipanic procedures reduce the strychnine-facilitated wild running of rats. *Behav. Brain Res.* **2003**, *147*, 157–162. [CrossRef]
9. Fless, D.A.; Salimov, R.M. An analysis of prespasmodic motor excitation in rats with audiogenic seizures. *Bull. Exptl. Biol. Med.* **1974**, *78*, 31–33.
10. Freitas, R.L.; Felippotti, T.T.; Coimbra, N.C. Neuroethological validation of an experimental apparatus to evaluate oriented and non-oriented escape behaviours: Comparison between the polygonal arena with a burrow and the circular enclosure of an open-field test. *Behav. Brain Res.* **2016**, *298*, 65–77. [CrossRef]
11. Faingold, C.L.; Walsh, E.J.; Maxwell, J.K.; Randall, M.E. Audiogenic seizure severity and hearing deficits in the genetically epilepsy-prone rat. *Exp. Neurol.* **1990**, *108*, 55–60. [CrossRef]
12. Faingold, C.L. Neuronal networks in the genetically epilepsy-prone rat. *Adv. Neurol.* **1999**, *79*, 311–321. [PubMed]
13. Garcia-Cairasco, N.; Rossetti, F.; Oliveira, J.A.; de Furtado, M.A. Neuroethological study of status epilepticus induced by systemic pilocarpine in Wistar audiogenic rats (WAR strain). *Epilepsy Behav.* **2004**, *5*, 455–463. [CrossRef] [PubMed]
14. Poletaeva, I.I.; Surina, N.M.; Kostina, Z.A.; Perepelkina, O.V.; Fedotova, I.B. The Krushinsky-Molodkina rat strain: The study of audiogenic epilepsy for 65 years. *Epilepsy Behav.* **2017**, *71*, 130–141. [CrossRef] [PubMed]
15. Noga, B.R.; Kriellaars, D.J.; Brownstone, R.M.; Jordan, L.M. Mechanism for activation of locomotor centers in the spinal cord by stimulation of the mesencephalic locomotor region. *J. Neurophysiol.* **2003**, *90*, 1464–1478. [CrossRef] [PubMed]
16. Ross, K.C.; Coleman, J.R. Developmental and genetic audiogenic seizure models: Behavior and biological substrates. *Neurosci. Biobehav. Rev.* **2000**, *24*, 639–653. [CrossRef]
17. Garcia-Cairasco, N.; Umeoka, E.H.L.; Cortes de Oliveira, J.A. The Wistar Audiogenic Rat (WAR) strain and its contributions to epileptology and related comorbidities: History and perspectives. *Epilepsy Behav.* **2017**, *71*, 250–273. [CrossRef] [PubMed]
18. Rossetti, F.; Cairrao, M.; Rodrigues, A.; de Oliveira, J.A.C.; Garcia-Cairasco, N. EEG wavelet analyses of the *striatum–substantia nigra pars reticulata–superior* colliculus circuitry: Audiogenic seizures and anticonvulsant drug administration in Wistar audiogenic rats (War strain). *Epilepsy Res.* **2006**, *72*, 192–208. [CrossRef] [PubMed]
19. Willott, J.F. Comparison of response properties of inferior colliculus neurons of two inbred mouse strains differing in susceptibility to audiogenic seizures. *J. Neurophysiol.* **1981**, *45*, 35–47. [CrossRef]
20. Parham, K.; Willott, J.F. Effects of inferior colliculus lesions on the acoustic startle response. *Behav. Neurosci.* **1990**, *104*, 831–840. [CrossRef] [PubMed]
21. Willott, J.F.; Demuth, R.M.; Lu, S.M. Excitability of auditory neurons in the dorsal and ventral cochlear nuclei of DBA/2 and C57BL/6 mice. *Exp. Neurol.* **1984**, *83*, 495–506. [CrossRef]
22. Chakravarty, D.N.; Faingold, C.L. Aberrant neuronal responsiveness in the genetically epilepsy-prone rat: Acoustic responses and influences of the central nucleus upon the external nucleus of inferior colliculus. *Brain Res.* **1997**, *761*, 263–270. [CrossRef]
23. de Oliveira, A.R.; Colombo, A.C.; Muthuraju, S.; Almada, R.C.; Brandao, M.L. Dopamine D2-Like Receptors Modulate unconditioned fear: Role of the inferior colliculus. *PLoS ONE* **2014**, *9*, e104228. [CrossRef]
24. Chung, S.H.; Johnson, M.S. Experimentally induced susceptibility to audiogenic seizure. *Exp. Neurol.* **1983**, *82*, 89–107. [CrossRef]
25. Bagri, A.; Sandner, G.; Di Scala, G. Aversive effects elicited by electrical stimulation of the inferior colliculus in normal and audiogenic seizure susceptible rats. *Neurosci. Lett.* **2005**, *379*, 180–184. [CrossRef]
26. Ribak, C.E.; Morin, C.L. The role of the inferior colliculus in a genetic model of audiogenic seizures. *Anat. Embryol.* **1995**, *191*, 279–295. [CrossRef] [PubMed]
27. Klein, B.D.; Fu, Y.H.; Ptacek, L.J.; White, H.S. c-Fos immunohistochemical mapping of the audiogenic seizure network and tonotopic neuronal hyperexcitability in the inferior colliculus of the Frings mouse. *Epilepsy Res.* **2004**, *62*, 13–25. [CrossRef]
28. Bandara, S.B.; Eubig, P.A.; Sadowski, R.N.; Schantz, S.L. Developmental PCB exposure increases audiogenic seizures and decreases glutamic acid decarboxylase in the inferior colliculus. *Toxicol. Sci.* **2016**, *149*, 335–345. [CrossRef] [PubMed]
29. Ishida, Y.; Nakahara, D.; Hashiguchi, H.; Nakamura, M.; Ebihara, K.; Takeda, R.; Nishimori, T.; Niki, H. Fos Expression in gabaergic cells and cells, immunopositive for NMDA and related emotions in mammals. *Braz. J. Med. Biol. Res.* **1994**, *27*, 811–829.

30. Makinson, C.D.; Dutt, K.; Lin, F.; Papale, L.A.; Shankar, A.; Barela, A.J.; Liu, R.; Goldin, A.L.; Escayg, A. An Scn1a epilepsy mutation in Scn8a alters seizure susceptibility and behavior. *Exp. Neurol.* **2016**, *275*, 46–58. [CrossRef] [PubMed]
31. Lee, Y.; Rodriguez, O.C.; Albanese, C.; Santos, V.R.; Cortes de Oliveira, J.A.; Donatti, A.L.F.; Fernandes, A.; Garcia-Cairasco, N.; N'Gouemo, P.; Forcelli, P.A. Divergent brain changes in two audiogenic rat strains: A voxel-based morphometry and diffusion tensor imaging comparison of the genetically epilepsy prone rat (GEPR-3) and the Wistar Audiogenic Rat (WAR). *Neurobiol. Dis.* **2018**, *111*, 80–90. [CrossRef] [PubMed]
32. Schenberg, L.C.; Povoa, R.M.F.; Costa, A.L.P.; Caldellas, A.V.; Tufik, S.; Bittencourt, A.S. Functional specializations within the tectum defense systems of the rat *Neurosci. Biobehav. Rev.* **2005**, *29*, 1279–1298. [CrossRef] [PubMed]
33. Ferreira-Netto, C.; Borelli, K.G.; Brandão, M.L. Distinct Fos expression in the brain following freezing behavior elicited by stimulation with NMDA of the ventral or dorsal inferior colliculus. *Exper. Neurol.* **2007**, *204*, 693–704. [CrossRef] [PubMed]
34. Xiong, X.R.; Liang, F.; Zingg, B.; Ji, X.-Y.; Ibrahim, L.A.; Tao, H.W.; Zhang, L.I. Auditory cortex controls sound-driven innate defense behaviour through corticofugal projections to inferior colliculus. *Nat. Commun.* **2015**, *6*, 7224. [CrossRef] [PubMed]
35. Capelli, P.; Pivetta, C.; Esposito, M.S.; Arber, S. Locomotor speed control circuits in the caudal brainstem. *Nature* **2017**, *551*, 373–377. [CrossRef] [PubMed]
36. Andreatini, R.; Blanchard, C.; Blanchard, R.; Brandão, M.L.; Carobrez, A.P.; Griebel, G.; Guimarães, F.S.; Handley, S.L.; Jenck, F.; Leite, J.R.; et al. The brain decade in debate: II. Panic or anxiety? From animal models to a neurobiological basis. *Braz. J. Med. Biol. Res.* **2001**, *34*, 145–154. [CrossRef] [PubMed]
37. Klein, S.; Nicolas, L.B.; Lopez-Lopez, C.; Jacobson, L.H.; McArthur, S.G.; Grundschober, C.; Prinssen, E.P. Examining face and construct validity of a noninvasive model of panic disorder in Lister-hooded rats. *Psychopharmacology* **2010**, *211*, 197–208. [CrossRef] [PubMed]
38. Schenberg, L.C.; Bittencourt, A.S.; Sudré, E.C.; Vargas, L.C. Modeling panic attacks. *Neurosci. Biobehav. Rev.* **2001**, *25*, 647–659. [CrossRef]
39. da Silva, J.A.; Biagioni, A.F.; Almada, R.C.; de Souza Crippa, J.A.; Hallak, J.E.C.; Zuardi, A.W.; Coimbra, N.C. Dissociation between the panicolytic effect of cannabidiol microinjected into the substantia nigra, pars reticulata, and fear-induced antinociception elicited by bicuculline administration in deep layers of the superior colliculus: The role of cb1-cannabinoid receptor in the ventral mesencephalon. *Eur. J. Pharmacol.* **2015**, *758*, 153–163. [PubMed]
40. da Silva, J.A.; Almada, R.C.; de Figueiredo, R.M.; Coimbra, N.C. Blockade of synaptic activity in the neostriatum and activation of striatal efferent pathways produce opposite effects on panic attack-like defensive behaviours evoked by GABAergic disinhibition in the deep layers of the superior colliculus. *Physiol. Behav.* **2018**, *196*, 104–111. [CrossRef] [PubMed]
41. Calvo, F.; Almada, R.C.; da Silva, J.A.; Medeiros, P.; da Silva Soares, R., Jr.; de Paiva, Y.B.; Marroni Roncon, C.; Coimbra, N.C. The Blockade of μ1- And κ-Opioid Receptors in the Inferior Colliculus Decreases the Expression of Panic Attack-Like Behav-iours Induced by Chemical Stimulation of the Dorsal Midbrain. *Neuropsychobiology* **2019**, *78*, 218—228. [CrossRef]
42. Tannure, R.M.; Bittencourt, A.S.; Schenberg, L.C. Short-term full kindling of the amygdala dissociates natural and periaqueductal gray-evoked flight behaviors of the rat. *Behav. Brain Res.* **2009**, *199*, 247–256. [CrossRef]
43. Pinto, H.P.P.; de Oliveira, L.E.L.; Carvalho, V.R.; Mourão, F.A.G.; de Oliveira Guarnieri, L.; Mendes, E.M.A.M.; de Castro Medeiros, D.; Moraes, M.F.D. Seizure susceptibility corrupts inferior colliculus acoustic integration. *Front Syst. Neurosci.* **2019**, *13*, 63. [CrossRef] [PubMed]
44. Pinto, H.P.; Carvalho, V.R.; Medeiros, D.C.; Almeida, A.F.; Mendes, E.M.; Moraes, M.F. Auditory processing assessment suggests that Wistar audiogenic rat neural networks are prone to entrainment. *Neuroscience* **2017**, *347*, 48–56. [CrossRef] [PubMed]
45. Brandão, M.L.; Tomaz, C.; Borges, P.C.; Coimbra, N.C.; Bagri, A. Defense reaction induced by microinjections of bicuculline into the inferior colliculus. *Physiol. Behav.* **1988**, *44*, 361–365. [CrossRef]
46. Kincheski, G.C.; Mota-Ortiz, S.R.; Pavesi, E.; Canteras, N.S.; Carobrez, A.P. The dorsolateral periaqueductal gray and its role in mediating fear learning to life threatening events. *PLoS ONE* **2012**, *7*, e50361. [CrossRef] [PubMed]
47. Canteras, N.S.; Graeff, F.G. Executive and modulatory neural circuits of defensive reactions: Implications for panic disorder. *Neurosci. Biobehav. Rev.* **2014**, *3*, 352–364. [CrossRef]
48. Brandao, M.L.; Zanoveli, J.M.; Ruiz-Martinez, R.C.; Oliveira, L.C.; Landeira-Fernandez, J. Different patterns of freezing behavior organized in the periaqueductal gray of rats: Association with different types of anxiety. *Behav. Brain Res.* **2008**, *188*, 1–13. [CrossRef]
49. Borelli, K.G.; Ferreira-Netto, C.; Brandão, M.L. Distribution of Fos immunoreactivity in the rat brain after freezing or escape elicited by inhibition of glutamic acid decarboxylase or antagonism of GABA-A receptors in the inferior colliculus. *Behav. Brain Res.* **2006**, *170*, 84–93. [CrossRef]
50. Barroca, N.C.B.; Guarda, M.D.; da Silva, N.T.; Colombo, A.C.; Reimer, A.E.; Brandão, M.L.; de Oliveira, A.R. Influence of aversive stimulation on haloperidol-induced catalepsy in rats. *Behav. Pharmacol.* **2019**, *30*, 229–238. [CrossRef] [PubMed]
51. Melo, L.L.; Santos, P.; Medeiros, P.; Mello, R.O.; Ferrari, E.A.; Brandão, M.L.; Maisonnette, S.S.; Francisco, A.; Coimbra, N.C. Glutamatergic neurotransmission mediated by NMDA receptors in the inferior colliculus can modulate haloperidol-induced catalepsy. *Brain Res.* **2010**, *1349*, 41–47. [CrossRef] [PubMed]
52. Fedotova, I.B.; Sourina, N.M.; Malikova, L.A.; Raevsky, K.S.; Poletaeva, I.I. The investigation of cataleptic muscle tonus changes in rats after audiogenic seizures. *Zh. Vyssh. Nerv. Deiat. Im. I P Pavlov.* **2008**, *58*, 620–627.

53. Kulikov, A.V.; Kozlachkova, E.Y.; Kudryavtseva, N.N.; Popova, N.K. Correlation between tryptophan hydroxylase activity in the brain and predisposition to pinch-induced catalepsy in mice. *Pharmacol. Biochem. Behav.* **1995**, *50*, 431–435. [CrossRef]
54. Kolpakov, V.G.; Kulikov, A.V.; Alekhina, T.A.; Chuguĭ, V.F.; Petrenko, O.I.; Barykina, N.N. Catatonia or depression: The GC rat strain as an animal model of psychopathology. *Genetika* **2004**, *40*, 827–834. [CrossRef] [PubMed]
55. Surina, N.M.; Fedotova, I.B.; Kulikov, A.V.; Poletaeva, I.I. Pinch-induced catalepsy in rats of various genetic groups with different predisposition to audiogenic epilepsy. *Zh. Vyssh. Nerv. Deiat. Im. I P Pavlov.* **2010**, *60*, 364–371.
56. Kulikova, E.A.; Bazovkina, D.V.; Akulov, A.E.; Tsybko, A.S.; Fursenko, D.V.; Kulikov, A.V.; Naumenko, V.S.; Ponimaskin, E.; Kondaurova, E.M. Alterations in pharmacological and behavioural responses in recombinant mouse line with an increased predisposition to catalepsy: Role of the 5-HT1A receptor. *Br. J. Pharmacol.* **2016**, *173*, 2147–2161. [CrossRef] [PubMed]
57. Faingold, C.L. Role of GABA abnormalities in the inferior colliculus pathophysiology—Audiogenic seizures. *Hear. Res.* **2002**, *168*, 223–237. [CrossRef]
58. Castellan-Baldan, L.; da Costa Kawasaki, M.; Ribeiro, S.J.; Calvo, F.; Corrêa, V.M.; Coimbra, N.C. Topographic and functional neuroanatomical study of GABAergic disinhibitory striatum-nigral inputs and inhibitory nigrocollicular pathways: Neural hodology recruiting the substantia nigra, pars reticulata, for the modulation of the neural activity in the inferior colliculus involved with panic-like emotions. *J. Chem. Neuroanat.* **2006**, *32*, 1–27. [CrossRef]
59. Ribak, C.E. An abnormal GABAergic system in the inferior colliculus provides a basis for audiogenic seizures in genetically epilepsy-prone rats. *Epilepsy Behav.* **2017**, *71*, 160–164. [CrossRef]
60. Graeff, F.G. Neuroanatomy and neurotransmitter regulation of defensive behaviors. *J. Cereb. Blood Flow Metab.* **1989**, *9*, 821–829. [CrossRef]
61. Nobre, M.J.; Sandner, G.; Brandão, M.L. Enhancement of Acoustic Evoked Potentials and Impairment of Startle Reflex Induced by Reduction of GABAergic Control of the Neural Substrates of Aversion in the Inferior Colliculus. *Hear. Res.* **2003**, *184*, 82–90. [CrossRef]
62. Miguel, T.L.; Pobbe, R.L.; Spiacci, A., Jr.; Zangrossi, H., Jr. Dorsal raphe nucleus regulation of a panic-like defensive behavior evoked by chemical stimulation of the rat dorsal periaqueductal gray matter. *Behav. Brain Res.* **2010**, *213*, 195–200. [CrossRef] [PubMed]
63. Reimer, A.E.; De Oliveira, A.R.; Brandao, M.L. Glutamatergic mechanisms of the dorsal periaqueductal gray matter modulate the expression of conditioned freezing and fear-potentiated startle. *Neuroscience* **2012**, *219*, 72–81. [CrossRef] [PubMed]
64. Muthuraju, S.; Talbot, T.; Brandão, M.L. Dopamine D2 receptors regulate unconditioned fear in deep layers of the superior colliculus and dorsal periaqueductal gray. *Behav. Brain Res.* **2016**, *297*, 116–123. [CrossRef] [PubMed]
65. Chou, X.-L.; Wang, X.; Zhang, Z.-G.; Shen, L.; Zingg, B.; Huang, J.; Wen, Z.; Mesik, L.; Zhang, L.; Tao, H.W. Inhibitory gain modulation of defense behaviors by zona incerta. *Nat. Commun.* **2018**, *9*, 1151. [CrossRef]
66. Casarotto, P.C.; de Bortoli, V.C.; Corrêa, F.M.; Resstel, L.B.; Zangrossi, H., Jr. Panicolytic-like effect of BDNF in the rat dorsal periaqueductal grey matter: The role of 5-HT and GABA. *Int. J. Neuropsychophar.* **2010**, *13*, 573–582. [CrossRef]
67. Cabral-Pereira, G.; Sánchez-Benito, D.; Díaz-Rodríguez, S.M.; Gonçalves, J.; Sancho, C.; Castellano, O.; Muñoz, L.J.; López, D.E.; Gómez-Nieto, R. Behavioral and molecular effects induced by cannabidiol and valproate administration in the GASH/Sal model of acute audiogenic seizures. *Front. Behav. Neurosci.* **2021**, *14*, 612624. [CrossRef] [PubMed]
68. Penny, J.E.; Brown, R.D.; Hodges, K.B.; Kupetz, S.A.; Glenn, D.W.; Jobe, P.C. Cochlear morphology of the audiogenic-seizure susceptible (AGS) or genetically epilepsy prone rat (GEPR). *Acta Otolaryngol.* **1983**, *95*, 1–12. [CrossRef] [PubMed]
69. Misawa, H.; Sherr, E.H.; Lee, D.J.; Chetkovich, D.M.; Tan, A.; Schreiner, C.E.; Bredt, D.S. Identification of a monogenic locus (jams1) causing juvenile audiogenic seizures in mice. *J. Neurosci.* **2002**, *22*, 10088–10093. [CrossRef] [PubMed]
70. Sánchez-Benito, D.; Gómez-Nieto, R.; Hernández-Noriega, S.; Murashima, A.A.B.; de Oliveira, J.A.C.; Garcia-Cairasco, N.; López, D.E.; Hyppolito, M.A. Morphofunctional alterations in the olivocochlear efferent system of the genetic audiogenic seizure-prone hamster GASH: Sal. *Epilepsy Behav.* **2017**, *71*, 193–206. [CrossRef] [PubMed]
71. Poletaeva, I.I.; Fedotova, I.B.; Sourina, N.M.; Kostina, Z.A. Audiogenic Seizures—Biological Phenomenon and Experimental Model of Human Epilepsies. In *Clinical and Genetic Aspects of Epilepsy*; Zaid Afawi, C., Ed.; InTechOpen: London, UK, 2011; pp. 115–148. ISBN 978-953-307-700-0.
72. Henry, K.R.; Buzzone, R. Auditory physiology and behavior in RB/1bg, RB/3bg, and their F1 hybrid mice (Mus musculus): Influence of genetics, age, and acoustic variables on audiogenic seizure thresholds and cochlear functions. *J. Comp. Psychol.* **1986**, *100*, 46–51. [CrossRef] [PubMed]
73. Solius, G.M.; Revishchin, A.V.; Pavlova, G.V.; Poletaeva, I.I. Audiogenic epilepsy and GABAergic system of the colliculus inferior in Krushinsky-Molodkina rats. *Dokl. Biochem. Biophys.* **2016**, *466*, 32–34. [CrossRef]
74. Romanova, L.G.; Zorina, Z.A.; Korochkin, L.I. A genetic, physiological, and biochemical investigation of audiogenic seizures in rats. *Behav. Genet.* **1993**, *23*, 483–489. [CrossRef] [PubMed]
75. Fedotova, I.B.; Kostyna, Z.A.; Poletaeva, I.I.; Kolpakov, V.G.; Barykina, N.N.; Aksenovich, T.I. Genetic analysis of the predisposition to audiogenic seizure fits in Krushinsky-Molodkina rat strain. *Genetika* **2005**, *41*, 1487–1494. [CrossRef]
76. Ribak, C.E.; Roberts, R.C.; Byun, M.Y.; Kim, H.L. Anatomical and behavioral analyses of the inheritance of audiogenic seizures in the progeny of genetically epilepsy-prone and Sprague-Dawley rats. *Epilepsy Res.* **1988**, *2*, 345–355. [CrossRef]

77. Kurtz, B.S.W.; Lehman, J.; Garlick, P.; Amberg, J.; Mishra, P.K.; Dailey, J.W.; Weber, R.; Jobe, P.C. Penetrance and expressivity of genes involved in the development of epilepsy in the genetically epilepsy-prone rat (GEPR). *J. Neurogenet.* **2001**, *15*, 233–244. [CrossRef] [PubMed]
78. Damasceno, S.; Fonseca, P.A.S.; Rosse, I.C.; Moraes, M.F.D.; de Oliveira, J.A.C.; Garcia-Cairasco, N.; Godard, A.L.B. Putative causal variant on Vlgr1 for the epileptic phenotype in the model Wistar Audiogenic Rat. *Front. Neurol.* **2021**, *12*, 647859. [CrossRef] [PubMed]
79. Revishchin, A.V.; Solus, G.M.; Poletaeva, I.I.; Pavlova, G.V. Audiogenic Epilepsy and Structural Features of Superior Colliculus in KM Rats. *Dokl. Biochem. Biophys.* **2018**, *478*, 47–49. [CrossRef] [PubMed]
80. Chernigovskaya, E.V.; Lebedenko, O.O.; Nidenfyur, A.V.; Nikitina, L.S.; Glazova, M.V. Analysis of ERK1/2 kinases in the inferior colliculus of rats genetically prone to audiogenic seizures during postnatal development. *Dokl. Biochem. Biophys.* **2017**, *476*, 296–298. [CrossRef] [PubMed]
81. Arida, R.M.; Scorza, F.A.; de Amorim Carvalho, R.; Cavalheiro, E.A. Proechimys guyannensis: An Animal Model of Resistance to Epilepsy. *Epilepsia* **2005**, *46*, 189–197. [CrossRef] [PubMed]
82. Popova, N.K.; Barykina, N.N.; Plyusnina, I.Z.; Alekhina, T.A.; Kolpakov, V.G. Expression of the Startle Reaction in Rats Genetically Predisposed Towards Different Types of Defensive Behavior. *Neurosci. Behav. Physiol.* **2000**, *30*, 321–325. [CrossRef] [PubMed]
83. Runke, D.; McIntyre, D.C.; St-Onge, V.; Gilby, K.L. Relation between startle reactivity and sucrose avidity in two rat strains bred for differential seizure susceptibility. *Exp. Neurol.* **2011**, *229*, 259–263. [CrossRef]
84. Laird, H.E.; Dailey, J.W.; Jobe, P.C. Neurotransmitter abnormalities in genetically epileptic rodents. *Fed. Proc.* **1984**, *43*, 2505–2509. [PubMed]
85. Jobe, P.C.; Dailey, J.W.; Reigel, C.E. Noradrenergic and serotonergic determinants of seizure susceptibility and severity in genetically epilepsy-prone rats. *Life Sci.* **1986**, *39*, 775–782. [CrossRef]
86. Browning, R.A.; Wade, D.R.; Marcinczyk, M.; Long, G.L.; Jobe, P.C. Regional brain abnormalities in norepinephrine uptake and dopamine beta-hydroxylase activity in the genetically epilepsy-prone rat. *J. Pharmacol. Exp. Ther.* **1989**, *249*, 229–235. [PubMed]
87. Dailey, J.W.; Lasley, S.M.; Burger, R.L.; Bettendorf, A.F.; Mishra, P.K.; Jobe, P.C. Amino acids, monoamines and audiogenic seizures in genetically epilepsy-prone rats: Effects of aspartame. *Epilepsy Res.* **1991**, *8*, 122–133. [CrossRef]
88. Medvedev, A.E.; Gorkin, V.Z.; Fedotova, I.B.; Semiokhina, A.F.; Glover, V.; Sandler, M. Increase of brain endogenous monoamine oxidase inhibitory activity (tribulin) in experimental audiogenic seizures in rats: Evidence for a monoamine oxidase A inhibiting component of tribulin. *Biochem. Pharmacol.* **1992**, *44*, 1209–1210. [CrossRef]
89. Jobe, P.C.; Mishra, P.K.; Browning, R.A.; Wang, C.; Adams-Curtis, L.E.; Ko, K.H.; Dailey, J.W. Noradrenergic abnormalities in the genetically epilepsy-prone rat. *Brain Res. Bull.* **1994**, *35*, 493–504. [CrossRef]
90. Clough, R.W.; Browning, R.A.; Maring, M.L.; Statnick, M.A.; Wang, C.; Jobe, P.C. Effects of intraventricular locus coeruleus transplants on seizure severity in genetically epilepsy-prone rats following depletion of brain norepinephrine. *J. Neural Transplant. Plast.* **1994**, *5*, 65–79. [CrossRef] [PubMed]
91. Statnick, M.A.; Dailey, J.W.; Jobe, P.C.; Browning, R.A. Abnormalities in brain serotonin concentration, high-affinity uptake, and tryptophan hydroxylase activity in severe-seizure genetically epilepsy-prone rats. *Epilepsia* **1996**, *37*, 311–321. [CrossRef] [PubMed]
92. Kosacheva, E.S.; Kudrin, V.S.; Fedotova, I.B.; Semiokhina, A.F.; Raevskiĭ, K.S. The effect of carbamazepine on the content of monoamines and their metabolites in the brain structures of rats with audiogenic epilepsy. *Eksp. Klin. Farmakol.* **1998**, *61*, 25–27. [PubMed]
93. Sorokin, A.I.; Kudrin, V.S.; Klodt, P.M.; Tuomisto, L.; Poletaeva, I.I.; Raevskiĭ, K.S. The interstrain differences in the effects of D-amphetamine and raclopride on dorsal striatum dopaminergic system in KM and Wistar rats (microdialysis study). *Genetika* **2004**, *40*, 846–849. [CrossRef] [PubMed]
94. Fedotova, I.B.; Semiokhina, A.F.; Arkhipova, G.V.; Burlakova, E.B. The possibilities of correcting some complex behavioral reactions in KM rats by using an antioxidant. *Zh. Vyssh. Nerv. Deiat. Im. I P Pavlov.* **1990**, *40*, 318–325.
95. Onodera, K.; Tuomisto, L.; Tacke, U.; Airaksinen, M. Strain differences in regional brain histamine levels in genetically epilepsy-prone and resistant rats. *Methods Find. Exp. Clin. Pharmacol.* **1992**, *14*, 13–16. [PubMed]
96. López-López, D.; Gómez-Nieto, R.; Herrero-Turrión, M.J.; García-Cairasco, N.; Sánchez-Benito, D.; Ludeña, M.D.; López, D.E. Overexpression of the immediate-early genes Egr1, Egr2, and Egr3 in two strains of rodents susceptible to audiogenic seizures. *Epilepsy Behav.* **2017**, *71*, 226–237. [CrossRef] [PubMed]
97. Szot, P.; Weinshenker, D.; White, S.S.; Robbins, C.A.; Rust, N.C.; Schwartzkroin, P.A.; Palmiter, R.D. Norepinephrine-deficient mice have increased susceptibility to seizure-inducing stimuli. *J. Neurosci.* **1999**, *19*, 10985–10992. [CrossRef] [PubMed]
98. Werner, F.M.; Coveñas, R. Classical neurotransmitters and neuropeptides involved in generalized epilepsy in a multi-neurotransmitter system: How to improve the antiepileptic effect? *Epilepsy Behav.* **2017**, *71*, 124–129. [CrossRef] [PubMed]
99. Gachon, F.; Fonjallaz, P.; Damiola, F.; Gos, P.; Kodama, T.; Zakany, J.; Duboule, D.; Petit, B.; Tafti, M.; Schibler, U. The loss of circadian PAR bZip transcription factors results in epilepsy. *Genes Dev.* **2004**, *18*, 1397–1412. [CrossRef] [PubMed]
100. Etheridge, S.L.; Ray, S.; Li, S.; Hamblet, N.S.; Lijam, N.; Tsang, M.; Greer, J.; Kardos, N.; Wang, J.; Sussman, D.J.; et al. Murine dishevelled 3 functions in redundant pathways with dishevelled 1 and 2 in normal cardiac outflow tract, cochlea, and neural tube development. *PLoS Genet.* **2008**, *4*, e1000259. [CrossRef] [PubMed]

101. Delfino-Pereira, P.; Bertti-Dutra, P.; de Lima Umeoka, E.H.; de Oliveira, J.A.C.; Santos, V.R.; Fernandes, A.; Marroni, S.S.; Del Vecchio, F.; Garcia-Cairasco, N. Intense olfactory stimulation blocks seizures in an experimental model of epilepsy. *Epilepsy Behav.* **2018**, *79*, 213–224. [CrossRef]
102. Poletaeva, I.I.; Surina, N.M.; Fedotova, I.B. The effects of toluene vapor inhalation on the intensity of audiogenic seizure fits in rats of Krushinsky–Molodkina strain. *Sechenov. Ross. Fisiol. J.* **2019**, *105*, 742–748.
103. Brosnan, R.J.; Pham, T.L. Carbon dioxide negatively modulates N-methyl-D-aspartate receptors. *Br. J. Anaesth.* **2008**, *101*, 673–679. [CrossRef] [PubMed]
104. Ohmori, I.; Hayashi, K.; Wang, H.; Ouchida, M.; Fujita, N.; Inoue, T.; Michiue, H.; Nishiki, T.; Matsui, H. Inhalation of 10% carbon dioxide rapidly terminates Scn1a mutation-related hyperthermia-induced seizures. *Epilepsy Res.* **2013**, *105*, 220–224. [CrossRef] [PubMed]
105. Inamura, K.; Smith, M.L.; Hansen, A.J.; Siesjö, B.K. Seizure-induced damage to substantia nigra and globus pallidus is accompanied by pronounced intra- and extracellular acidosis. *Synapse* **2002**, *46*, 100–107. [CrossRef] [PubMed]
106. Garcia-Gomes, M.S.A.; Zanatto, D.A.; Galvis-Alonso, O.Y.; Mejia, J.; Antiorio, A.T.F.B.; Yamamoto, P.K.; Olivato, M.C.M.; Sandini, T.M.; Flório, J.C.; Lebrun, I.; et al. Behavioral and neurochemical characterization of the spontaneous mutation tremor, a new mouse model of audiogenic seizures. *Epilepsy Behav.* **2020**, *105*, 106945. [CrossRef]
107. Totola, L.T.; Takakura, A.C.; Oliveira, J.A.; Garcia-Cairasco, N.; Moreira, T.S. Impaired central respiratory chemoreflex in an experimental genetic model of epilepsy. *J. Physiol.* **2017**, *595*, 983–999. [CrossRef]
108. Schimitel, F.G.; De Almeida, G.M.; Pitol, D.N.; Armini, R.S.; Tufik, S.; Schenberg, L.C. Evidence of a suffocation alarm system within the periaqueductal gray matter of the rat. *Neuroscience* **2012**, *200*, 59–73. [CrossRef] [PubMed]
109. N'Gouemo, P.; Faingold, C.L.; Morad, M. Calcium channel dysfunction in inferior colliculus neurons of the genetically epilepsy-prone rat. *Neuropharmacology* **2009**, *56*, 665–675. [CrossRef] [PubMed]
110. N'Gouemo, P.; Yasuda, R.; Faingold, C.L. Seizure susceptibility is associated with altered protein expression of voltage-gated calcium channel subunits in inferior colliculus neurons of the genetically epilepsy-prone rat. *Brain Res.* **2010**, *1308*, 153–157. [CrossRef]
111. Ptácek, L.J. Channelopathies: Ion channel disorders of muscle as a paradigm for paroxysmal disorders of the nervous system. *Neuromuscul. Disord.* **1997**, *7*, 250–255. [CrossRef]
112. Wei, F.; Yan, L.M.; Su, T.; He, N.; Lin, Z.J.; Wang, J.; Shi, Y.W.; Yi, Y.H.; Liao, W.P. Ion Channel Genes and Epilepsy: Functional Alteration, Pathogenic Potential, and Mechanism of Epilepsy. *Neurosci. Bull.* **2017**, *33*, 455–477. [CrossRef] [PubMed]
113. Bartolini, E.; Campostrini, R.; Kiferle, L.; Pradella, S.; Rosati, E.; Chinthapalli, K.; Palumbo, P. Epilepsy and brain channelopathies from infancy to adulthood. *Neurol. Sci.* **2020**, *41*, 749–761. [CrossRef] [PubMed]
114. Menezes, L.F.S.; Sabiá, E.F., Jr.; Tibery, D.V.; Carneiro, L.D.A.; Schwartz, E.F. Epilepsy-Related Voltage-Gated Sodium Channelopathies: A Review. *Front. Pharmacol.* **2020**, *11*, 1276. [CrossRef] [PubMed]
115. Gould, T.D.; Gottesman, I.I. Psychiatric endophenotypes and the development of valid animal models. *Genes Brain Behav.* **2006**, *5*, 113–119. [CrossRef] [PubMed]
116. Traub, R.D.; Whittington, M.A.; Hall, S.P. Does epileptiform activity represent a failure of neuromodulation to control central pattern generator-like neocortical behavior? *Front. Neural Circuits* **2017**, *11*, 78. [CrossRef] [PubMed]

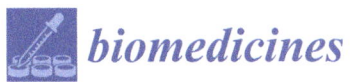

Article

Blockade of TASK-1 Channel Improves the Efficacy of Levetiracetam in Chronically Epileptic Rats

Ji-Eun Kim and Tae-Cheon Kang *

Department of Anatomy and Neurobiology and Institute of Epilepsy Research, College of Medicine, Hallym University, Chuncheon 24252, Korea; jieunkim@hallym.ac.kr
* Correspondence: tckang@hallym.ac.kr; Tel.: +82-33-248-2524; Fax: +82-33-248-2525

Abstract: Tandem of P domains in a weak inwardly rectifying K^+ channel (TWIK)-related acid sensitive K^+-1 channel (TASK-1) is an outwardly rectifying K^+ channel that acts in response to extracellular pH. TASK-1 is upregulated in the astrocytes (particularly in the CA1 region) of the hippocampi of patients with temporal lobe epilepsy and chronically epilepsy rats. Since levetiracetam (LEV) is an effective inhibitor for carbonic anhydrase, which has a pivotal role in buffering of extracellular pH, it is likely that the anti-epileptic action of LEV may be relevant to TASK-1 inhibition, which remains to be elusive. In the present study, we found that LEV diminished the upregulated TASK-1 expression in the CA1 astrocytes of responders (whose seizure activities were responsive to LEV), but not non-responders (whose seizure activities were not controlled by LEV) in chronically epileptic rats. ML365 (a selective TASK-1 inhibitor) only reduced seizure duration in LEV non-responders, concomitant with astroglial TASK-1 downregulation. Furthermore, ML365 co-treatment with LEV decreased the duration, frequency and severity of spontaneous seizures in non-responders to LEV. To the best of our knowledge, our findings suggest, for the first time, that the up-regulation of TASK-1 expression in CA1 astrocytes may be involved in refractory seizures in response to LEV. This may be a potential target to improve responsiveness to LEV.

Keywords: astrocyte; intractable epilepsy; ML365; pharmacoresistant epilepsy; refractory seizure

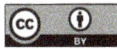

1. Introduction

Epilepsy is a chronic neurological disease that is characterized by the presence of spontaneous aberrant neuronal discharges which manifest as seizures. The causes of epileptic seizure generation (ictogenesis) are imbalance of excitatory/inhibitory transmissions, channelopathies, neuroinflammation, and aberrant synaptic plasticity [1–4]. Since shifts in activity-dependent intracellular and extracellular pH regulate the initiation and cessation of seizure activity [5–7], impaired acid-base balance also contributes to an augmented capability to generate epileptic discharges. Indeed, recurrent epileptiform activity results in biphasic pH shifts, consisting of an initial extracellular alkalinization followed by a slower acidification in the CA1 region of the hippocampus [7]. Extracellular alkalinization decreases the inhibitory conductance through γ-aminobutyric acid type A receptor ($GABA_A$ receptor) [8] and increases the N-methyl-D-aspartate (NMDA) receptor-mediated excitatory current [9,10]. Thus, activity-dependent extracellular alkaline shifts initiate the seizure activity, while extracellular acidification terminates the epileptiform activity [6,7].

Astrocytes play an important role in the redistribution of K^+ in extracellular space (K^+ buffering) that is involved in the control of resting membrane potential and neuronal firing. When K^+ buffering becomes hindered, an accumulation of extracellular K^+ leads to hyperexcitability of neurons by inhibiting K^+ efflux from neurons during repolarization. Interestingly, astrocytes in the CA1 region (CA1 astrocytes) have lost barium (Ba^{2+})-sensitive K^+ buffering in the epileptic hippocampi of humans and rats, unlike those in the dentate gyrus [11,12]. Furthermore, the ratio of inward-to-outward K$^+$ conductance in astrocytes is significantly lower in the hippocampus of temporal lobe epilepsy (TLE) patients [13]. Therefore, the dysfunction of astrocyte-mediated extracellular K$^+$ homeostasis is an important factor in the pathogenesis of epilepsy.

Tandem of P domains in a weak inwardly rectifying K$^+$ channel (TWIK)-related acid sensitive K$^+$-1 channel (TASK-1) is an outwardly rectifying K$^+$ channel that acts in response to extracellular pH. Low extracellular pH (6.0–6.4) completely inhibits TASK-1 current, whereas high extracellular pH (7.2–8.2) potentiates it [14,15]. TASK-1 is upregulated in astrocytes (particularly in the CA1 region) of the hippocampi of TLE patients and chronically epileptic rats [16,17]. Furthermore, conventional antiepileptic drugs (AEDs, currently termed as anti-seizure medication (ASM)) reduce astroglial TASK-1 expression in seizure-prone gerbils (a genetic epilepsy model) [18]. Thus, it is plausible that TASK-1 upregulation can contribute to seizure activity by increasing astroglial K$^+$ outward rectification in response to extracellular alkalinization.

More than ~10–30% of TLE patients show intractable seizures that are uncontrolled by AEDs [19]. Therefore, pharmacoresistances to AEDs are a major clinical problem in the medication of TLE patients. The anti-epileptic properties of levetiracetam (LEV, 2S-(oxo-1-pyrrolidinyl)butanamide, Keppra®) are relevant to the high-affinity binding to synaptic vesicle protein 2A (SV2A) that may affect presynaptic neurotransmitter release. Although LEV treatment often results in seizure-free conditions in TLE patients who show refractory seizures to other AEDs, LEV does not mitigate spontaneous seizures in approximately 30% of TLE patients at the beginning of the pharmacotherapy [20]. Similar to the case of TLE patients, ~25–40% of pilocarpine-induced chronically epileptic rats do not show a significant response to LEV [21,22]. On the other hand, LEV also leads to a pH shift by inhibiting the transmembrane HCO$_3^-$-mediated acid extrusion and carbonic anhydrase, like other AEDs [23–27]. Thus, it is likely that the anticonvulsive potency of LEV may be closely relevant to the induction of extracellular acidification, which would inhibit the upregulated TASK-1 in the epileptic hippocampus. In the present study, therefore, we performed a comparative analysis of TASK-1 expression in the hippocampi of responders (whose seizure activities were responsive to LEV) and non-responders (whose seizure activities were uncontrolled by LEV) in chronically epileptic rats, and validated the effect of ML365 (a selective TASK-1 inhibitor) co-treatment with LEV on refractory seizures in response to LEV to extend our understanding of the underlying mechanisms of pharmacoresistant epilepsy.

2. Materials and Methods

2.1. Experimental Animals and Chemicals

In the present study, we used male Sprague-Dawley (SD) rats (7 weeks old). Rats were housed in a controlled environment at a humidity of $55 \pm 5\%$ and a temperature of 22 ± 2 °C on a 12 h light/dark cycle and provided with food and water ad libitum [22,28,29]. All animal studies were performed in accordance with protocols approved by the Institutional Animal Care and Use Committee of Hallym University (No. Hallym 2018-2, 26 April 2018; No. Hallym 2018-21, 8 June 2018; and Hallym 2021-3, 27 April 2021). All reagents, unless otherwise noted, were obtained from Sigma-Aldrich (St. Louis, MO, USA).

2.2. Generation of Chronically Epileptic Rats

To generate chronically epileptic rats, we applied the status epilepticus (SE) model. For SE induction, animals were treated with LiCl (127 mg/kg) via intraperitoneal injection (i.p.) 24 h prior to pilocarpine treatment. Animals were given atropine methylbromide (5 mg/kg i.p.) 20 min before pilocarpine (30 mg/kg). Two h after SE onset, all rats received diazepam (Hoffman la Roche, Neuilly sur-Seine, France; 10 mg/kg, i.p.) to cease SE and was repeated as needed. The control rats were treated with the same volume of saline in place of pilocarpine. SE-experiencing rats were video monitored 8 h a day to select for the chronically epileptic rats showing the occurrence of spontaneous seizures (Racine's scale ≥ 3 more than once) [22,28–30].

2.3. Electrode Implantation and ML365 Infusion

The control and epilepsy rats were anesthetized with isoflurane anesthesia (3% induction, 1.5–2% for surgery, and 1.5% maintenance in a 65:35 mixture of $N_2O:O_2$) and placed in a stereotaxic frame. Thereafter, a monopolar stainless-steel electrode (#MS303-1-AIU-SPC, diameter 0.01 inch, Plastics One, Roanoke, VA, USA) was implanted in the right hippocampus at the following coordinates: 3.8 mm posterior, 2.0 mm lateral and −2.6 mm depth to bregma. A brain infusion kit 1 (Alzet, Cupertino, CA, USA) was also inserted into some animals for the infusion of vehicle or ML365 (a specific TASK-1 inhibitor, 400 nM [31]) into the right lateral ventricle at the following coordinates: 1 mm posterior, 1.5 mm lateral and 3.5 mm depth to the bregma. The electrode and brain infusion kits were secured to the exposed skull with dental acrylic [22,28,29].

2.4. Drug Trial Protocols

Figure 1 illustrates the experimental design in the present study, which is a modified drug trial methodology based on our previous studies [22,28,29].

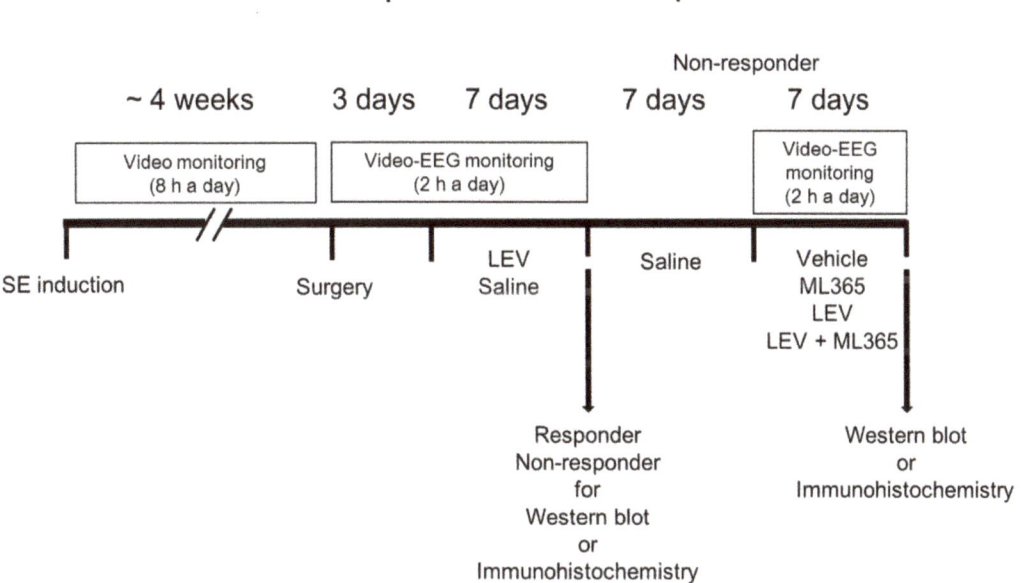

Figure 1. Scheme of the experimental design in the present study.

2.4.1. Experiment I

Baseline seizure activity in chronically epileptic rats were recorded over a 3-day period. Electroencephalographic (EEG) signals were acquired with a DAM 80 differential amplifier (0.1–1000 Hz bandpass; World Precision Instruments, Sarasota, FL, USA) 2 h a day at the same time over a 7-day period. Thereafter, animals received LEV (500 mg/kg, i.p., UCB Korea, Seoul, Korea) or saline (vehicle) once a day (at 6:00 p.m.) over a 7-day period [22,28,29]. The EEG data were digitized and analyzed using a LabChart Pro v7 (ADInstruments, Bella Vista, New South Wales, Australia). Racine's scale was applied to quantify behavioral seizure severity, as aforementioned. Animals whose seizure frequency was unaffected by LEV during recording, as compared to the pre-treatment stage, were defined as non-responders (Figure 1).

2.4.2. Experiment II

After saline treatment over a 7-day period, non-responders in experiment I were infused vehicle or ML365 (400 nM [31]) by connecting Alzet 1007D osmotic pump (Alzet, Cupertino, CA, USA). The pump was inserted into a subcutaneous pocket in the dorsal region. Some animals were also administered LEV (500 mg/kg, i.p., UCB Korea, Seoul, Korea) once a day.

2.5. Western Blot

After recording (18 h after the last drug treatment), animals were sacrificed by decapitation. Thereafter, the hippocampi were rapidly dissected and homogenized in lysis buffer. The lysis buffer contained protease inhibitor cocktail (Roche Applied Sciences, Branford, CT, USA) and phosphatase inhibitor cocktail (PhosSTOP®, Roche Applied Science, Branford, CT, USA). The protein concentration was determined using a Micro BCA Protein Assay Kit (Pierce Chemical, Rockford, IL, USA). An equal amount (10 µg each) was loaded on a bis-tris sodium dodecyl sulfate-polyacrylamide gel (SDS-PAGE). The proteins were separated by electrophoresis and transferred to membranes. The membranes were blocked with tris-buffered saline (TBS; in mM 10 Tris, 150 NaCl, pH 7.5, and 0.05% Tween 20) containing 2% bovine serum albumin and then incubated with primary antibodies (Table 1) overnight at 4 °C. The proteins were visualized using an electrochemiluminescence (ECL) Western Blotting System (GE Healthcare Korea, Seoul, Korea). For data normalization, β-actin was used as an internal reference. An ImageQuant LAS4000 system (GE Healthcare Korea, Seoul, Korea) was used to detect and quantify the Western blot data [22,28,29].

Table 1. Primary antibodies used in the present study.

Antigen	Host	Manufacturer (Catalog Number)	Dilution
Glia fibrillary acidic protein (GFAP)	Mouse	Millipore (MAB3402)	1:4000 (IH)
Neuronal nuclear antigen (NeuN)	Guinea pig	Millipore (ABN90P)	1:2000 (IH)
TASK-1	Rabbit	Millipore (AB5250)	1:50 (IH) 1:200 (WB)
β-actin	Mouse	Sigma (A5316)	1:5000 (WB)

IH, immunohistochemistry; WB, Western blot.

2.6. Immunohistochemistry

Animals were transcardially perfused and fixed with 4% paraformaldehyde under deep anesthesia with urethane (1.5 g/kg, i.p.). The brains were then removed and post-fixed in the same fixative overnight and left in 30% sucrose in phosphate buffer (PB) until sunk. Coronal sections (30 µm) of the brain samples were cut using a cryostat. Sections were placed in a plate, rinsed with phosphate-buffered saline (PBS) for over 10 min, and subsequently blocked for 30 min at room temperature in 10% goat serum (Vector, Burlingame, CA, USA). After blocking, samples were incubated with primary antibodies overnight at 4 °C. Sections were then washed for over 10 min three times with PBS and incubated with appropriate secondary antibodies (1:200, Vector, Burlingame, CA, USA) for 1 h at room temperature. After washing, sections were mounted in Vectashield mounting media with 4′,6-diamidino-2-phenyulindole (DAPI, Vector, Burlingame, CA, USA). The brain sections incubated with either preimmune serum (for GFAP) or the primary antibody reacted with the control peptide (for TASK-1) were used as negative controls [16]. Immunoreaction was observed using an Axio Scope microscope (Carl Zeiss Korea, Seoul, Korea). Five hippocampal sections from each animal were randomly captured and the areas of interest (1×10^5 μm^2) were selected from the stratum radiatum and the stratum pyramidale of the CA1 region. Thereafter, fluorescent intensity and the number of double-stained cells was measured using AxioVision Rel. 4.8 and ImageJ software. The quantification of TASK-1 fluorescent intensity and double-stained cells was performed in the left hippocampus to avoid the interfering effect of reactive astrogliosis induced by electrode implantation. The investigators were blinded to experimental groups in performing morphological analysis and immunohistochemical experiments [28,29].

2.7. Data Analysis

In the present study, the effects of each compound on seizures were analyzed based on the following seizure parameters: Seizure frequency was number of seizures in each animal during the 2 h recording. Seizure duration was the overall time spent in convulsive and non-convulsive seizures in each animal during the 2 h recording. Seizure severity was the behavioral seizure score in each animal during the 2 h recording. Total seizure frequency was the total seizure occurrence (number of seizures) in each animal over a 7-day period. Total seizure duration was the overall time spent in convulsive and non-convulsive seizures in each animal over a 7-day period. Average seizure severity was the average behavioral seizure core in each animal over a 7-day period. Seizure parameters were assessed by different investigators who were blind to the classification of animal groups and treatments. All data are presented as the means ± standard deviation (SD) or standard error of mean (SEM). After the Shapiro–Wilk W-test was used to evaluate the values on normality, the Student's t-test (for total seizure duration, immunohistochemistry and Western blot data), the Mann–Whitney U test (total seizure frequency and average seizure severity), a repeated measures ANOVA (seizure duration over a 7-day period), the Friedman test (seizure frequency and seizure severity over a 7-day period) and a one-way ANOVA followed by Bonferroni's post hoc comparisons (for immunohistochemistry and Western blot data) were applied to determine the statistical significance of the data. A p-value less than 0.05 was considered statistically significant.

3. Results

3.1. Effects of LEV on Spontaneous Epileptic Seizures

First, we explored the efficacy of LEV on spontaneous seizure activity in chronically epileptic rats. In vehicle-treated epileptic rats ($n = 14$), total seizure frequency (number of seizures), total electroencephalographic (EEG) seizure duration and average seizure severity (behavioral seizure core) were 11.3 ± 2.1, 681 ± 145 s, and 3.4 ± 0.6 over a 7-day period, respectively (Figure 2A–C). About 57% of the LEV-treated group ($n = 70$) were identified as responders whose seizure frequency ($\chi^2_{(7)} = 19.4$, $p = 0.007$, Friedman test), seizure duration ($F_{(7,483)} = 4.1$, $p < 0.001$, repeated measures ANOVA), and seizure severity ($\chi^2_{(7)} = 17.8$, $p = 0.013$, Friedman test) were effectively alleviated by LEV treatment over a 7-day period (Figure 2A,B). In this group, total seizure frequency, total seizure duration and average seizure severity were also attenuated to 4.4 ± 1.2 ($Z = 3.2$, $p = 0.002$ vs. vehicle, Mann–Whitney U-test), 349 ± 65 s ($t_{(82)} = 3.9$, $p = 0.002$ vs. vehicle, Student t-test), and 2 ± 0.3 ($Z = 2.4$, $p = 0.01$ vs. vehicle, Mann–Whitney U test) over a 7-day period, respectively (Figure 2C). LEV did not influence seizure activity in 52 out of 122 rats (~43% in LEV-treated rats). Thus, they were identified as non-responders (Figure 2A–C).

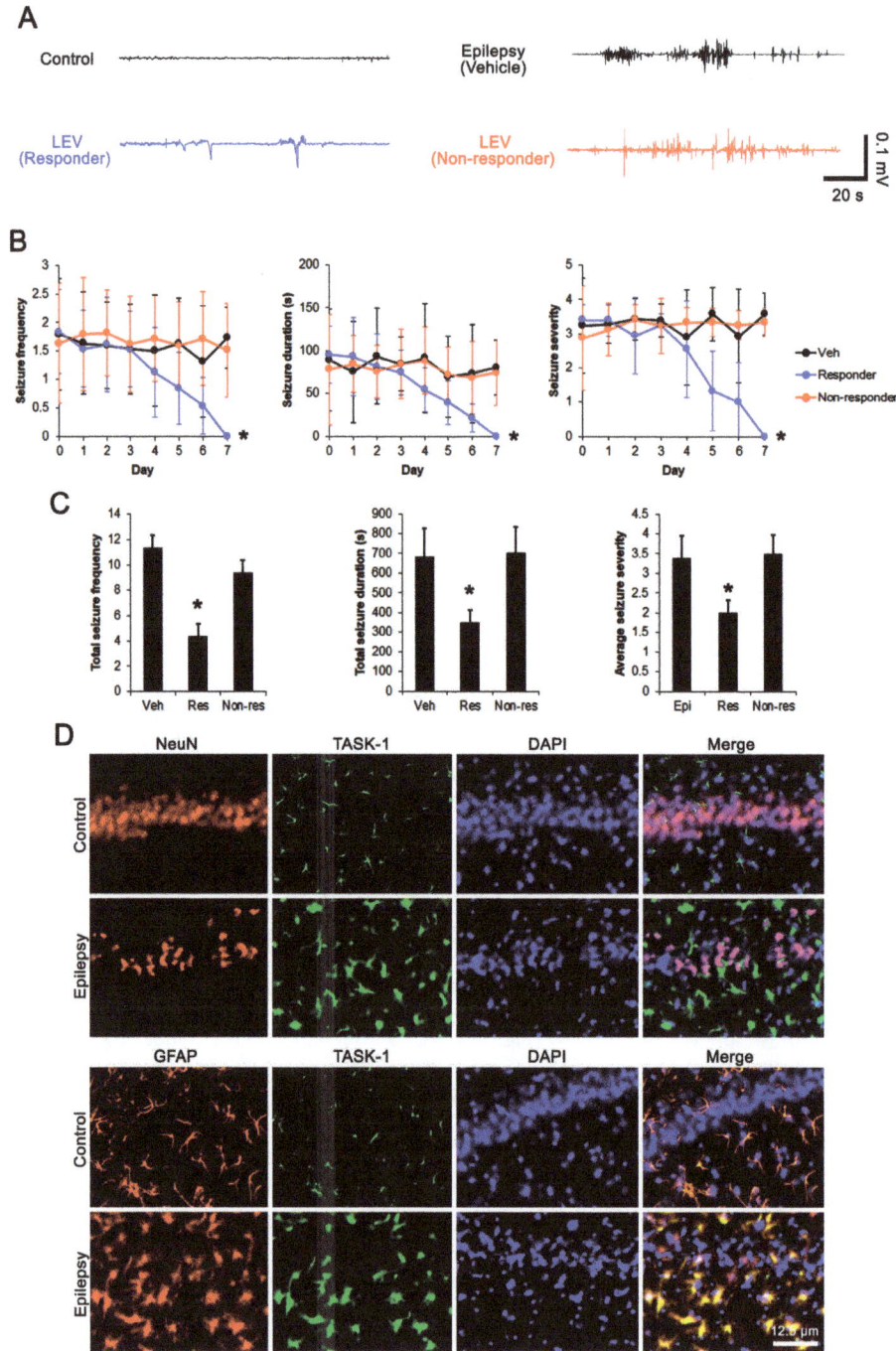

Figure 2. The effects of levetiracetam (LEV) on spontaneous seizure activities in chronically epileptic rats and the localization TASK-1 in the hippocampus of the control and chronically epileptic rats. LEV effectively attenuated spontaneous seizure activity on EEG in responders (**A**) at 4 days after

treatment, accompanied by reductions in seizure frequency (Friedman test), seizure duration (repeated measures ANOVA), seizure severity (seizure score, Friedman test), total seizure frequency (Mann–Whitney U test), total seizure duration (Student's t-test) and average behavioral seizure score (seizure severity; Mann–Whitney U test) over a 7-day period (**B,C**; *, $p < 0.05$ vs. vehicle (Veh)-treated animals; error bars, SD). However, the non-responders did not respond to LEV treatment (**B,C**). Double immunofluorescent data reveal that TASK-1 expression is observed in GFAP-positive astrocytes, but not in NeuN-positive neurons in both control and chronically epileptic rats (**D**).

3.2. Effects of LEV on TASK-1 Expression in the Epileptic Hippocampus

Consistent with previous studies [16,17,32], TASK-1 expression was rarely observed in CA1 neurons in both control and epileptic rats (Figure 2D). In contrast, TASK-1 expression was prominently detected in the astrocytes within the stratum radiatum and stratum lacunosum-moleculare of the CA1 region of the control rats ($n = 7$). TASK-1 expression was also detected in the astrocytes in the molecular layer and the hilus of the dentate gyrus of control rats (Figures 2D and 3A). In chronically epileptic rats ($n = 7$), TASK-1 expression was obviously detected in most of the reactive CA1 astrocytes, showing hypertrophy and hyperplasia of cell bodies and processes (Figure 2D). TASK-1 expression was rarely observed in reactive astrocytes within the dentate gyrus (Figure 3A). TASK-1 fluorescent intensity was increased to 1.62-fold of control level ($t_{(12)} = 14.4$, $p < 0.001$, Student's t-test, Figure 3A,B). However, the fraction of TASK-1 positive astrocytes in total astrocytes of chronically epileptic rats was similar to that in control animals (Figure 3C). As compared to the vehicle-treated animals ($n = 7$), responders to LEV ($n = 7$) showed a reduction in TASK-1 fluorescent intensity ($F_{(2,17)} = 49.7$, $p < 0.001$, one-way ANOVA), while the TASK-1 intensity in non-responders to LEV ($n = 6$) was unaffected by LEV treatment (Figure 3A,B). Thus, the fraction of TASK-1 positive astrocytes in total astrocytes was decreased in responders, as compared to the vehicle-treated animals ($F_{(2,17)} = 5.4$, $p = 0.015$, one-way ANOVA, Figure 3C). Compatible with the immunohistochemical data, the Western blot revealed that TASK-1 density was elevated to 1.65-fold of control level in chronically epileptic rats ($t_{(12)} = 11.9$, $p < 0.001$, $n = 7$, Student's t-test, Figure 3C,D). In responders ($n = 7$), LEV reduced TASK-1 density in the hippocampus ($F_{(2,17)} = 37.1$, $p < 0.001$, one-way ANOVA) but not in the non-responders ($n = 6$ Figure 3C,D, Supplementary Figure S1). Together with the effects of LEV on seizure activity, these findings indicate that the upregulated TASK-1 expression in CA1 astrocytes may be relevant to spontaneous seizure activity and affect the responsiveness to LEV.

3.3. Effects of ML365 on the Spontaneous Seizures and TASK-1 Expression in Chronically Epileptic Rats

To directly investigate the role of TASK-1 in spontaneous seizure activity, we applied ML365 (a selective TASK-1 inhibitor) to non-responders to LEV. In vehicle-treated non-responders to LEV ($n = 10$), the total seizure frequency, total EEG seizure duration and average seizure severity over a 7-day period were 14.4 ± 3.3, 751 ± 197 s, and 3.2 ± 0.5, respectively (Figure 4A–C). In ML365-treated non-responders to LEV ($n = 10$), seizure duration was gradually decreased over a 7-day period ($F_{(7,63)} = 3.326$, $p = 0.004$, repeated measures ANOVA; Figure 4A,B). In this group, the total seizure duration was also diminished to 519 ± 55 s over a 7-day period ($t_{(8)} = 2.5$, $p = 0.035$ vs. vehicle, Student's t-test; Figure 4C). Furthermore, ML365 reduced the TASK-1 fluorescent intensity to 0.73-fold of the vehicle levels ($t_{(8)} = 8.8$, $p < 0.001$ vs. vehicle, Student's t-test, $n = 5$). In addition, ML365 diminished the fraction of TASK-1 positive astrocytes of the total astrocytes ($t_{(8)} = 2.7$, $p = 0.027$, Student's t-test, Figure 5C). Consistent with the immunohistochemical study, the Western blot data showed a reduction in TASK-1 density to 0.71-fold of the vehicle levels ($t_{(8)} = 6.4$, $p < 0.001$ vs. vehicle, Student's t-test, $n = 5$) in ML365-treated non-responders (Figure 5D,E, Supplementary Figure S1). These findings indicate that TASK-1 in reactive

CA1 astrocytes may be involved in the prolongation of seizure duration rather than seizure generation (ictogenesis) in non-responders to LEV.

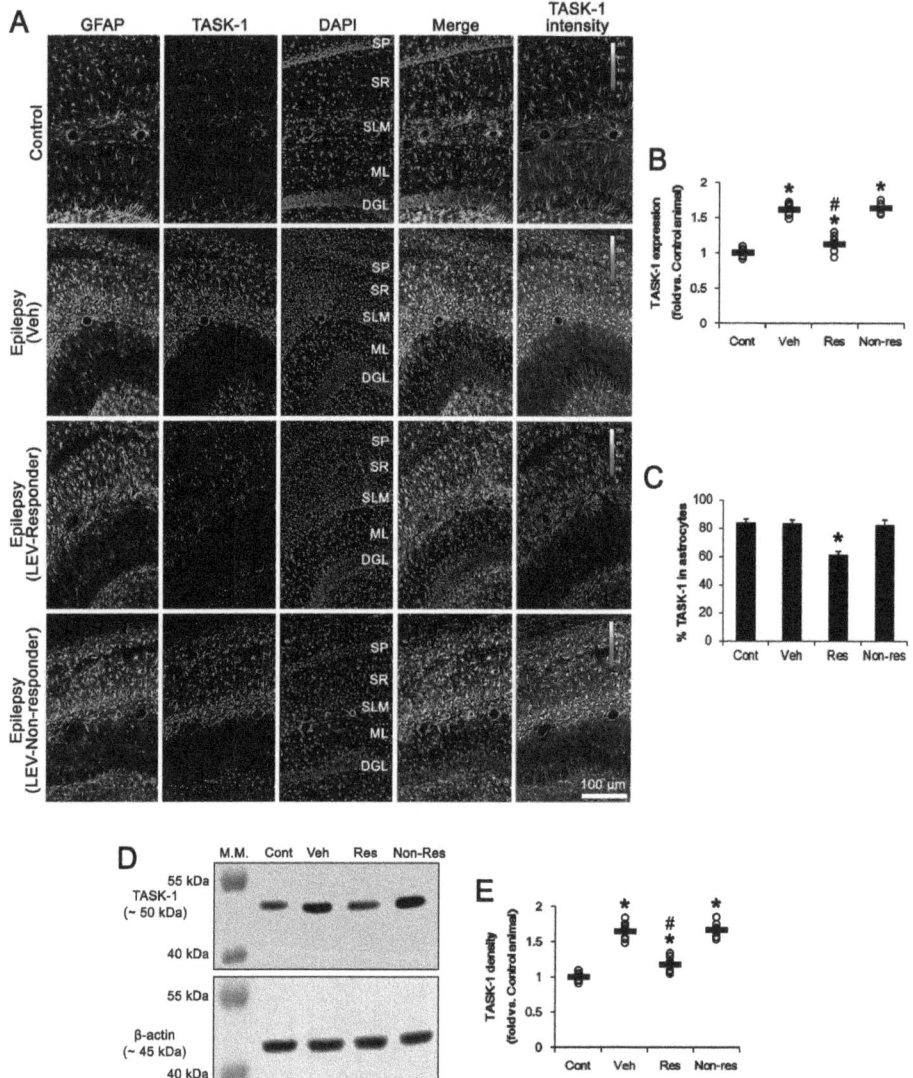

Figure 3. The effect of levetiracetam (LEV) on TASK-1 expression in chronically epileptic rats. As compared to control animals, TASK-1 expression is upregulated in CA1 astrocytes of epileptic rats. LEV significantly attenuated TASK-1 upregulation in responders, but not non-responders. (**A**) Representative photos of the TASK-1 expression in the hippocampus. SP, stratum pyramidale; SR, stratum radiatum; SLM, stratum lacunosum-moleculare; ML, molecular layer of the dentate gyrus; DGL, dentate granule cell layer. (**B**) Quantitative analyses of the effect of LEV on TASK-1 expression based on the immunohistochemical data (*,#, $p < 0.05$ vs. the control and vehicle (Veh)-treated animals, respectively; one-way ANOVA with *post hoc* Bonferroni's multiple comparison, open circles indicate each individual value, horizontal bars indicate the mean value, error bars indicate the SEM). (**C**) Quantitative analyses on the effect of LEV on the fraction of TASK-1 positive astrocytes in total

astrocytes (*, $p < 0.05$ vs. control animals; one-way ANOVA with post hoc Bonferroni's multiple comparison; error bars, SEM). (**D,E**) Representative images for Western blot of TASK-1 protein expression in the hippocampal tissues and quantifications of TASK-1 level based on Western blot results (*,#, $p < 0.05$ vs. control and vehicle (Veh)-treated animals, respectively; one-way ANOVA with post hoc Bonferroni's multiple comparison).

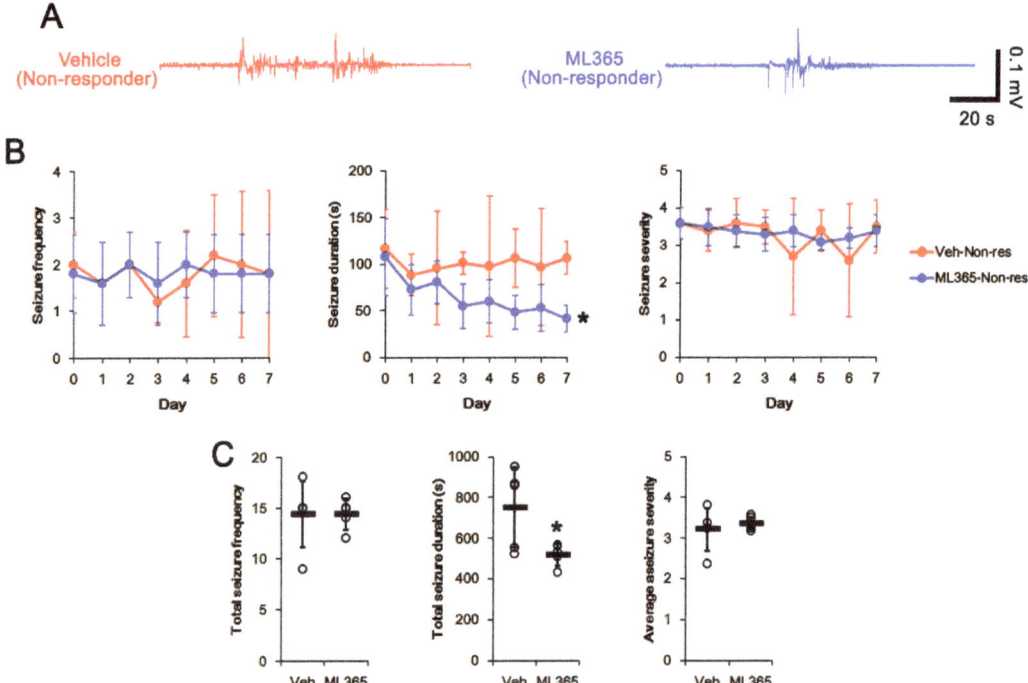

Figure 4. The effects of ML365 on spontaneous seizure activities in non-responders to levetiracetam (LEV). ML365 diminished only seizure duration. (**A**) Representative EEG signal in each group at 4 days after treatment. (**B**) Quantitative analyses of the effects of LEV on seizure frequency (Friedman test), seizure duration (repeated measures ANOVA) and seizure severity (seizure score, Friedman test) over a 7-day period (*, $p < 0.05$ vs. vehicle (Veh)-treated animals; error bars, SD). (**C**) Quantitative analyses of total seizure frequency (Mann–Whitney U test), total seizure duration (Student's t-test) and average behavioral seizure score (seizure severity, Mann–Whitney U test) over a 7-day period (*, $p < 0.05$ vs. vehicle (Veh)-treated animals; open circles, each individual value; horizontal bars, mean value; error bars, SD).

3.4. Effect of ML365 Co-Treatment on Refractory Seizures in Non-Responders to LEV

When considering the effect of ML365 on seizure activity and TASK-1 expression in CA1 astrocyte (Figures 4 and 5), it is likely that ML365 co-treatment may improve the efficacy of LEV in non-responders. Thus, we validated the effects of ML365 co-treatment on intractable seizures in non-responders to LEV. As compared to vehicle co-treatment ($n = 10$), ML365 co-treatment ($n = 10$) gradually reduced seizure frequency ($\chi^2_{(7)} = 18.9$, $p = 0.009$, Friedman test), seizure duration ($F_{(7,63)} = 25.1$, $p < 0.001$, repeated measures ANOVA) and seizure severity ($\chi^2_{(7)} = 15.6$, $p = 0.029$, Friedman test) in non-responders to LEV over a 7-day period (Figure 6A,B), although it could not completely inhibit spontaneous seizure activity (Figure 6A,B). ML365 co-treatment also diminished total seizure frequency ($Z = 2.7$, $p = 0.007$ vs. vehicle co-treatment, Mann–Whitney U test), total seizure duration ($t_{(8)} = 15.7$,

$p < 0.001$ vs. vehicle co-treatment, Student's t-test) and average seizure severity ($Z = 2.6$, $p = 0.009$ vs. vehicle co-treatment, Mann–Whitney U test) in non-responders to LEV over a 7-day period (Figure 6C). In addition, ML365 co-treatment decreased TASK-1 fluorescent intensity to 0.73-fold of the vehicle co-treatment animal level ($t_{(8)} = 7$, $p < 0.001$ vs. vehicle co-treatment, Student's t-test, $n = 5$) in non-responders. ML365 co-treatment reduced the fraction of TASK-1 positive astrocytes of the total astrocytes ($t_{(8)} = 2.9$, $p = 0.019$, Student's t-test, Figure 7A–C). TASK-1 density also diminished to 0.7-fold of the vehicle co-treated animal level ($t_{(8)} = 6$, $p < 0.001$ vs. vehicle co-treatment, Student's t-test, $n = 5$) in non-responders (Figure 7D,E, Supplementary Figure S1). Taken together, our findings suggest that TASK-1 inhibition by ML365 may improve the efficacy of LEV in non-responders.

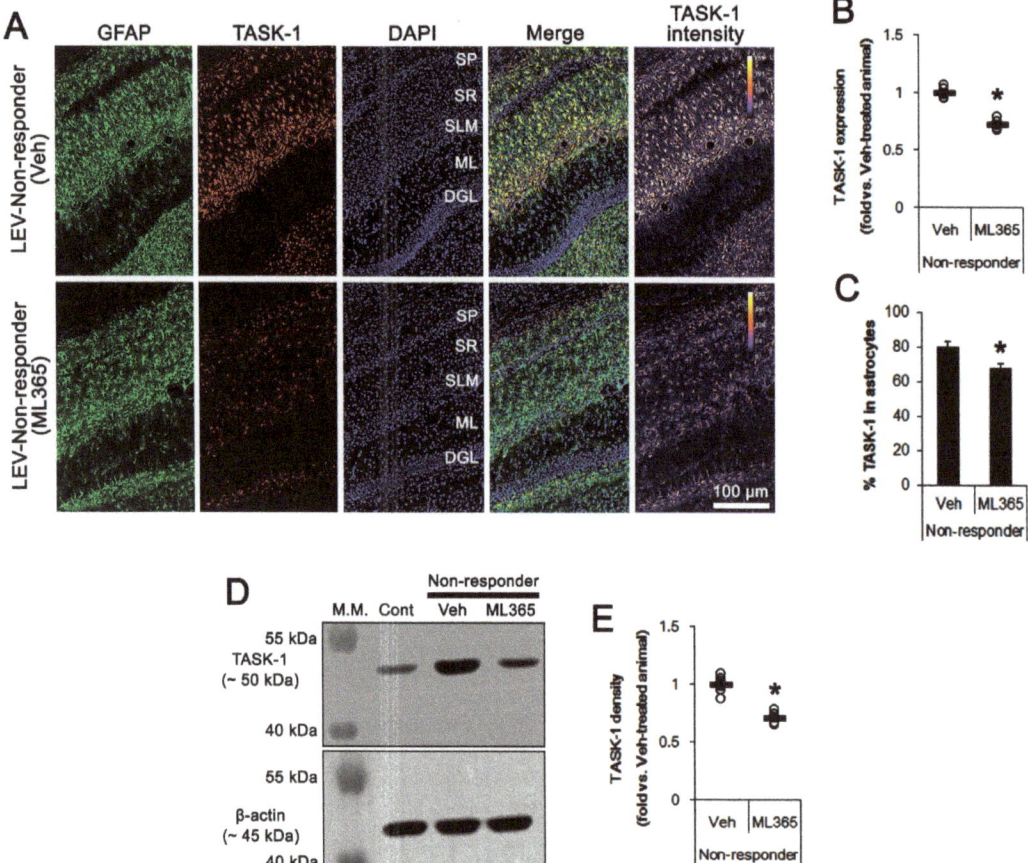

Figure 5. The effect of ML365 on TASK-1 expression in non-responders to levetiracetam (LEV). As compared to the vehicle (Veh), ML365 reduces TASK-1 expression in CA1 astrocytes within the hippocampus of non-responders. (**A**) Representative photos of TASK-1 expression in the hippocampus (SP, stratum pyramidale; SR, stratum radiatum; SLM, stratum lacunosum-moleculare; ML, molecular layer of the dentate gyrus; DGL, dentate granule cell layer). (**B**) Quantitative analyses of the effect of ML365 on TASK-1 expression based on immunohistochemical data. Open circles indicate each individual value. Horizontal bars indicate the mean value. Error bars indicate SEM (*, $p < 0.05$ vs. vehicle-treated animals; Student's t-test). (**C**) Quantitative analyses of the effect of

ML365 on the fraction of TASK-1 positive astrocytes in total astrocytes (*, $p < 0.05$ vs. control animals; Student's t-test; error bars, SEM). (**D**) Representative images for Western blot of TASK-1 protein expression in the hippocampal tissues. (**E**) Quantification of TASK-1 levels based on Western blots (*, $p < 0.05$ vs. vehicle-treated animals; Student's t-test).

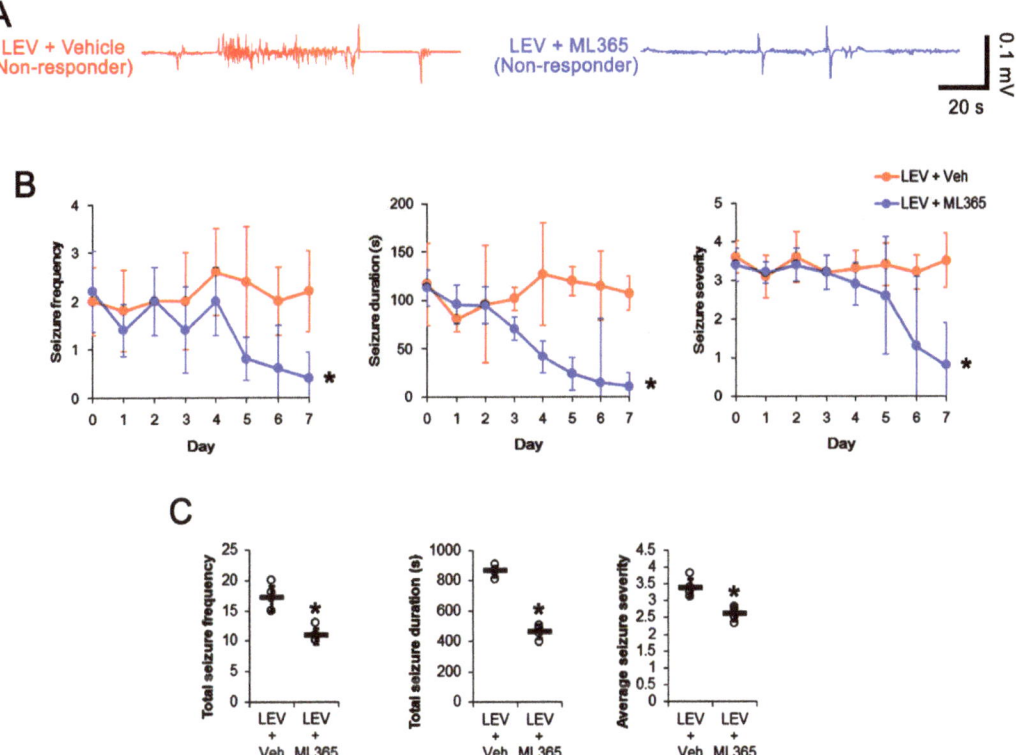

Figure 6. The effect of ML365 co-treatment with levetiracetam (LEV) on spontaneous seizure activities in non-responders to LEV. ML365 co-treatment improved the efficacy of LEV in non-responders. (**A**) Representative EEG signal in each group at 4 days after treatment. (**B**) Quantitative analyses of the effects of ML365 co-treatment on seizure frequency (Friedman test), seizure duration (repeated measures ANOVA) and seizure severity (seizure score, Friedman test) over a 7-day period (*, $p < 0.05$ vs. vehicle (Veh)-treated animals; error bars, SD). (**C**) Quantitative analyses of total seizure frequency (Mann–Whitney U test), total seizure duration (Student's t-test) and average behavioral seizure score (seizure severity, Mann–Whitney U test) over a 7-day period (*, $p < 0.05$ vs. vehicle (Veh)-treated animals; open circles, each individual value; horizontal bars, mean value; error bars, SD).

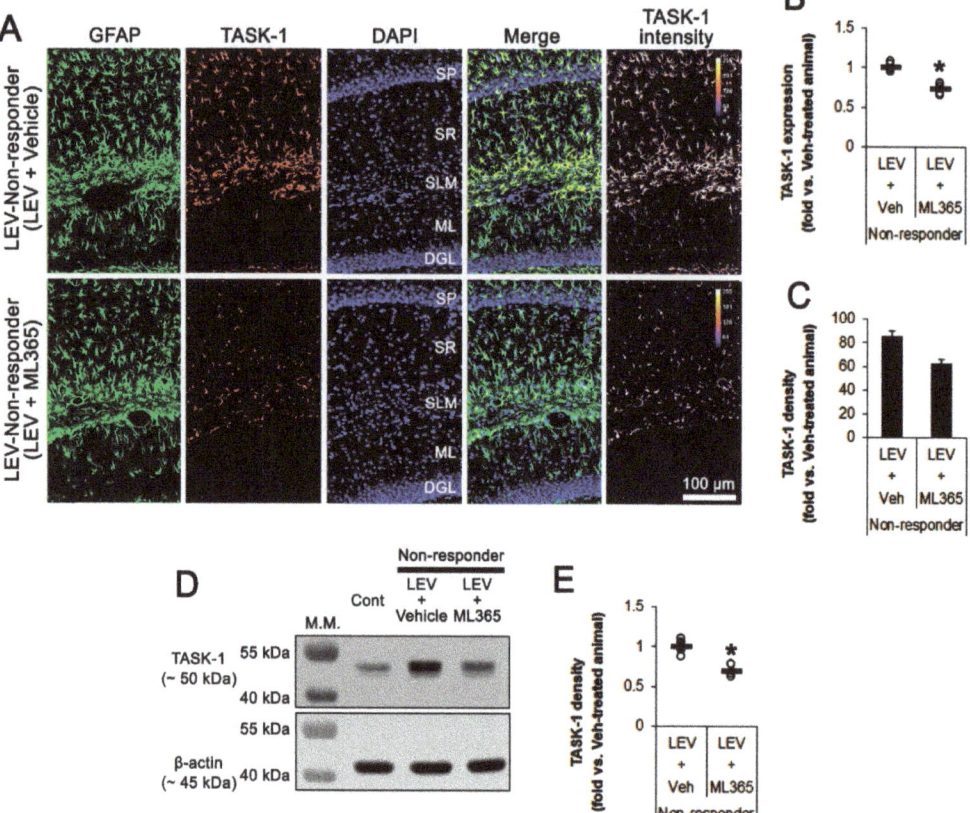

Figure 7. The effect of ML365 co-treatment with levetiracetam (LEV) on TASK-1 expression in non-responders to LEV. ML365 co-treatment reduced TASK-1 expression in CA1 astrocytes within the hippocampus of non-responders. (**A**) Representative photos of TASK-1 expression in the hippocampus (SP, stratum pyramidale; SR, stratum radiatum; SLM, stratum lacunosum-moleculare; ML, molecular layer of the dentate gyrus; DGL, dentate granule cell layer). (**B**) Quantitative analyses of the effect of ML365 co-treatment on TASK-1 expression based on immunohistochemical data. Open circles indicate each individual value. Horizontal bars indicate the mean value. Error bars indicate SEM (*, $p < 0.05$ vs. LEV-treated animals; Student's *t*-test). (**C**) Quantitative analyses of the effect of ML365 co-treatment on the fraction of TASK-1 positive astrocytes in total astrocytes (*, $p < 0.05$ vs. control animals; Student's *t*-test; error bars, SEM). (**D**) Representative images for Western blots of TASK-1 protein expression in the hippocampal tissues. (**E**) Quantifications of TASK-1 levels based on Western blot results (*, $p < 0.05$ vs. LEV-treated animals; Student's *t*-test).

4. Discussion

The major findings of the present study are that (1) LEV reduced TASK-1 expression in reactive CA1 astrocytes of responders, (2) TASK-1 inhibition by ML365 shortened seizure duration in non-responders, and (3) ML365 co-treatment with LEV effectively attenuated seizure activity in non-responders.

In the present study, 43% of chronically epileptic rats did not show a significant response to LEV. These results are consistent with previous studies that demonstrated the ratio of non-responders to LEV in TLE patients and chronically epileptic rats [20–22,33]. Basically, the anti-epileptic effects of LEV are relevant to the binding to SV2A [20]. However,

LEV also leads to intracellular acidification in neurons, which is coupled with extracellular pH shift [23,34]. Furthermore, LEV inhibits carbonic anhydrase, which leads to extracellular acidification [24–27]. Since extracellular acidification ceases the seizure activity [7–10,34], it is likely that extracellular acidic shifts may be one of the anti-epileptic potencies of LEV. Therefore, our findings suggest that the impairment of extracellular acidic shifts may be one of the causes of the low efficacy of LEV in non-responders.

Seizure activity increases the extracellular K^+ concentration due to K^+ efflux from neurons during repolarization, accompanied by an initial extracellular alkalinization. Thus, astrocyte-mediated K^+ buffering plays an important role in ictogenesis and seizure termination to regulate extracellular K^+ level [7,11,12,35]. Indeed, the low ratio of inward-to-outward K^+ conductance in astrocytes is reported in the hippocampus of TLE patients [13]. Since extracellular alkalinization potentiates TASK-1-mediated outward K^+ currents [14,15,36], TASK-1 may participate in a rise of extracellular K^+ concentration during or following seizure activity. In the present study, TASK-1 expression was increased in reactive CA1 astrocytes of chronically epileptic rats. Furthermore, LEV decreased seizure activity in responders, concomitant with TASK-1 downregulation in CA1 astrocytes. Considering astroglial roles in neuronal hyperexcitability [37,38], it is likely that aberrant elevation of extracellular K^+ concentration, induced by upregulated TASK-1, may affect seizure activity in the epileptic hippocampus, which would be abolished by LEV-induced extracellular acidification. Conversely, LEV may ameliorate seizure activity by directly regulating astroglial TASK-1 expression independent of extracellular pH shifts, since LEV reduces delayed rectifier K^+ current [39] and activates renal outer medullary inwardly rectifying K^+ channel-1 (ROMK1, also known as KCNJ1 or Kir1.1) [40]. The present data also reveal that ML365 effectively diminished TASK-1 expression in CA1 astrocytes and decreased seizure duration in non-responders. In addition, ML365 co-treatment increased the efficacy of LEV. These findings indicate that the inhibition of TASK-1-mediated outwardly K^+ rectification may overcome the ineffectiveness of LEV in extracellular acidic shifts and/or the direct regulation of TASK-1 expression in non-responders. Therefore, the present data suggest that TASK-1 is a potential therapeutic target for improving the responsiveness to LEV in non-responders.

On the other hand, the localization of TASK-1 in the hippocampus has been still controversial; TASK-1 expression is mainly observed in astrocytes of the hippocampus [16,32], whereas neuronal TASK-1 expression has been also reported [41]. Although the basis remains unclear, this discrepancy may be attributable to the age of animals used in the studies (adult [16,32], the present study vs. young [41]). Indeed, TASK-1 mRNA expression peaks by 7 days postnatal, and then gradually declines by 28 days postnatal in the mouse hippocampus [42]. Conversely, it is plausible that functional levels of TASK-1 expression on neurons would be extremely too low to be detectable with immunohistochemistry. If present on neurons, however, extracellular acidic shifts induced by LEV would result in prolonged depolarization by inhibiting TASK-1-mediated K^+ efflux from neurons. Furthermore, actions of LEV or ML365 on TASK-1 would increase the excitability of principal neurons and interneurons. Under these conditions, the delayed repolarization would impair the fast-spiking capability of interneurons, and lead to uncontrolled epileptiform discharges in principal neurons due to reduced GABAergic inhibition [43]. Similar to chronically epileptic rats, TASK-1 expression is rarely observed in principal neurons of TLE patients but is predominantly detected in astrocytes [17]. In addition, the massive degeneration of hippocampal neurons (particularly, CA1 pyramidal cells and interneurons) are observed in chronically epileptic rats [28,29]. Therefore, our findings suggest that LEV or ML365 may diminish spontaneous seizures by inhibiting TASK-1 in CA1 astrocytes rather than neurons in chronically epileptic rats.

In the present study, we could not access the underlying mechanisms of the modulation of astroglial TASK-1 expression. However, it is worth considering that serum- and glucocorticoid-inducible kinase (SGK)-mediated signaling pathway may be involved in astroglial TASK-1 regulation. This is because SGK1 activity is lower in chronically epileptic rats as compared to the controls [44], and SGK inhibits TASK-1 current and its surface expression [45]. Further studies are needed to elucidate the role of SGK-mediated signaling pathway in astroglial TASK-1 regulation.

5. Conclusions

In the present study, we demonstrated, for the first time, that LEV ameliorated spontaneous seizure activity in responders by reducing the upregulated TASK-1 expression in CA1 astrocytes. Furthermore, ML365 co-treatment improved the efficacy of LEV in non-responders. Therefore, our findings suggest that the dysregulation of TASK-1 function may be one of the causes of refractory seizures to LEV, and TASK-1 inhibition is a potential therapeutic target for improving the responsiveness to LEV in non-responders.

Supplementary Materials: The following supporting information can be downloaded at: https://www.mdpi.com/article/10.3390/biomedicines10040787/s1, Figure S1: Full-length gel images of the Western blot data in Figures 3C, 5C and 7C.

Author Contributions: T.-C.K. designed the experiments. J.-E.K. and T.-C.K. performed the experiments described in the manuscript. J.-E.K. and T.-C.K. analyzed the data, and wrote the manuscript. All authors have read and agreed to the published version of the manuscript.

Funding: This study was supported by a grant of Hallym University (No. HRF-202202-002).

Institutional Review Board Statement: The animal study protocol was approved by the Institutional Animal Care and Use Committee of Hallym University (No. Hallym 2018-2, 26 April 2018; No, Hallym 2018-21, 8 June 2018 and Hallym 2021-3, 27 April 2021).

Informed Consent Statement: Not applicable.

Data Availability Statement: Not applicable.

Conflicts of Interest: The authors declare no conflict of interest. The funders had no role in the design of the study; in the collection, analyses, or interpretation of data; in the writing of the manuscript; or in the decision to publish the results.

References

1. Menezes, L.F.S.; Sabiá Júnior, E.F.; Tibery, D.V.; Carneiro, L.D.A.; Schwartz, E.F. Epilepsy-Related Voltage-Gated Sodium Channelopathies: A Review. *Front. Pharmacol.* **2020**, *11*, 1276. [CrossRef] [PubMed]
2. Van Loo, K.M.J.; Becker, A.J. Transcriptional Regulation of Channelopathies in Genetic and Acquired Epilepsies. *Front. Cell. Neurosci.* **2020**, *13*, 587. [CrossRef] [PubMed]
3. Dejakaisaya, H.; Kwan, P.; Jones, N.C. Astrocyte and glutamate involvement in the pathogenesis of epilepsy in Alzheimer's disease. *Epilepsia* **2021**, *62*, 1485–1493. [CrossRef] [PubMed]
4. Tan, T.H.; Perucca, P.; O'Brien, T.J.; Kwan, P.; Monif, M. Inflammation, ictogenesis, and epileptogenesis: An exploration through human disease. *Epilepsia* **2021**, *62*, 303–324. [CrossRef] [PubMed]
5. Chow, S.Y.; Li, J.; Woodbury, D.M. Water and electrolyte contents, cell pH, and membrane potential of primary cultures of astrocytes from DBA, C57, and SW mice. *Epilepsia* **1992**, *33*, 393–401. [CrossRef]
6. Xiong, Z.Q.; Saggau, P.; Stringer, J.L. Activity-dependent intracellular acidification correlates with the duration of seizure activity. *J. Neurosci.* **2000**, *20*, 1290–1296. [CrossRef]
7. Xiong, Z.Q.; Stringer, J.L. Extracellular pH responses in CA1 and the dentate gyrus during electrical stimulation, seizure discharges, and spreading depression. *J. Neurophysiol.* **2000**, *83*, 3519–3524. [CrossRef]
8. Pasternack, M.; Bountra, C.; Voipio, J.; Kaila, K. Influence of extracellular and intracellular pH on GABA-gated chloride conductance in crayfish muscle fibres. *Neuroscience* **1992**, *47*, 921–929. [CrossRef]
9. Tang, C.M.; Dichter, M.; Morad, M. Modulation of the N-methyl-D-aspartate channel by extracellular H+. *Proc. Natl. Acad. Sci. USA* **1990**, *87*, 6445–6449. [CrossRef]
10. Traynelis, S.F.; Cull-Candy, S.G. Proton inhibition of N-methyl-D-aspartate receptors in cerebellar neurons. *Nature* **1990**, *345*, 347–350. [CrossRef]
11. Gabriel, S.; Kivi, A.; Kovacs, R.; Lehmann, T.N.; Lanksch, W.R.; Meencke, H.J.; Heinemann, U. Effects of barium on stimulus-induced changes in [K+]o and field potentials in dentate gyrus and area CA1 of human epileptic hippocampus. *Neurosci. Lett.* **1998**, *249*, 91–94. [CrossRef]

12. Gabriel, S.; Eilers, A.; Kivi, A.; Kovacs, R.; Schulze, K.; Lehmann, T.N.; Heinemann, U. Effects of barium on stimulus induced changes in extracellular potassium concentration in area CA1 of hippocampal slices from normal and pilocarpine-treated epileptic rats. *Neurosci. Lett.* **1998**, *242*, 9–12. [CrossRef]
13. Hinterkeuser, S.; Schröder, W.; Hager, G.; Seifert, G.; Blümcke, I.; Elger, C.E.; Schramm, J.; Steinhäuser, C. Astrocytes in the hippocampus of patients with temporal lobe epilepsy display changes in potassium conductances. *Eur. J. Neurosci.* **2000**, *12*, 2087–2096. [CrossRef]
14. Duprat, F.; Lesage, F.; Fink, M.; Reyes, R.; Heurteaux, C.; Lazdunski, M. TASK, a human background K+ channel to sense external pH variations near physiological pH. *EMBO J.* **1997**, *16*, 5464–5471. [CrossRef]
15. Niemeyer, M.I.; González-Nilo, F.D.; Zúñiga, L.; González, W.; Cid, L.P.; Sepúlveda, F.V. Gating of two-pore domain K+ channels by extracellular pH. *Biochem. Soc. Trans.* **2006**, *34*, 899–902. [CrossRef]
16. Kim, J.E.; Kwak, S.E.; Choi, S.Y.; Kang, T.C. Region-specific alterations in astroglial TWIK-related acid-sensitive K+-1 channel immunoreactivity in the rat hippocampal complex following pilocarpine-induced status epilepticus. *J. Comp. Neurol.* **2008**, *510*, 463–474. [CrossRef]
17. Kim, J.E.; Yeo, S.I.; Ryu, H.J.; Chung, C.K.; Kim, M.J.; Kang, T.C. Changes in TWIK-related acid sensitive K+-1 and -3 channel expressions from neurons to glia in the hippocampus of temporal lobe epilepsy patients and experimental animal model. *Neurochem. Res.* **2011**, *36*, 2155–2168. [CrossRef]
18. Kim, D.S.; Kim, J.E.; Kwak, S.E.; Choi, H.C.; Song, H.K.; Kim, Y.I.; Choi, S.Y.; Kang, T.C. Up-regulated astroglial TWIK-related acid-sensitive K+ channel-1 (TASK-1) in the hippocampus of seizure-sensitive gerbils: A target of anti-epileptic drugs. *Brain Res.* **2007**, *1185*, 346–358. [CrossRef]
19. Juvale, I.I.A.; Che Has, A.T. Possible interplay between the theories of pharmacoresistant epilepsy. *Eur. J. Neurosci.* **2021**, *53*, 1998–2026. [CrossRef]
20. Lynch, J.M.; Tate, S.K.; Kinirons, P.; Weale, M.E.; Cavalleri, G.L.; Depondt, C.; Murphy, K.; O'Rourke, D.; Doherty, C.P.; Shianna, K.V.; et al. No major role of common SV2A variation for predisposition or levetiracetam response in epilepsy. *Epilepsy Res.* **2009**, *83*, 44–51. [CrossRef]
21. Glien, M.; Brandt, C.; Potschka, H.; Löscher, W. Effects of the novel antiepileptic drug levetiracetam on spontaneous recurrent seizures in the rat pilocarpine model of temporal lobe epilepsy. *Epilepsia* **2002**, *43*, 350–357. [CrossRef]
22. Ko, A.R.; Kang, T.C. Blockade of endothelin B receptor improves the efficacy of levetiracetam in chronic epileptic rats. *Seizure* **2015**, *31*, 133–140. [CrossRef]
23. Leniger, T.; Thöne, J.; Bonnet, U.; Hufnagel, A.; Bingmann, D.; Wiemann, M. Levetiracetam inhibits Na+-dependent Cl-/HCO3- exchange of adult hippocampal CA3 neurons from guinea-pigs. *Br. J. Pharmacol.* **2004**, *142*, 1073–1080. [CrossRef]
24. Bonnet, U.; Bingmann, D.; Speckmann, E.J.; Wiemann, M. Levetiracetam mediates subtle pH-shifts in adult human neocortical pyramidal cells via an inhibition of the bicarbonate-driven neuronal pH-regulation—Implications for excitability and plasticity modulation. *Brain Res.* **2019**, *1710*, 146–156. [CrossRef]
25. Aribi, A.M.; Stringer, J.L. Effects of antiepileptic drugs on extracellular pH regulation in the hippocampal CA1 region in vivo. *Epilepsy Res.* **2002**, *49*, 143–151. [CrossRef]
26. Koç, E.R.; Erken, G.; Bilen, C.; Sackes, Z.; Gencer, N. The effects of anti-epileptic drugs on human erythrocyte carbonic anhydrase I and II isozymes. *Arch. Physiol. Biochem.* **2014**, *120*, 131–135. [CrossRef]
27. Theparambil, S.M.; Hosford, P.S.; Ruminot, I.; Kopach, O.; Reynolds, J.R.; Sandoval, P.Y.; Rusakov, D.A.; Barros, L.F.; Gourine, A.V. Astrocytes regulate brain extracellular pH via a neuronal activity-dependent bicarbonate shuttle. *Nat. Commun.* **2020**, *11*, 5073. [CrossRef]
28. Kim, J.E.; Lee, D.S.; Park, H.; Kang, T.C. Src/CK2/PTEN-Mediated GluN2B and CREB Dephosphorylations Regulate the Responsiveness to AMPA Receptor Antagonists in Chronic Epilepsy Rats. *Int. J. Mol. Sci.* **2020**, *21*, 9633. [CrossRef]
29. Kim, J.E.; Lee, D.S.; Park, H.; Kim, T.H.; Kang, T.C. Inhibition of AKT/GSK3β/CREB Pathway Improves the Responsiveness to AMPA Receptor Antagonists by Regulating GRIA1 Surface Expression in Chronic Epilepsy Rats. *Biomedicines* **2021**, *9*, 425. [CrossRef]
30. Racine, R.J. Modification of seizure activity by electrical stimulation. II. Motor seizure. *Electroencephalogr. Clin. Neurophysiol.* **1972**, *32*, 281–294. [CrossRef]
31. Flaherty, D.P.; Simpson, D.S.; Miller, M.; Maki, B.E.; Zou, B.; Shi, J.; Wu, M.; McManus, O.B.; Aubé, J.; Li, M.; et al. Potent and selective inhibitors of the TASK-1 potassium channel through chemical optimization of a bis-amide scaffold. *Bioorg. Med. Chem. Lett.* **2014**, *24*, 3968–3973. [CrossRef] [PubMed]
32. Kindler, C.H.; Pietruck, C.; Yost, C.S.; Sampson, E.R.; Gray, A.T. Localization of the tandem pore domain K+ channel TASK-1 in the rat central nervous system. *Brain Res. Mol. Brain Res.* **2000**, *80*, 99–108. [CrossRef]
33. Grimminger, T.; Pernhorst, K.; Surges, R.; Niehusmann, P.; Priebe, L.; von Lehe, M.; Hoffmann, P.; Cichon, S.; Schoch, S.; Becker, A.J. Levetiracetam resistance: Synaptic signatures & corresponding promoter SNPs in epileptic hippocampi. *Neurobiol. Dis.* **2013**, *60*, 115–125. [PubMed]
34. Chesler, M. The regulation and modulation of pH in the nervous system. *Prog. Neurobiol.* **1990**, *34*, 401–427. [CrossRef]
35. Xiong, Z.Q.; Stringer, J.L. Regulation of extracellular pH in the developing hippocampus. *Brain Res. Dev. Brain Res.* **2000**, *122*, 113–117. [CrossRef]

36. Ma, L.; Zhang, X.; Zhou, M.; Chen, H. Acid-sensitive TWIK and TASK two-pore domain potassium channels change ion selectivity and become permeable to sodium in extracellular acidification. *J. Biol. Chem.* **2012**, *287*, 37145–37153. [CrossRef]
37. Kim, J.E.; Kang, T.C. CDDO-Me Attenuates Astroglial Autophagy via Nrf2-, ERK1/2-SP1- and Src-CK2-PTEN-PI3K/AKT-Mediated Signaling Pathways in the Hippocampus of Chronic Epilepsy Rats. *Antioxidants* **2021**, *10*, 655. [CrossRef]
38. Binder, D.K.; Yao, X.; Zador, Z.; Sick, T.J.; Verkman, A.S.; Manley, G.T. Increased seizure duration and slowed potassium kinetics in mice lacking aquaporin-4 water channels. *Glia* **2006**, *53*, 631–636. [CrossRef]
39. Madeja, M.; Margineanu, D.G.; Gorji, A.; Siep, E.; Boerrigter, P.; Klitgaard, H.; Speckmann, E.J. Reduction of voltage-operated potassium currents by levetiracetam: A novel antiepileptic mechanism of action? *Neuropharmacology* **2003**, *45*, 661–671. [CrossRef]
40. Lee, C.H.; Lee, C.Y.; Tsai, T.S.; Liou, H.H. PKA-mediated phosphorylation is a novel mechanism for levetiracetam, an antiepileptic drug, activating ROMK1 channels. *Biochem. Pharmacol.* **2008**, *76*, 225–235. [CrossRef]
41. Zhou, M.; Xu, G.; Xie, M.; Zhang, X.; Schools, G.P.; Ma, L.; Kimelberg, H.K.; Chen, H. TWIK-1 and TREK-1 are potassium channels contributing significantly to astrocyte passive conductance in rat hippocampal slices. *J. Neurosci.* **2009**, *29*, 8551–8564. [CrossRef]
42. Aller, M.I.; Wisden, W. Changes in expression of some two-pore domain potassium channel genes (KCNK) in selected brain regions of developing mice. *Neuroscience* **2008**, *151*, 1154–1172. [CrossRef]
43. Cammarota, M.; Losi, G.; Chiavegato, A.; Zonta, M.; Carmignoto, G. Fast spiking interneuron control of seizure propagation in a cortical slice model of focal epilepsy. *J. Physiol.* **2013**, *591*, 807–822. [CrossRef]
44. Kim, J.E.; Lee, D.S.; Park, H.; Kim, T.H.; Kang, T.C. AMPA receptor antagonists facilitate NEDD4-2-mediated GRIA1 ubiquitination by regulating PP2B-ERK1/2-SGK1 pathway in chronic epilepsy rats. *Biomedicines* **2021**, *9*, 1069. [CrossRef]
45. Rinné, S.; Kiper, A.K.; Schmidt, C.; Ortiz-Bonnin, B.; Zwiener, S.; Seebohm, G.; Decher, N. Stress-Kinase Regulation of TASK-1 and TASK-3. *Cell Physiol. Biochem.* **2017**, *44*, 1024–1037. [CrossRef]

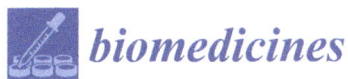

Article

AMPA Receptor Antagonists Facilitate NEDD4-2-Mediated GRIA1 Ubiquitination by Regulating PP2B-ERK1/2-SGK1 Pathway in Chronic Epilepsy Rats

Ji-Eun Kim *, Duk-Shin Lee, Hana Park, Tae-Hyun Kim and Tae-Cheon Kang *

Department of Anatomy and Neurobiology, Institute of Epilepsy Research, College of Medicine, Hallym University, Chuncheon 24252, Korea; dslee84@hallym.ac.kr (D.-S.L.); M19050@hallym.ac.kr (H.P.); hyun1028@hallym.ac.kr (T.-H.K.)
* Correspondence: jieunkim@hallym.ac.kr (J.-E.K.); tckang@hallym.ac.kr (T.-C.K.); Tel.: +82-33-248-2522 (J.-E.K.); +82-33-248-2524 (T.-C.K.); Fax: +82-33-248-2525 (J.-E.K. & T.-C.K.)

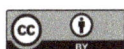

Citation: Kim, J.-E.; Lee, D.-S.; Park, H.; Kim, T.-H.; Kang, T.-C. AMPA Receptor Antagonists Facilitate NEDD4-2-Mediated GRIA1 Ubiquitination by Regulating PP2B-ERK1/2-SGK1 Pathway in Chronic Epilepsy Rats. *Biomedicines* 2021, 9, 1069. https://doi.org/10.3390/biomedicines9081069

Academic Editor: Prosper N'Gouemo

Received: 23 July 2021
Accepted: 19 August 2021
Published: 23 August 2021

Publisher's Note: MDPI stays neutral with regard to jurisdictional claims in published maps and institutional affiliations.

Copyright: © 2021 by the authors. Licensee MDPI, Basel, Switzerland. This article is an open access article distributed under the terms and conditions of the Creative Commons Attribution (CC BY) license (https://creativecommons.org/licenses/by/4.0/).

Abstract: The neural precursor cell expressed by developmentally downregulated gene 4-2 (NEDD4-2) is a ubiquitin E3 ligase that has a high affinity toward binding and ubiquitinating glutamate ionotropic receptor α-amino-3-hydroxy-5-methyl-4-isoxazolepropionic acid (AMPA) type subunit 1 (GRIA1, also referred to GluR1 or GluA1). Since dysregulation of GRIA1 surface expression is relevant to the responsiveness to AMPA receptor (AMPAR) antagonists (perampanel and GYKI 52466) in chronic epilepsy rats, it is likely that NEDD4-2 may be involved in the pathogenesis of intractable epilepsy. However, the role of NEDD4-2-mediated GRIA1 ubiquitination in refractory seizures to AMPAR antagonists is still unknown. In the present study, both AMPAR antagonists recovered the impaired GRIA1 ubiquitination by regulating protein phosphatase 2B (PP2B)-extracellular signal-regulated kinase 1/2 (ERK1/2)-serum and glucocorticoid-regulated kinase 1 (SGK1)-NEDD4-2 signaling pathway in responders (whose seizure activities are responsive to AMPAR), but not non-responders (whose seizure activities were uncontrolled by AMPAR antagonists). In addition, cyclosporin A (CsA, a PP2B inhibitor) co-treatment improved the effects of AMPAR antagonists in non-responders, independent of AKT signaling pathway. Therefore, our findings suggest that dysregulation of PP2B-ERK1/2-SGK1-NEDD4-2-mediated GRIA1 ubiquitination may be responsible for refractory seizures and that this pathway may be a potential therapeutic target for improving the treatment of intractable epilepsy in response to AMPAR antagonists.

Keywords: 3-phosphoinositide-dependent protein kinase-1; AKT; cyclosporin A; GluA1; GluR1; intractable epilepsy; PDK1; refractory seizure

1. Introduction

Epilepsy is a brain function disorder characterized by recurrent and unprovoked seizures. The prevalence of epilepsy in the general population is approximately 0.6–0.8% [1]. Initial/acute prolonged seizure (status epilepticus, SE), trauma, stroke or infections are postulated as precipitating factors of epilepsy [2]. Mesial temporal lobe epilepsy (MTLE) is the most common form of epilepsy and a medically intractable syndrome that is partially or totally uncontrolled by conventional anti-epileptic drug (AED) treatments [3]. Although disturbances in glutamatergic/GABAergic transmissions and the related signaling pathways are associated with the pathogenesis of MTLE in humans, the underlying mechanisms of MTLE remain largely unclear.

The pilocarpine model (including LiCI-pilocarpine model) serves as a reliable animal model of intractable epilepsy. The profiles of spontaneous recurrent seizures in this model resemble those of human MTLE. This model shows limbic seizures that become secondarily generalized, evolving to SE, which lasts for several hours (acute period). The SE is followed by a latent "seizure-free" period (about 15–30 days) and by a chronic period characterized by the presence of spontaneous recurrent seizures. The lesions of mesial temporal structures, including a well-known hippocampal sclerosis, in this model are also similar to those of human MTLE patients [4,5]. Therefore, the pilocarpine model provides the opportunity to investigate the pathogenesis of MTLE.

The α-amino-3-hydroxy-5-methyl-4-isoxazolepropionic acid receptor (AMPAR) is one of the major subtypes of ionotropic glutamate receptors. AMPARs are comprised of combinations of glutamate ionotropic receptor AMPA type subunit 1 (GRIA1, also referred to GluR1 or GluA1)—GRIA4, which are assembled as homo- or heterotetramers [6]. The regulation of AMPAR trafficking is critical for homeostatic regulation of synaptic strength and the pathogenesis of epilepsy [7]. Indeed, AMPAR antagonists inhibit seizure activity in chronic epilepsy rats, accompanied by reduced GRIA1 surface expression in the hippocampus [4,8–10].

The neural precursor cell expressed by developmentally downregulated gene 4-2 (NEDD4-2) is a ubiquitin E3 ligase that has a high affinity toward binding and ubiquitinating membrane proteins [11]. Some neuronal membrane receptors/channels have been identified as substrates of NEDD4-2: voltage-gated Na^+ channel (Na_v)1.6 [12], voltage-gated K^+ channels K_v7/KCNQ [13–15] and neurotrophin receptor TrkA [16]. NEDD4-2 also regulates neuronal activity and seizure susceptibility through ubiquitination of the GRIA1 subunit of AMPAR [11,17]. Therefore, it is likely that NEDD4-2 may be involved in the fine-tuning of AMPAR-mediated neuronal excitation. Indeed, at least three missense mutations in the NEDD4-2 gene are identified through genomic mutation screening in patients with epilepsy [18–20]. Furthermore, NEDD4-2 plays an important role in seizure progression in response to kainic acid through regulation of AMPAR ubiquitination [11,17,21,22].

On the other hand, multifactorial events are involved in the underlying mechanisms of pharmacoresistant epilepsy: (1) a reduced yield of AED concentration in the brain by hyper-activation of drug efflux transporter or sustained inflammatory conditions [23,24], (2) dysfunctions of ion/neurotransmitter channels of transporters [25], and (3) abnormal neural networks [25]. Interestingly, GRIA1 surface expression is higher in the hippocampus of chronic epilepsy rats than that of normal rats, which is attenuated by AMPAR antagonists (such as perampanel and GYKI 52466) in responders whose seizure activities are reduced by them [4,10,26]. Since ubiquitination of GRIA1 is linked to AMPAR surface expression and trafficking [27–29], it is postulated that AMPAR antagonists may modulate NEDD4-2 activity that is required for limiting GluA1 surface expression and functionality of AMPAR in the epileptic hippocampus. However, little data are available to describe whether NEDD4-2-mediated GRIA1 ubiquitination is changed, and this alteration is relevant to the generation of refractory seizures to AMPAR antagonists in a chronic epilepsy model. In the present study, therefore, we investigated the effects of AMPAR antagonists on NEDD4-2-mediated GRIA1 regulation in responders and non-responders (whose seizure activities were uncontrolled by AMPAR antagonists) of a LiCl-pilocarpine epilepsy rat model to elucidate the role of NEDD4-2 in MTLE.

Here, we demonstrate that the anti-convulsive effects of AMPAR antagonists are closely related to the regulation of GRIA1 ubiquitination via protein phosphatase 2B (PP2B)-extracellular signal-regulated kinase 1/2 (ERK1/2)-serum and glucocorticoid-regulated kinase 1 (SGK1)-NEDD4-2 signaling pathway. In addition, impairment of this signaling pathway resulted in refractory seizures to AMPAR antagonists, which was improved by cyclosporin A (CsA, a PP2B inhibitor) co-treatment. Therefore, our findings suggest that the PP2B-ERK1/2-SGK1-NEDD4-2 pathway may be a potential therapeutic strategy to improve the treatment of intractable MTLE in response to AMPAR antagonists.

2. Materials and Methods

2.1. Experimental Animals and Chemicals

Male Sprague Dawley (SD) rats (seven weeks old) were provided with a commercial diet and water ad libitum under controlled temperature, humidity and lighting conditions (22 ± 2 °C, 55 ± 5% and a 12:12 light/dark cycle with lights). Animal protocols were approved by the Institutional Animal Care and Use Committee of Hallym University (Code number: #Hallym 2018-2, 26 April 2018, #Hallym 2018-21, 8 June 2018 and #Hallym 2021-3, 27 April 2021). All reagents were purchased from Sigma-Aldrich (St. Louis, MO, USA), except where noted.

2.2. Generation of Chronic Epilepsy Rats

Animals were intraperitoneally (i.p.) given LiCl (127 mg/kg) 24 h before pilocarpine treatment. On the next day, animals were treated with pilocarpine (30 mg/kg, i.p.) 20 min after atropine methylbromide (5 mg/kg i.p.). Two hours after SE on-set, animals were administered diazepam (Valium; Hoffman la Roche, Neuilly sur-Seine, France; 10 mg/kg, i.p.) as needed. Control animals received saline in place of pilocarpine. Animals were video-monitored 8 h a day for general behavior and occurrence of spontaneous seizures by four weeks after SE (Figure 1). We classified chronic epilepsy rats that showed behavioral seizures with seizure score ≥ 3 more than once.

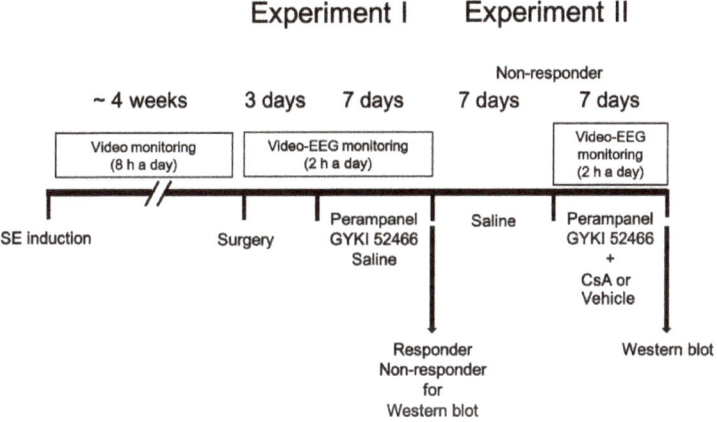

Figure 1. Scheme of the experimental design in the present study.

2.3. Surgery

Control and epilepsy rats were implanted with monopolar stainless steel electrodes (Plastics One, Roanoke, VA, USA) in the right hippocampus (stereotaxic coordinates was -3.8 mm posterior; 2.0 mm lateral; -2.6 mm depth to bregma) under isoflurane anesthesia (3% induction, 1.5–2% for surgery, and 1.5% maintenance in a 65:35 mixture of $N_2O:O_2$). Some animals were also implanted with a brain infusion kit 1 (Alzet, Cupertino, CA, USA) to infuse with vehicle or cyclosporin A (CsA, a PP2B inhibitor, 250 µM) into the right lateral ventricle (1 mm posterior; 1.5 mm lateral; -3.5 mm depth to the bregma, see below). The CsA concentration did not affect spontaneous seizure activities in chronic epilepsy rats [30]. Throughout surgery, the core temperature of each rat was maintained at 37–38 °C. Electrodes were secured to the exposed skull with dental acrylic.

2.4. Drug Trials, EEG Analysis and Quantification of Behavioral Seizure Activity

2.4.1. Experiment I

Figure 1 illustrates the design of the drug trial methodology, which was a modified protocol based on previous studies [10,26,30,31]. After baseline seizure activity was determined over three days, perampanel (8 mg/kg, i.p, Eisai Korea Inc., Seoul, Korea), GYKI 52466 (10 mg/kg, i.p.) or saline (vehicle) was daily administered at 6:00 PM over a one-week period [4,30]. Electroencephalographic (EEG) signals were detected with a DAM 80 differential amplifier (0.1–3000 Hz bandpass; World Precision Instruments, Sarasota, FL, USA) 2 h a day at the same time over a one-week period. The data were digitized (1000 Hz) and analyzed using LabChart Pro v7 (ADInstruments, Bella Vista, New South Wales,

Australia). Behavioral seizure severity was evaluated according to Racine's scale [32]: 1, immobility, eye closure, twitching of vibrissae, sniffing, facial clonus; 2, head nodding associated with more severe facial clonus; 3, clonus of one forelimb; 4, rearing, often accompanied by bilateral forelimb clonus; and 5, rearing with loss of balance and falling accompanied by generalized clonic seizures. After recording (18 h after the last drug treatment), animals were used for Western blot.

2.4.2. Experiment II

Some non-responders in experiment I were given saline (i.p.) over a seven-day period. Thereafter, perampanel or GYKI 52466 was daily administered by the aforementioned method. Non-responders were also connected with Alzet 1007D osmotic pump (Alzet, Cupertino, CA, USA) containing vehicle or CsA (250 µM). The pump was placed in a subcutaneous pocket in the dorsal region. After recording (18 h after the last drug treatment), animals were used for Western blot.

2.5. Co-Immunoprecipitation

The hippocampal tissues were lysed in radioimmunoprecipitation assay buffer (RIPA: 50 mM Tris–HCl pH 8.0; 1% Nonidet P-40; 0.5% deoxycholate; 0.1% SDS, Thermo Fisher Scientific Korea, Seoul, South Korea) containing a protease inhibitor cocktail (Roche Applied Sciences, Branford, CT, USA), phosphatase inhibitor cocktail (PhosSTOP®, Roche Applied Science, Branford, CT, USA) and 1 mM sodium orthovanadate. Protein concentrations were calibrated by BCA protein assay (Pierce Chemical, Rockford, IL, USA) and equal amounts of total proteins were incubated with NEDD4-2, SGK1 or GluA1 antibody (Table 1) and protein G sepharose beads at 4 °C overnight. Beads were collected by centrifugation, eluted in 2× SDS sample buffer, and boiled at 95 °C for 5 min. Thereafter, Western blots for ubiquitin were performed.

2.6. Western Blot

Animals were sacrificed by decapitation, and their hippocampi were obtained and homogenized in lysis buffer containing protease inhibitor cocktail (Roche Applied Sciences, Branford, CT, USA) and phosphatase inhibitor cocktail (PhosSTOP®, Roche Applied Science, Branford, CT, USA). Thereafter, total protein concentration was calibrated using a Micro BCA Protein Assay Kit (Pierce Chemical, Rockford, IL, USA). Western blot was performed by the standard protocol: Sample proteins (10 µg) were separated on a Bis-Tris sodium dodecyl sulfate-poly-acrylamide gel (SDS-PAGE) and transferred to membranes. Membranes were incubated with 2% bovine serum albumin (BSA) in Tris-buffered saline (TBS; in mM 10 Tris, 150 NaCl, pH 7.5, and 0.05% Tween 20), and then reacted with primary antibodies (Table 1) overnight at 4 °C. After washing, membranes were incubated in a solution containing horseradish peroxidase (HRP)-conjugated secondary antibodies for 1 h at room temperature. Immunoblots were detected and quantified using an ImageQuant LAS4000 system (GE Healthcare Korea, Seoul, Korea). Optical densities of proteins were calculated with the corresponding amount of β-actin.

2.7. Data Analysis

The Shapiro–Wilk W-test was used to evaluate the normality values. Mann–Whitney U-test, Wilcoxon signed rank test, Student's t-test, and paired Student's t-test were applied to determine statistical significance of data. Comparisons among groups were also performed using repeated measures ANOVA, Friedman test and one-way ANOVA followed by Bonferroni's post hoc comparisons. A p-value less than 0.05 was considered to be significant.

Table 1. Primary antibodies used in the present study.

Antigen	Host	Manufacturer (Catalog Number)	Dilution Used
NEDD4-2	Rabbit	Abcam (ab131167): IP Abcam (ab46521): WB	1:100 (IP) 1:1000 (WB)
GRIA1	Mouse	Synaptic systems (#182011)	1:100 (IP) 1:1000 (WB)
p-NEDD4-2 S342	Rabbit	Cell signaling (#12146)	1:1000 (WB)
p-NEDD4-2 S448	Rabbit	Abcam (ab168349)	1:1000 (WB)
SGK1	Rabbit	ST John's Laboratory (STJ25513)	1:100 (IP) 1:1000 (WB)
p-SGK1 S78	Rabbit	Thermo (PA5-38392)	1:1000 (WB)
p-SGK1 S422	Rabbit	Abcam (ab55281)	1:1000 (WB)
Ubiquitin	Rabbit	Abcam(ab7780)	1:1000 (WB)
ERK1/2	Rabbit	Biorbyt (Orb160960)	1:1000 (WB)
p-ERK1/2	Rabbit	Bioss (bs-3330R)	1:1000 (WB)
PDK1	Rabbit	Cell signaling(#3062)	1:1000 (WB)
p-PDK1 S241	Rabbit	Cell signaling (#3061)	1:1000(WB)
AKT	Rabbit	Cell signaling (#9272)	1:1000 (WB)
pAKT S473	Rabbit	Cell signalling (#4060)	1:1000 (WB)
PP2A	Rabbit	Cell signaling (#2038)	1:5000 (WB)
p-PP2A Y308	Rabbit	Sigma (SAB4503975)	1:1000 (WB)
PP2B	Rabbit	Millipore (07-068-I)	1:1000 (WB)
p-PP2B S197	Rabbit	Badrilla (A010-80)	1:1000 (WB)
β-actin	Mouse	Sigma (#A5316)	1:5000 (WB)

IP, immunoprecipitation; WB, Western blot.

3. Results

3.1. AMPAR Antagonists Attenuate Spontaneous Seizure Activity in Responders

In epileptic rats, the total seizure frequency (number of seizures), the total electroencephalographic (EEG) seizure duration and average seizure severity (behavioral seizure core) were 12.6 ± 2.9, 945.8 ± 102 s and 3.7 ± 0.5 over a one-week period, respectively ($n = 7$, Figure 2A–C). In responders (showing the significant reduction in seizure activities), perampanel gradually reduced seizure frequency ($\chi^2_{(1)} = 5.1$, $p = 0.024$, Friedman test, $n = 7$), seizure duration ($F_{(1,12)} = 6.8$, $p = 0.022$, repeated measures ANOVA, $n = 7$) and the seizure severity ($\chi^2_{(1)} = 5.6$, $p = 0.018$ Friedman test, $n = 7$) over a one-week period (Figure 2A,B). The total seizure frequency was 6.57 ± 1.72 ($z = 3.07$, $p = 0.002$ vs. vehicle, Mann–Whitney U-test, $n = 7$), the total seizure duration was 538.3 ± 127 s ($t_{(12)} = 8.54$, $p < 0.001$ vs. vehicle, Student t-test, $n = 7$), and the average seizure severity was 1.9 ± 0.4 over a one-week period ($z = 3.14$, $p = 0.002$ vs. vehicle, Mann–Whitney U-test, $n = 7$; Figure 2C). Six out of thirteen rats in the perampanel-treated group were identified as non-responders whose seizure activities were uncontrolled by perampanel (total seizure frequency, 11.5 ± 1.9; total seizure duration, 909 ± 103.9 s; average seizure severity, 3.8 ± 0.2; Figure 2B,C).

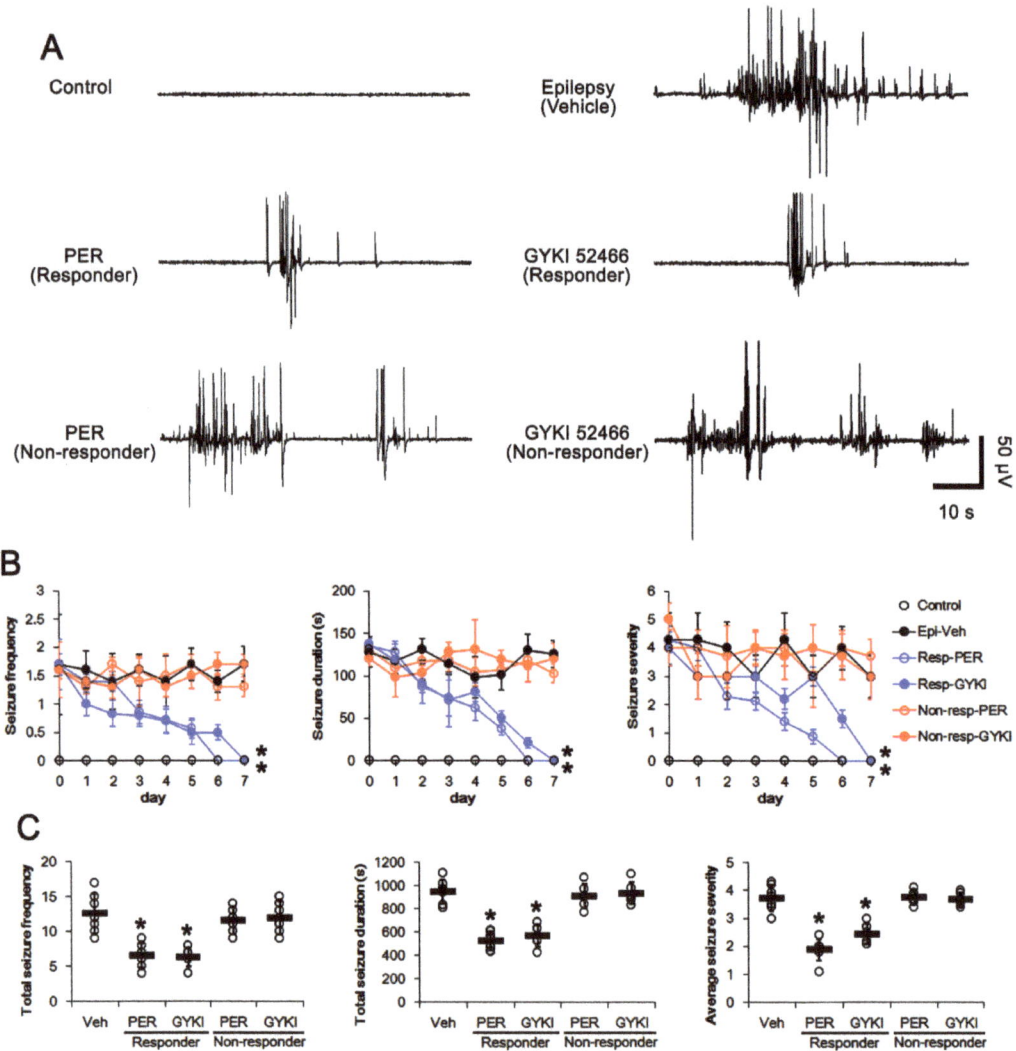

Figure 2. The effects of perampanel (PER) and GYKI 52466 (GYKI) on spontaneous seizure activities in chronic epilepsy rats. Both α-amino-3-hydroxy-5-methylisoxazole-4-propionic acid receptor (AMPAR) antagonists effectively attenuate spontaneous seizure activities in responders. (**A**) Representative electroencephalograms (EEG) in each group at 2 days after treatment. (**B**) Quantitative analyses of the chronological effects of AMPAR antagonists on seizure frequency, seizure duration and seizure severity (seizure score) over a seven-day period. Error bars indicate SD (* $p < 0.05$ vs. vehicle (Veh)-treated animals; Friedman test for seizure frequency and seizure severity; repeated measures ANOVA for seizure duration). (**C**) Quantitative analyses of seizure frequency, total seizure duration and average behavioral seizure score (seizure severity) over a seven-day period. Open circles indicate each individual value. Horizontal bars indicate mean value. Error bars indicate SD (* $p < 0.05$ vs. vehicle (Veh)-treated animals; Mann–Whitney U-test for seizure frequency and seizure severity; Student t-test for seizure duration).

GYKI 52466 also decreased seizure frequency ($\chi^2_{(1)} = 4.6$, $p = 0.033$, Friedman test, $n = 6$), total seizure duration ($F_{(1,11)} = 5.9$, $p = 0.033$, repeated measures ANOVA, $n = 6$), and seizure severity ($\chi^2_{(1)} = 4.7$, $p = 0.031$, Friedman test, $n = 6$) in responders over a one-week period (Figure 2A,B). In responders to GYKI 52466, the total seizure frequency was 6.3 ± 1.4 (z = 3.01, p = 0.001 vs. vehicle, Mann–Whitney U-test, n = 6), the total seizure duration was 571.2 ± 94.1 s ($t_{(11)}$ = 6.82, p < 0.001 vs. vehicle, Student t-test, n = 6), and the average seizure severity was 2.5 ± 0.4 over a one-week period (z = 2.94, p = 0.003 vs. vehicle, Mann–Whitney U-test, n = 6; Figure 2C). Six out of twelve rats in the GYKI 52466-treated group were identified as non-responders (total seizure frequency, 12 ± 2.4; total seizure duration, 935.2 ± 95.3 s; average seizure severity, 3.7 ± 0.2; Figure 2B,C).

3.2. AMPAR Antagonists Facilitates NEDD4-2-Mediated GRIA1 Ubiquitination by Enhancing NEDD4-2 S448 Phosphorylation in Responders

NEDD4-2 plays an important role in the regulation of seizure susceptibility, and its phosphorylation level is closely related to the maintenance of its stability, which modulates AMPAR functionality [17,33]. Thus, we explored whether AMPAR antagonists affect NEDD4-2 protein expression and its phosphorylation levels.

Consistent with previous studies [34], NEDD4-2 protein level was 39% lower in the epileptic hippocampus ($t_{(12)}$ = 14.2, p < 0.001 vs. control animals, Student t-test; Figure 3A,B and Figure S1), as compared to control animals. Compatible with its protein level, NEDD4-2 S342 and NEDD4-2 S448 phosphorylation levels were decreased to 0.61 ($t_{(12)}$ = 13.3, p < 0.001 vs. control animals, Student t-test) and 0.65 times ($t_{(12)}$ = 12.9, p < 0.001 vs. control animals, Student t-test) the control level in the vehicle-treated epilepsy rats, respectively (Figure 3A,C,D and Figure S1). The NEDD4-2 S342 and S448 phosphorylation ratios in epilepsy rats were similar to those in control animals (Figure 3E,F and Figure S1).

In responders to perampanel and GYKI 52466, NEDD4-2 protein levels were increased to 0.78 and 0.77 times the control level, respectively ($F_{(2,17)}$ = 35.8, p < 0.001 vs. vehicle, one-way ANOVA; Figure 3A,B and Figure S1). NEDD4-2 S342 phosphorylation level was unaffected by both AMPAR antagonists ($F_{(2,17)}$ = 1.4, p = 0.28 vs. vehicle, one-way ANOVA; Figure 3A,C and Figure S1). Due to upregulation of NEDD4-2 protein level induced by AMPAR antagonists, S342 phosphorylation ratios were reduced to 0.84 and 0.83 times the control level in perampanel and GYKI 52466-treated epilepsy rats, respectively ($F_{(2,17)}$ = 8.3, p = 0.003 vs. vehicle, one-way ANOVA; Figure 3A, E and Figure S1). However, perampanel and GYKI 52466 increased NEDD4-2 S448 phosphorylation level to 0.84 and 0.83 times the control level, respectively ($F_{(2,17)}$ = 47.9, p < 0.001 vs. vehicle, one-way ANOVA; Figure 3A,D). In contrast to NEDD4-2 S342 phosphorylation ratio, neither AMPAR antagonist altered NEDD4-2 S448 phosphorylation ratios ($F_{(2,17)}$ = 0.01, p = 0.99 vs. vehicle, one-way ANOVA; Figure 3A,F and Figure S1). In non-responders to perampanel and GYKI 52466, NEDD4-2 protein level and its S342 and S448 phosphorylation levels/ratios were unchanged by each compound (Figure 3A–F and Figure S1). Since phosphorylation stabilize NEDD4-2 against ubiquitination [17,35], we also investigated the effects of AMPAR antagonists on NEDD4-2 ubiquitination. In epileptic hippocampuses, NEDD4-2 ubiquitination (ubiquitin (Ub)-NEDD4-2 binding) was increased to 3.07 times the control level ($t_{(12)}$ = 11.2, p < 0.001 vs. control animals, Student t-test; Figure 3A,G and Figure S1), while GRIA1 ubiquitination was reduced to 0.58 times the control level ($t_{(12)}$ = 13.1, p < 0.001 vs. control animals, Student t-test; Figure 3A,H). In responders to perampanel and GYKI 52466, NEDD4-2 ubiquitination was reduced to 1.67 and 1.76 times the control level, respectively ($F_{(2,17)}$ = 38.8, p < 0.001 vs. vehicle, one-way ANOVA; Figure 3A,G and Figure S1). In contrast, GRIA1 ubiquitination was increased to 0.8 and 0.76 times the control level, respectively ($F_{(2,17)}$ = 20.7, p < 0.001 vs. vehicle, one-way ANOVA; Figure 3A,H and Figure S1). In non-responders to perampanel and GYKI 52466, ubiquitination of NEDD4-2 and GRIA1 were unaffected by each AMPAR antagonist (Figure 3A,G,H and Figure S1). Therefore, our findings indicate that the regulation of NEDD4-2-mediated GRIA1 ubiquitination may be relevant to the responsiveness to AMPAR antagonists that inhibit spontaneous seizure activity.

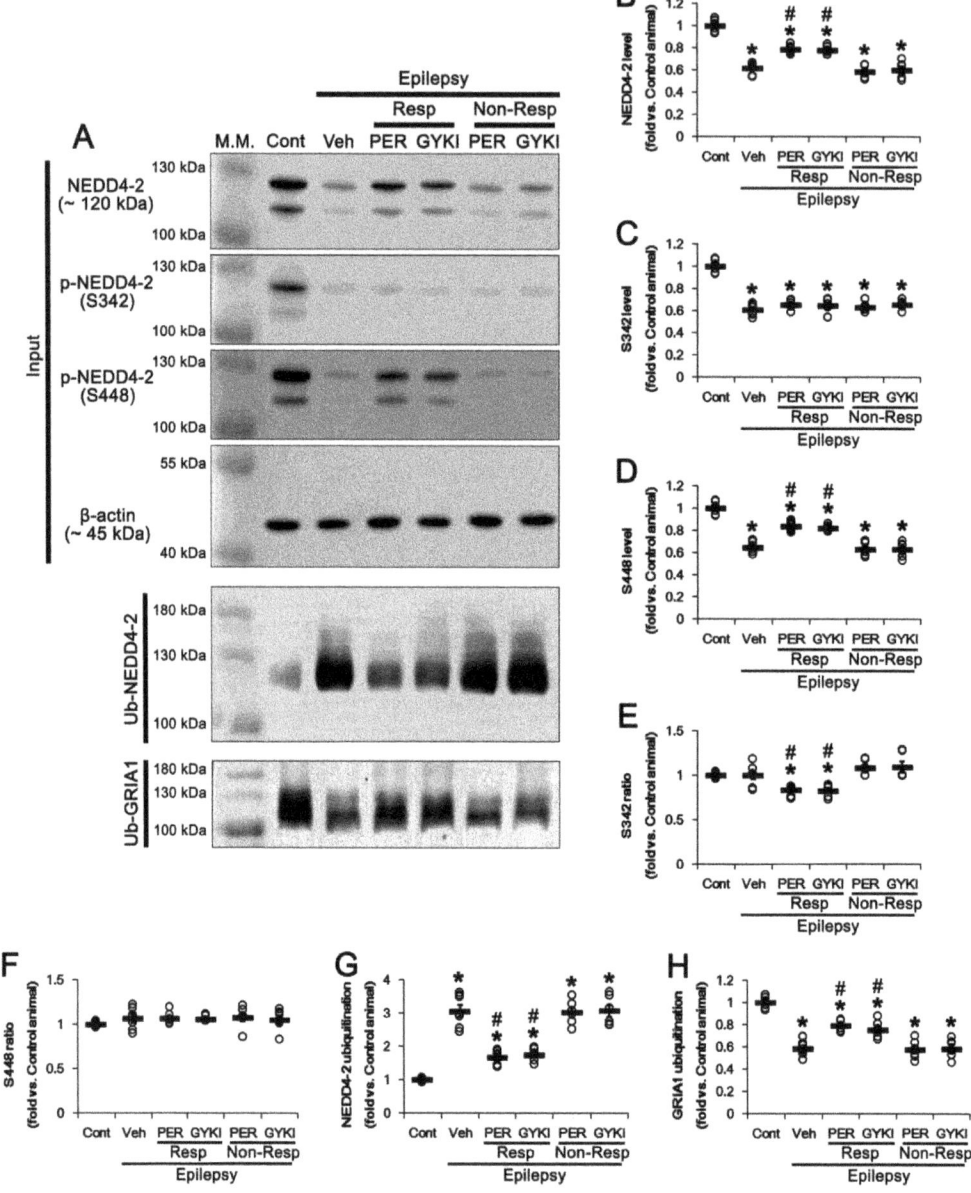

Figure 3. The effects of perampanel (PER) and GYKI 52466 (GYKI) on total NEDD4-2 protein expression/phosphorylation and ubiquitination of NEDD4-2 and GRIA1. (**A**) Representative images for Western blot of NEDD4-2 protein expression/phosphorylation and ubiquitination of NEDD4-2 and GRIA1 in the hippocampal tissues. (**B–F**) Quantifications of NEDD4-2 level (**B**), p-NEDD4-2 S342 level (**C**), p-NEDD4-2 S448 level (**D**), p-NEDD4-2 S342/NEDD4-2 ratio (**E**) and p-NEDD4-2 S448/NEDD4-2 ratio (**F**) in the hippocampal tissues. (**G–H**) Quantifications of the bindings of NEDD4-2 (**G**) and GRIA1 (**H**) with ubiquitin (Ub) in the hippocampal tissues. Open circles indicate each individual value. Horizontal bars indicate mean value. Error bars indicate SEM (*,# $p < 0.05$ vs. control and vehicle (Veh)-treated animals, respectively; one-way ANOVA with post hoc Bonferroni's multiple comparison).

3.3. AMPAR Antagonists Enhance SGK1 S78 Phosphorylation, but Not Protein Level, in Responders

Serum and glucocorticoid-regulated kinase 1 (SGK1) plays a key role in NEDD4-2 phosphorylation, and SGK1 and NEDD4-2 regulate one another in a reciprocal manner: SGK1-mediated NEDD4-2 phosphorylation increases SGK1 ubiquitination by NEDD4-2 [36]. Therefore, we investigated the effects of AMPAR antagonists on SGK1-NEDD4-2 interactions in chronic epilepsy rats.

In the epileptic hippocampus, SGK1 protein level was increased to 1.26 times the control level ($t_{(12)}$ = 7.5, $p < 0.001$ vs. control animals, Student t-test; Figure 4A,B and Figure S2). SGK1 S78 and S422 phosphorylation levels were decreased to 0.61 ($t_{(12)}$ = 14.9, $p < 0.001$ vs. control animals, Student t-test) and 0.43 times ($t_{(12)}$ = 18.5, $p < 0.001$ vs. control animals, Student t-test) the control level in epilepsy rats, respectively (Figure 4A,C,D). The SGK1 S78 and S422 phosphorylation ratios in epilepsy rats were reduced to 0.48 ($t_{(12)}$ = 24.3, $p < 0.001$ vs. control animals, Student t-test) and 0.34 times ($t_{(12)}$ = 25.8, $p < 0.001$ vs. control animals, Student t-test) the control level (Figure 4E,F and Figure S2).

In responders, both AMPAR antagonists restored SGK1 protein levels to control level ($F_{(2,17)}$ = 29.7, $p < 0.001$ vs. vehicle, one-way ANOVA; Figure 4A,B). Perampanel and GYKI 52466 also increased SGK1 S78 phosphorylation level to 0.79 and 0.75 times the control level, respectively ($F_{(2,17)}$ = 18.6, $p < 0.001$ vs. vehicle, one-way ANOVA; Figure 4A,C and Figure S2). The SGK1 S78 phosphorylation ratios were increased to 0.77- and 0.73 times the control level in perampanel and GYKI 52466-treated animals, respectively ($F_{(2,17)}$ = 36.5, $p < 0.001$ vs. vehicle, one-way ANOVA; Figure 4A,E). However, neither AMPAR antagonist affected the S422 phosphorylation level ($F_{(2,17)}$ = 0.1, $p = 0.92$ vs. vehicle, one-way ANOVA; Figure 4A,C,D and Figure S2) or its phosphorylation ratio ($F_{(2,17)}$ = 1.7, $p = 0.22$ vs. vehicle, one-way ANOVA; Figure 4E,F and Figure S2).

Unlike NEDD4-2, SGK1 ubiquitination was reduced to 0.52 times the control level in the epileptic hippocampus ($t_{(12)}$ = 14.4, $p < 0.001$ vs. control animals, Student t-test; Figure 4A,G). In responders to perampanel and GYKI 52466, SGK1 ubiquitination were 0.78 and 0.77 times the control level, respectively ($F_{(2,17)}$ = 19.6, $p < 0.001$ vs. vehicle, one-way ANOVA; Figure 4A,G and Figure S2). In non-responders to perampanel and GYKI 52466, SGK1 protein level, its S78 and S422 phosphorylation levels/ratios, and SGK1 ubiquitination were unaffected by each compound (Figure 4A–G and Figure S2). These findings indicate that AMPAR antagonists may selectively enhance SGK1 78 phosphorylation, which phosphorylates NEDD4-2 S448 site. Furthermore, considering NEDD4-2-mediated SGK1 ubiquitination [36], it is likely that upregulation of NEDD4-2 phosphorylation induced by AMPAR antagonists will lead to SGK1 ubiquitination.

3.4. AMPAR Antagonists Increases ERK1/2, but Reduces PDK1, Phosphorylation in Responders

Mitogen-activated protein kinase (MAPK)/extracellular signal-regulated kinase 1/2 (ERK1/2) and phosphatidylinositol 3-kinases (PI3K)/3-phosphoinositide-dependent protein kinase-1 (PDK1)/AKT pathways phosphorylate SGK1 at S78 and S422 sites, respectively [37–40]. In addition, PI3K/PDK1/AKT cascade directly phosphorylates NEDD4-2 [41]. Thus, we explored the effects of AMPAR antagonists on PDK1 and AKT activities (phosphorylation).

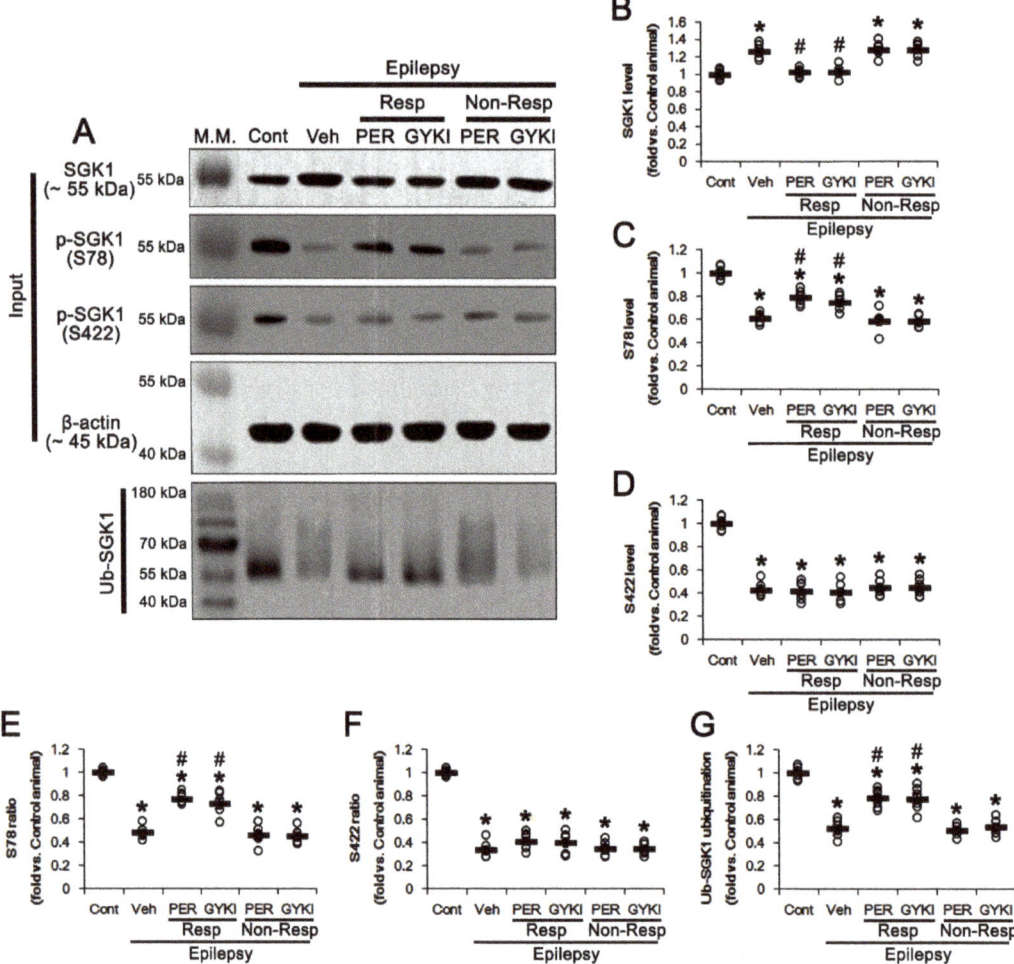

Figure 4. The effects of perampanel (PER) and GYKI 52466 (GYKI) on total SGK1 protein expression/phosphorylation and SGK1 ubiquitination. (**A**) Representative images for Western blot of SGK1 protein expression/phosphorylation and SGK1 ubiquitination in the hippocampal tissues. (**B–F**) Quantifications of SGK1 level (**B**), p-SGK1 S78 level (**C**), p-SGK1 S422 level (**D**), p-SGK1 S78/SGK1 ratio (**E**) and p-SGK1 S422/SGK1 ratio (**F**) in the hippocampal tissues. (**G**) Quantifications of the binding of SGK1 with ubiquitin (Ub) in the hippocampal tissues. Open circles indicate each individual value. Horizontal bars indicate mean value. Error bars indicate SEM (*,# $p < 0.05$ vs. control and vehicle (Veh)-treated animals, respectively; one-way ANOVA with post hoc Bonferroni's multiple comparison).

In the present study, ERK1/2 phosphorylation level and its ratio were decreased to 0.51 ($t_{(12)}$ = 11.6, $p < 0.001$ vs. control animals, Student t-test) and 0.52 times ($t_{(12)}$ = 10.9, $p < 0.001$ vs. control animals, Student t-test) the control level in epilepsy rats, respectively, without altering ERK1/2 protein level (Figure 5A–D and Figure S3). In contrast, PDK1 phosphorylation level and its ratio were increased to 1.55 ($t_{(12)}$ = 10.0, $p < 0.001$ vs. control animals, Student t-test) and 1.57 times ($t_{(12)}$ = 8.7, $p < 0.001$ vs. control animals, Student t-test) the control level in epilepsy rats, respectively, while PDK1 protein level was unchanged (Figure 5A,E–G and Figure S3). AKT phosphorylation level and its ratio were also increased to 1.8 ($t_{(12)}$ = 8.9, $p < 0.001$ vs. control animals, Student t-test) and 1.81 times ($t_{(12)}$ = 8.4,

$p < 0.001$ vs. control animals, Student t-test) the control level in epilepsy rats, respectively, without changing AKT protein level (Figure 5A,H–J and Figure S3).

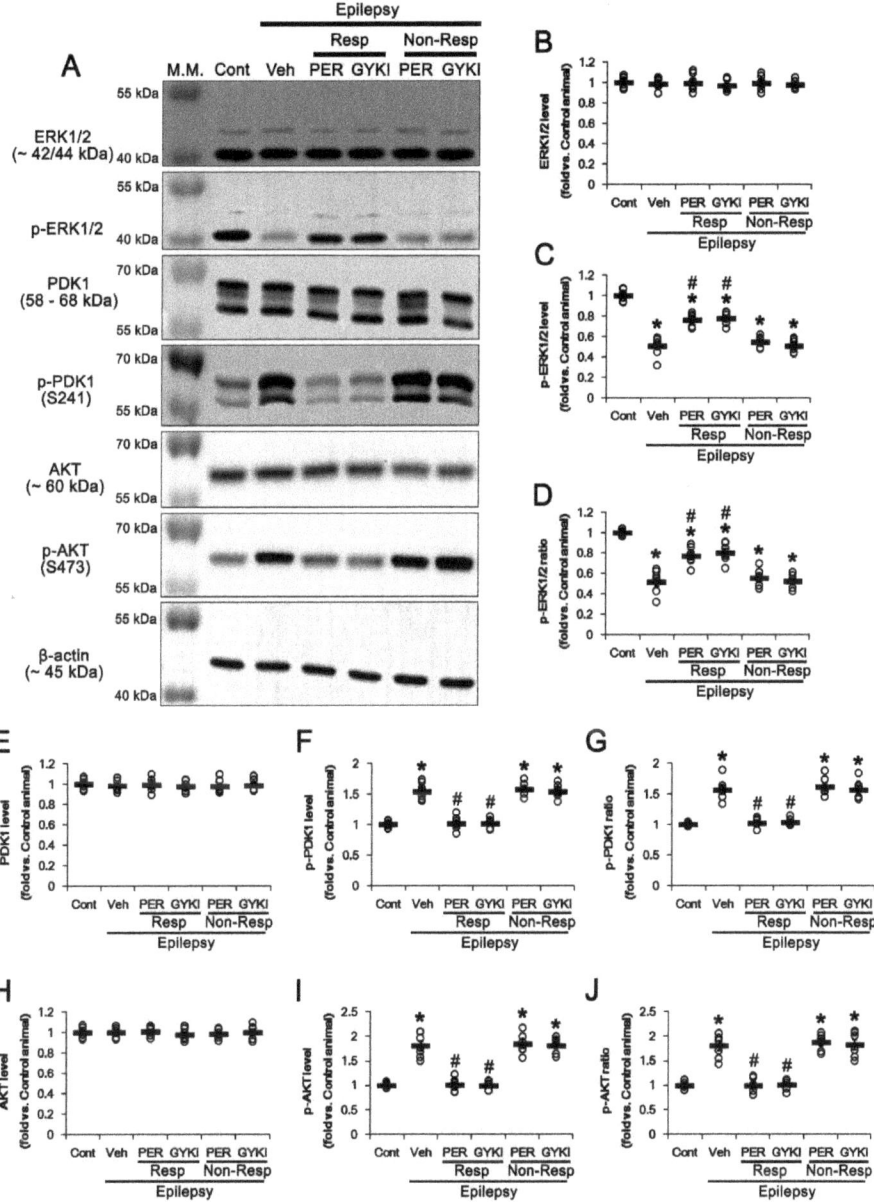

Figure 5. The effects of perampanel (PER) and GYKI 52466 (GYKI) on protein and phosphorylation levels of ERK1/2, PDK1 and AKT. (**A**) Representative images for Western blot of protein and phosphorylation levels of ERK1/2, PDK1 and AKT. (**B–J**) Quantifications of ERK1/2 level (**B**), p-ERK1/2 level (**C**), p-ERK1/2 ratio (**D**), PDK1 level (**E**), p-PDK1 level (**F**), p-PDK1 ratio (**G**), AKT level (**H**), p-AKT level (**I**) and p-AKT ratio (**J**) in the hippocampal tissues. Open circles indicate each individual value. Horizontal bars indicate mean value. Error bars indicate SEM (*,# $p < 0.05$ vs. control and vehicle (Veh)-treated animals, respectively; one-way ANOVA with post hoc Bonferroni's multiple comparison).

In responders, neither AMPAR antagonist affected ERK1/2 protein levels ($F_{(2,17)} = 0.3$, $p = 0.78$ vs. vehicle, one-way ANOVA; Figure 5A,B and Figure S3). However, perampanel and GYKI 52466 enhanced ERK1/2 phosphorylation level to 0.76 and 0.78 times the control level, respectively ($F_{(2,17)} = 26.9$, $p < 0.001$ vs. vehicle, one-way ANOVA; Figure 5A,C and Figure S3). The ERK1/2 phosphorylation ratios were also increased to 0.77 and 0.8 times the control level, respectively ($F_{(2,17)} = 15.6$, $p < 0.001$ vs. vehicle, one-way ANOVA; Figure 5A,D and Figure S3). In contrast to ERK1/2, both AMPAR antagonists restored PDK1 phosphorylation level ($F_{(2,17)} = 50.5$, $p < 0.001$ vs. vehicle, one-way ANOVA), PDK1 phosphorylation ratio ($F_{(2,17)} = 49.6$, $p < 0.001$ vs. vehicle, one-way ANOVA), AKT phosphorylation level ($F_{(2,17)} = 52$, $p < 0.001$ vs. vehicle, one-way ANOVA) and AKT phosphorylation ratio ($F_{(2,17)} = 45.4$, $p < 0.001$ vs. vehicle, one-way ANOVA) to control level without affecting their protein levels (Figure 5A,E–J and Figure S3). In non-responders, perampanel and GYKI 52466 did not result in these phenomena (Figure 5A–J and Figure S3). These findings indicate that AMPAR antagonists may increase NEDD4-2 S448 phosphorylation via ERK1/2-mediated SGK1 activation, independent of PI3K/PDK1/AKT signaling pathway.

3.5. Effects of AMPAR Antagonists on Protein Phosphatase Phosphorylation

Protein phosphatase 2A (PP2A) and protein phosphatase 2B (PP2B) inhibit ERK1/2 kinase activity by dephosphorylating threonine and tyrosine residues [42,43]. In our previous study [30], perampanel increases PP2B, but not PP2A, phosphorylation ratio (inactivation), while their expressions/phosphorylation ratios in epileptic animals are lower than those in normal animals. Since PP2A leads to SGK1 inactivation [44], we confirmed whether both AMPAR antagonists activate ERK1/2-medaited SGK1 S78 phosphorylation by inhibiting PP2B, but not PP2A.

Consistent with our previous study [30], the present study showed that PP2A protein level was 0.5 times the control level in the epileptic hippocampus ($t_{(12)} = 16.3$, $p < 0.001$ vs. control animals, Student t-test; Figure 6A,B and Figure S4). PP2A phosphorylation level and its ratio were 0.28 ($t_{(12)} = 26$, $p < 0.001$ vs. control animals, Student t-test) and 0.58 times ($t_{(12)} = 8$, $p < 0.001$ vs. control animals, Student t-test) the control level in epilepsy rats, respectively (Figure 6A,C,D and Figure S4). Similarly, PP2B protein level was reduced to 0.49 times the control level in the epileptic hippocampus ($t_{(12)} = 12.6$, $p < 0.001$ vs. control animals, Student t-test; Figure 6A,E and Figure S4). PP2B phosphorylation level and its ratio were decreased to 0.26 ($t_{(12)} = 30.3$, $p < 0.001$ vs. control animals, Student t-test) and 0.55 times ($t_{(12)} = 12.9$, $p < 0.001$ vs. control animals, Student t-test) the control level in epilepsy rats, respectively (Figure 6A,F,G and Figure S4). Since phosphorylation negatively regulates PP2A and PP2B activities [45,46], these findings indicate that PP2A and PP2B activities may be enhanced in the epileptic hippocampus as compensatory responses to downregulation of their protein levels.

In responders, neither AMPAR antagonist affected PP2A protein levels ($F_{(2,17)} = 0.3$, $p = 0.73$ vs. vehicle, one-way ANOVA), PP2A phosphorylation levels ($F_{(2,17)} = 0.1$, $p = 0.93$ vs. vehicle, one-way ANOVA) or its phosphorylation ratio ($F_{(2,17)} = 0.11$, $p = 0.89$ vs. vehicle, one-way ANOVA; Figure 6A–D and Figure S4). In contrast, perampanel and GYKI 52466 increased PP2B phosphorylation level to 0.45 and 0.44 times the control level (m, $p < 0.001$ vs. vehicle, one-way ANOVA), respectively, without altering its protein level (Figure 6A,E,F and Figure S4). Thus, PP2B phosphorylation ratios were enhanced to 0.88 and 0.89 times the control level in perampanel- and GYKI 52466-treated animals, respectively ($F_{(2,17)} = 32.7$, $p < 0.001$ vs. vehicle, one-way ANOVA; Figure 6A,G and Figure S4). In non-responders, perampanel and GYKI 52466 did not affect the protein and phosphorylation levels of these phosphatases (Figure 6A–G and Figure S4). These findings indicate that AMPAR antagonists may increase PP2B, but not PP2A, phosphorylation (inactivation), which would affect the ERK1/2-SGK1-NEDD4-2 signaling pathway.

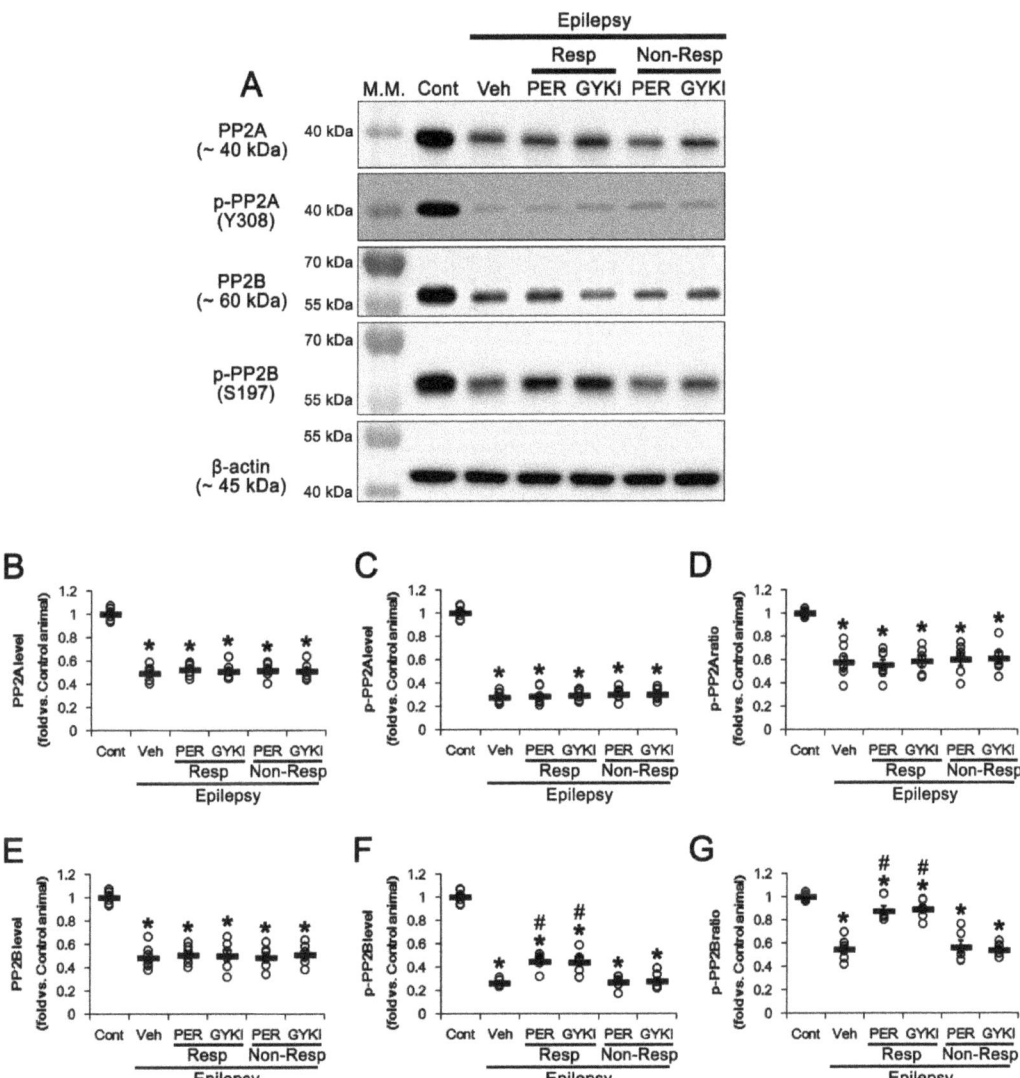

Figure 6. The effects of perampanel (PER) and GYKI 52466 (GYKI) on protein and phosphorylation levels of PP2A and PP2B. (**A**) Representative images for Western blot of protein and phosphorylation levels of PP2A and PP2B. (**B–G**) Quantifications of PP2A level (**B**), p-PP2A level (**C**), p-PP2A ratio (**D**), PP2B level (**E**), p-PP2B level (**F**) and p-PP2B ratio (**G**). Open circles indicate each individual value. Horizontal bars indicate mean value. Error bars indicate SEM (*,# $p < 0.05$ vs. control and vehicle (Veh)-treated animals, respectively; one-way ANOVA with post hoc Bonferroni's multiple comparison).

3.6. Co-Treatment of PP2B Inhibitor Increases the Efficacies of AMPAR Antagonists in Non-Responders

To confirm the role of the PP2B-ERK1/2-SGK1-NEDD4-2 signaling pathway in GRIA1 ubiquitination and refractory seizures to AMPAR antagonists, cyclosporin A (CsA, a PP2B inhibitor) was co-treated with perampanel or GYKI 52466 in non-responders. In non-responders to perampanel, total seizure frequency was 12.4 ± 3.1, total seizure duration was 946.4 ± 153.1 s, and average seizure severity was 4 ± 0.4 over a one-week period ($n = 5$, Figure 7A–C). In non-responders to GYKI 52466, total seizure frequency was 12 ± 2.7, total seizure duration was 908.8 ± 146.9 s, and average seizure severity was 3.8 ± 0.3 over a one-week period ($n = 5$, Figure 7A–C).

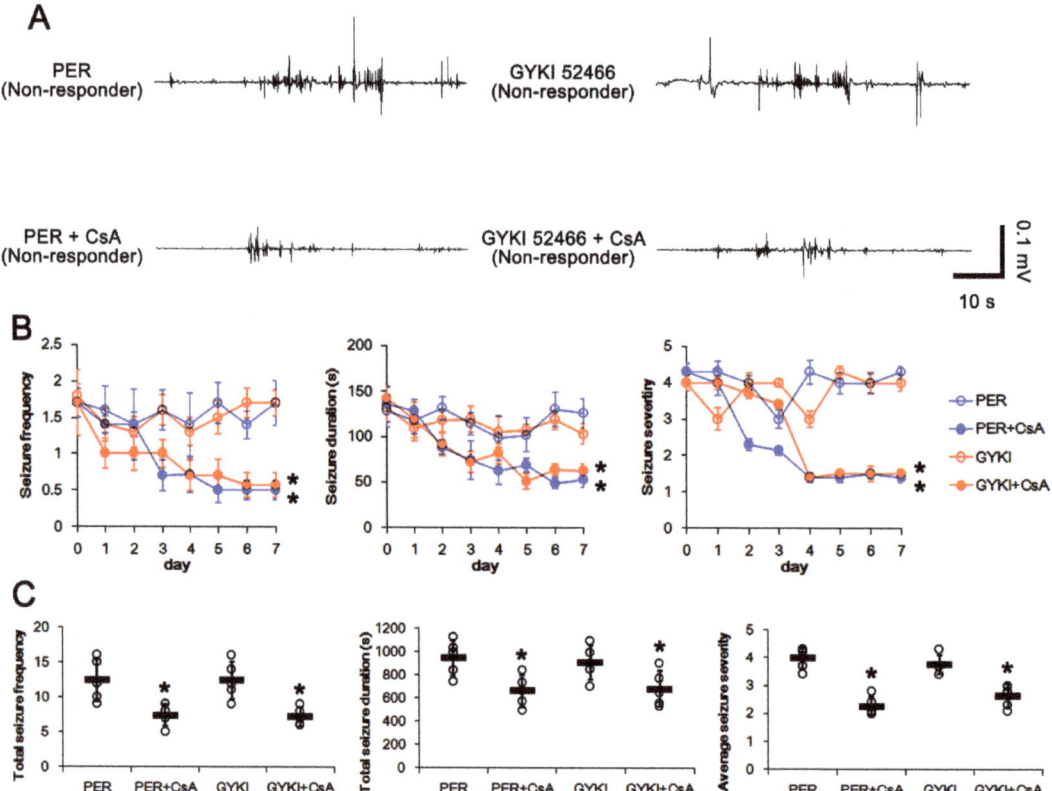

Figure 7. The effects of CsA co-treatment with perampanel (PER) and GYKI 52466 (GYKI) on spontaneous seizure activities in non-responders. CsA co-treatment effectively improves the anti-epileptic effects of both AMPAR antagonists in non-responders. (**A**) Representative electroencephalograms (EEG) in each group at two days after CsA co-treatment. (**B**) Quantitative analyses of the chronological effects of CsA co-treatment with AMPAR antagonists on seizure frequency, seizure duration and seizure severity (seizure score) over seven-day period. Error bars indicate SD (* $p < 0.05$ vs. vehicle (Veh)-treated animals; Friedman test for seizure frequency and seizure severity; repeated measures ANOVA for seizure duration). (**C**) Quantitative analyses of seizure frequency, total seizure duration and average behavioral seizure score (seizure severity) in seven-day period. Open circles indicate each individual value. Horizontal bars indicate mean value. Error bars indicate SD (* $p < 0.05$ vs. vehicle (Veh)-treated animals; Wilcoxon signed rank test for seizure frequency and seizure severity; paired Student t-test for seizure duration).

CsA co-treatment gradually decreased seizure frequency ($\chi^2_{(3)} = 8.4$, $p = 0.038$, Friedman test, $n = 5$), total seizure duration ($F_{(3,16)} = 4.2$, $p = 0.023$, repeated measures ANOVA, $n = 5$), and seizure severity ($\chi^2_{(3)} = 9.7$, $p = 0.021$, Friedman test, $n = 5$) in both perampanel- and GYKI 52466-treated groups over a one-week period (Figure 7A,B). In non-responders to perampanel, CsA co-treatment reduced the total seizure frequency to 7.4 ± 1.5 ($z = 2.02$, $p = 0.043$, Wilcoxon signed rank test, $n = 5$; Figure 7A,C), the total seizure duration to 660 ± 136.8 s ($t_{(4)} = 3.58$, $p = 0.02$, paired Student t-test, $n = 5$; Figure 7A,C), and average seizure severity to 2.3 ± 0.3 ($z = 2.03$, $p = 0.042$, Wilcoxon signed rank test, $n = 5$; Figure 7A,C). In non-responders to GYKI 52466, CsA co-treatment also attenuated the seizure frequency to 7.5 ± 1.3 ($z = 2.04$, $p = 0.041$, Wilcoxon signed rank test, $n = 5$;

Figure 7A,C), the total seizure duration to 680.8 ± 153.1 s ($t_{(4)}$ = 3.2, p = 0.03, paired Student t-test, n = 5; Figure 7A,C), and the seizure severity to 2.6 ± 0.4 (z = 2.02, p = 0.043 vs. vehicle, Wilcoxon signed rank test, n = 5; Figure 7A,C). Taken together, these findings indicate that dysregulation of the PP2B-ERK1/2-SGK1-NEDD4-2 signaling pathway may play an important role in the generation of refractory seizures to AMPAR antagonists.

3.7. CsA Co-Treatment Facilicates GRIA1 Ubiquitination in Non-Responders to AMPAR Antagonists

Next, we investigated whether CsA co-treatment influences ERK1/2- or AKT-mediated SGK1-NEDD4-2 regulation in non-responders to AMPAR antagonists.

CsA co-treatment did not affect ERK1/2 protein level in non-responders (Figure 8A,B). However, CsA co-treatment enhanced ERK1/2 phosphorylation to 0.82 and 0.78 times the control level in non-responders to perampanel ($t_{(8)}$ = 4.73, p = 0.001, Student t-test) and GYKI 52466 ($t_{(8)}$ = 4.9, p = 0.001, Student t-test), respectively (Figure 8A,B and Figure S5). Thus, CsA co-treatment increased ERK1/2 phosphorylation ratio in non-responders to perampanel ($t_{(8)}$ = 4.67, p = 0.002, Student t-test) and GYKI 52466 ($t_{(8)}$ = 5.88, p < 0.001, Student t-test), respectively (Figure 8A,B and Figure S5). CsA co-treatment restored the increased SGK1 protein level to control level in non-responders to perampanel ($t_{(8)}$ = 6.8, p < 0.001, Student t-test) and GYKI 52466 ($t_{(8)}$ = 6.2, p < 0.001, Student t-test), respectively (Figure 8A,C and Figure S5). However, CsA co-treatment enhanced SGK1 S78 phosphorylation to 0.78 and 0.77 times the control level in non-responders to perampanel ($t_{(8)}$ = 4, p = 0.004, Student t-test) and GYKI 52466 ($t_{(8)}$ = 4.8, p = 0.001, Student t-test), respectively (Figure 8A,C and Figure S5). CsA co-treatment increased the SGK1 S78 phosphorylation ratio to 0.77 and 0.74 times the control level in non-responders to perampanel ($t_{(8)}$ = 5.9 p < 0.001, Student t-test) and GYKI 52466 ($t_{(8)}$ = 5.8, p < 0.001, Student t-test; Figure 8A,C and Figure S5), respectively. In addition, CsA co-treatment increased NEDD4-2 protein level to 0.83- and 0.77 times the control level in non-responders to perampanel ($t_{(8)}$ = 6.7, p < 0.001, Student t-test) and GYKI 52466, respectively ($t_{(8)}$ = 5.1, p < 0.001, Student t-test; Figure 8A,D and Figure S5). CsA co-treatment enhanced NEDD4-2 S448 phosphorylation to 0.8 and 0.74 times the control level in non-responders to perampanel ($t_{(8)}$ = 7, p < 0.001, Student t-test) and GYKI 52466 ($t_{(8)}$ = 4, p = 0.004, Student t-test), respectively (Figure 8A,D and Figure S5). However, CsA co-treatment did not change AKT protein level and its phosphorylation level/ratio (Figure 8A,E and Figure S5). These findings indicate that the PP2B inhibition may improve anti-convulsive effects of AMPAR antagonists in non-responders by regulating ERK1/2-SGK1-NEDD4-2 signaling pathway without affecting AKT activity.

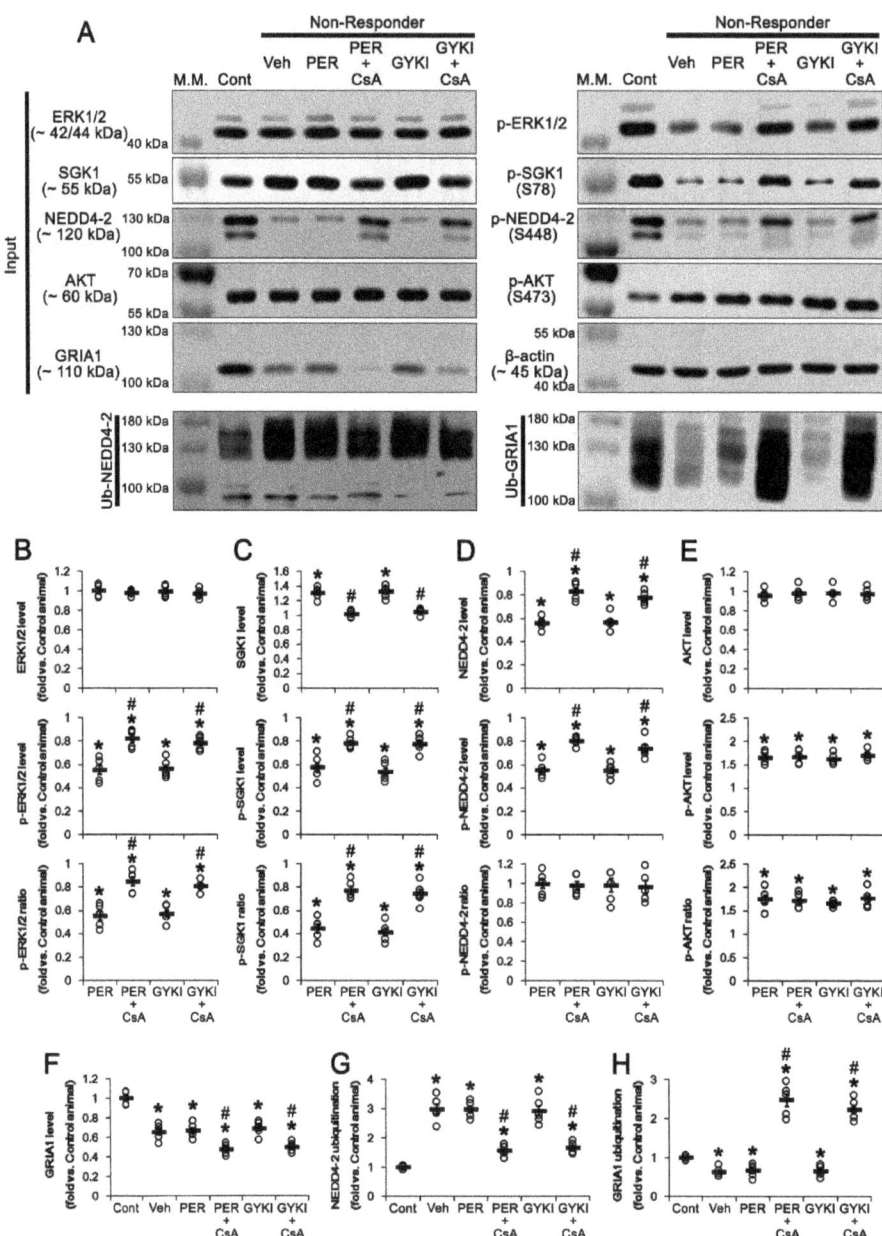

Figure 8. The effects of CsA co-treatment with perampanel (PER) and GYKI 52466 (GYKI) on expression/phosphorylation levels of ERK1/2, SGK1, NEDD4-2 and AKT, and ubiquitination of NEDD4-2 and GRIA1. (**A**) Representative images for Western blot of ERK1/2, SGK1, NEDD4-2 and AKT and ubiquitination of NEDD4-2 and GRIA1 in the hippocampal tissues. (**B–E**) Quantifications of protein level, phosphorylation level and phosphorylation ratio of ERK1/2 (**B**), SGK1 (**C**), NEDD4-2 (**D**) and AKT (**E**) in the hippocampal tissues. (**F–H**) Quantifications of GRIA1 level (**F**) and the bindings of NEDD4-2 (**G**) and GRIA1 (**H**) with ubiquitin (Ub) in the hippocampal tissues. Open circles indicate each individual value. Horizontal bars indicate mean value. Error bars indicate SEM (*,# $p < 0.05$ vs. control and vehicle (Veh)-treated animals, respectively; one-way ANOVA with post hoc Bonferroni's multiple comparison).

3.8. CsA Co-Treatment Reversely Regulates Ubiquitination of NEDD4-2 and GRIA1 in Non-Responders

Finally, we investigated whether PP2B inhibition affects ubiquitination of NEDD4-2 and GRIA1 in the hippocampus of non-responders, since perampanel reduces total GRIA1 protein level in responders and NEDD4-2 phosphorylation facilitates GRIA1 ubiquitination [4,10,17,26,30].

The present study shows that the total GRIA1 protein level in the epileptic hippocampus was 0.66 times the control level ($t_{(8)}$ = 7.3, p < 0.001 vs. control animals, Student t-test; Figure 8A,F and Figure S5). AMPAR antagonists did not affect GRIA1 protein level in non-responders (Figure 8A,F). CsA co-treatment decreased GRIA1 protein level to 0.48 and 0.5 times the control level in non-responders to perampanel ($t_{(8)}$ = 4.5, p = 0.002, Student t-test) and GYKI 52466 ($t_{(8)}$ = 4.7, p = 0.001, Student t-test), respectively (Figure 8A,F). Consistent with NEDD4-2 S448 phosphorylation, CsA co-treatment also reduced NEDD4-2 ubiquitination to 1.57 and 1.67 times the control level in non-responders to perampanel ($t_{(8)}$ = 9.2, p < 0.001, Student t-test) and GYKI 52466 ($t_{(8)}$ = 5.7, p = 0.004, Student t-test), respectively (Figure 8A,G and Figure S5). GRIA1 ubiquitination in the epileptic hippocampus was 0.64 times the control level ($t_{(8)}$ = 5.7, p < 0.001 vs. control animals, Student t-test; Figure 8A,H and Figure S5). AMPAR antagonists did not affect GRIA1 ubiquitination in non-responders (Figure 8A,H and Figure S5). However, CsA co-treatment increased GRIA1 ubiquitination to 2.48 and 2.23 times the control level in non-responders to perampanel ($t_{(8)}$ = 9, p < 0.001, Student t-test) and GYKI 52466 ($t_{(8)}$ = 11.5, p < 0.001, Student t-test), respectively (Figure 8A,H and Figure S5). These findings indicate that CsA may increase the responsiveness to AMPAR antagonists in non-responders by increasing NEDD4-2-mediated GRIA1 ubiquitination.

4. Discussion

Although the pathogenesis of MTLE has been studied for decades, the underlying mechanisms of intractable MTLE are still elusive. Recently, the dysregulation of ubiquitination has been considered as a potential factor for the generation of refractory epilepsy, since ubiquitination is involved in the modulation of synaptic function [47,48]. Ubiquitination is a posttranslational modification that degrades proteins through a sequential reaction by the ubiquitin-activating enzyme (E1), ubiquitin-conjugating enzyme (E2) and ubiquitin ligase enzyme (E3) [47,48]. Among E3 ubiquitin ligases, NEDD4-2 has been focused on for its dysregulation of cellular trafficking/endocytosis and lysosomal degradation of ion channels and transporters in MTLE [17,34]. Under physiological conditions, NEDD4-2 contributes to the elevation of spontaneous neuronal activity, particularly spontaneous spike frequency, when the AMPAR is activated [11]. Indeed, *NEDD4-2^{andi}* mice (in whom one of the major forms of NEDD4-2 in the brain is selectively deficient) are less sensitive to AMPAR activation but very sensitive to AMPAR inhibition. Briefly, the direct AMPAR stimulation by AMPA treatment elevates the synchrony of neuronal activity in wild-type mice more than *NEDD4-2^{andi}* mice. In contrast, *NEDD4-2^{andi}* mice are very sensitive to 2,3-dihydroxy-6-nitro-7-sulphamoyl-benzo(F)quinoxaline (NBQX, an AMPAR antagonist) with regard to spontaneous spike frequency, although average spontaneous spike amplitude and electrode burst activity do not differ after AMPA or NBQX treatment for either genotype [11]. Paradoxically, *NEDD4-2^{andi}* mice show a higher seizure susceptibility than kainic acid, which is recovered by the genetically reducing GRIA1 level [11]. Furthermore, kainic acid-induced seizure activity increases NEDD4-2 ubiquitination without altered GRIA1 surface expression [17]. In addition, the upregulated NEDD4-2 ubiquitination increases the latency of seizure onset and seizure progression in response to kainic acid, accompanied by reduced GRIA1 ubiquitination [17]. Therefore, it is likely that the dysregulated GRIA1/AMPAR-mediated intracellular signaling pathway, rather than the direct AMPAR functionality, may contribute to the dysfunction of NEDD4-2-mediated GRIA1 ubiquitination in the epileptic hippocampus. In the present study, NEDD4-2 protein level was lower in the epileptic hippocampus than that in the normal one, concomitant with decreased phosphorylation levels. AMPAR antagonists effectively increased NEDD4-2 protein and its S448 phosphorylation level in responders, but not in non-responders. Furthermore, AMPAR inhibitions decreased NEDD4-2 ubiquitination in responders. Since NEDD4-2 itself is a substrate of the ubiquitin-proteasome system, which is negatively regulated by phosphorylation [17,49], AMPAR antagonists may increase NEDD4-2 protein level by inhibiting its ubiquitination. Compatible with NEDD4-2 protein level, furthermore, GRIA1 ubiquitination was reduced in epilepsy rats as compared to control animals, which was restored by both AMPAR antagonists in responders. Although it could not be excluded that the higher clearance of AMPAR antagonists by multidrug efflux systems or the lower affinities of AMPAR antagonists on GRIA1 due to allosteric changes of AMPAR [23–25] would decrease the efficacies of AMPAR antagonists in non-responders, our findings indicate that maladaptive regulation of intracellular signaling pathways for NEDD4-2-mediated GRIA1 ubiquitination may be one of the important factors in pharmacoresistant seizures to AMPAR antagonists.

The binding of NEDD4-2 to substrates is differently regulated by phosphorylation. In the unphosphorylated state, NEDD4-2 binds to epithelial Na$^+$ channels (ENaC), Na$_V$1.6, KCNQ2/3 and KCNQ3/5, and facilitates their ubiquitination [12–15]. In the phosphorylated condition, however, NEDD4-2 preferentially potentiates the degradations of SGK1, GRIA1 and glutamate transporter-1 (GLT-1) [11,17,36,50]. Thus, it is likely that the phosphorylation status may contribute to switching the downstream substrate specificity of NEDD4-2, which is pending further investigation. SGK1 is a serine–threonine kinase that plays an important role in NEDD4-2 phosphorylation [51]. Interestingly, the enhanced SGK1-mediated NEDD4-2 phosphorylation decreases SGK1 protein levels in a dose-dependent manner by increasing SGK1 ubiquitination/degradation in the 26S proteasome. Thus, SGK1 and NEDD4-2 regulate one another in a reciprocal manner [36]. SGK1 protein level is upregulated in the temporal neocortex of patients with pharmacoresistant epilepsy and chronic epilepsy rats [52]. Consistent with this report, the present study shows that SGK1 protein level was increased, while its ubiquitination was reduced, in the epileptic hippocampus as compared to the normal (control) hippocampus. Furthermore, AMPAR antagonists restored SGK1 level to control level by increasing its ubiquitination and NEDD4-2 protein level in responders. Considering the reciprocal SGK1-NEDD4-2 interactions [36], these findings indicate that SGK1 upregulation may be relevant to the NEDD4-2 degradation in the epileptic hippocampus, which would be attenuated by AMPAR antagonists.

SGK1 is activated by phosphorylating S78 and S422 sites through MAPK-ERK1/2 and PI3K-PDK1-AKT pathways, respectively [37–40]. NEDD4-2 can also be directly phosphorylated by AKT [41]. Consistent with previous studies [4,10,30], the epileptic hippocampus showed upregulated PDK1-AKT phosphorylation and downregulated ERK1/2 phosphorylation, which were reversely regulated by AMPAR antagonists. However, both SGK1 S78 and S422 phosphorylation ratios were lower in epilepsy rats than those in control animals. In addition, AMPAR antagonists enhanced S78, but not S422, phosphorylation level in responders, although they inhibited the PDK1-AKT signaling pathway. Taken together, our findings suggest that reduced ERK1/2 activity (phosphorylation) may lead to dysregulation of SGK1-mediated NEDD4-2 activation, independent of PI3K-PDK1-AKT signaling cascade.

In the present study, PP2A and PP2B expressions in chronic epilepsy rats were lower than those in control animals. Furthermore, their phosphorylation ratios were also reduced in epilepsy animals. Since phosphorylation inhibits protein phosphatase activities [45,46], it is likely that the reduced phosphorylation ratios of PP2A and PP2B may be compensatory responses for maintenance of their activities against downregulation of expressions. Consistent with our previous study [30], furthermore, both AMPAR antagonists elevated PP2B phosphorylation in responders, indicating the decreased PP2B phosphatase activity. Considering that PP2A and PP2B deactivate ERK1/2 kinase activity [42,43], these findings indicate that AMPAR antagonists may enhance ERK1/2 phosphorylation by inhibiting PP2B activity. Indeed, CsA co-treatment improved the anti-epileptic effects of AMPAR antagonists in non-responders, concomitant with the increases in ERK1/2 and SGK1 S78 phosphorylation, NEDD4-2 protein level, NEDD4-2 S448 phosphorylation and ubiquitination of NEDD4-2 and GRIA1. Taken together, these findings indicate that dysregulation of PP2B-ERK1/2-SGK1 signaling pathway may play an important role in the generation of refractory seizures to AMPAR antagonists via impaired NEDD4-2-mediated GRIA1 ubiquitination.

PP2A also leads to SGK1 inactivation [44]. In the present study, however, neither AMPAR antagonist affected PP2A expression or its phosphorylation. Recently, we have reported that AMPAR antagonists inhibit casein kinase 2 (CK2) that binds to PP2A and increases PP2A activity [53]. Thus, the possibility that AMPAR antagonists may reduce CK2-PP2A-mediated SGK1 dephosphorylation in a phosphorylation-independent manner cannot be excluded.

Under physiological conditions, AMPARs contain the GRIA2 subunit, which are permeable to Na^+ and K^+, but not Ca^{2+} [54]. In chronic epilepsy rats, membrane GRIA1/GRIA2 ratio is significantly higher than that in control animals, indicating a preponderance of GRIA2-lacking (Ca^{2+}-permeable) AMPAR [4,10,26]. A higher expression of Ca^{2+}-permeable AMPAR in the epileptic hippocampus results in a subsequent elevated Ca^{2+} influx followed by PP2B activation [55–57]. AMPAR antagonists decrease GRIA1/GRIA2 ratio in responders by reducing GRIA1, but not GRIA2, surface expression [4,10,26]. The present study also demonstrates that AMPAR antagonists increased GRIA1 ubiquitination in responders, which indicates the decreased Ca^{2+}-permeable AMPAR level. Furthermore, the hyper-activation of AKT-glycogen synthase kinase 3β (GSK3β)-Ca^{2+}/cAMP response element-binding protein (CREB) pathway leads to increased Ca^{2+}-permeable AMPAR in non-responders [20,26], suggesting that dysregulation of AKT/GSK3β/CREB-mediated GRIA1 surface expression may also be responsible for the prolonged PP2B activation. Therefore, it is plausible that the increased Ca^{2+}-permeable AMPAR expression would be a fundamental reason for the lack of response to the AMPAR antagonists in the non-responders. However, the present data show that the lower efficacies of AMPAR antagonists to the PP2B-ERK1/2-SGK1-NEDD4-2-mediated GRIA1 ubiquitination and the inhibition of spontaneous seizure activities (presumably due to the higher clearance of AMPAR antagonists or the lower affinities of AMPAR antagonists on GRIA1 [23–25]) in non-responders were improved by CsA co-treatment. If the upregulated GRIA2-lacking AMPAR expression resulted in refractory seizures to AMPAR antagonists, CsA co-treatment would not inhibit seizure activity in non-responders, since a lack of effects of CsA on neuronal excitability and seizure activity is well known [30,58,59]. Therefore, our findings suggest that the upregulated GRIA2-lacking AMPAR expression in non-responders may not be a primary cause of intractable seizures to AMPAR antagonists (although it may be relevant to ictogenesis), but may be a consequence of the irresponsiveness to AMPAR antagonists. Moreover, PP2B inhibition may enhance the efficacies of AMPAR antagonists in non-responders by recovering the dysregulation of ERK1/2-SGK1-NEDD4-2-mediated GRIA1 ubiquitination and secondarily reducing Ca^{2+}-permeable AMPAR expression.

On the other hand, deubiquitination (the removal of ubiquitin moieties) also plays a role in AMPAR-mediated neurotransmission [60,61]. Ubiquitin-specific protease (USP) 46, a deubiquitinating enzyme, inhibits GRIA1 ubiquitination, accompanied by a decreased rate in GRIA1 degradation and an increase in AMPAR synaptic accumulation [60]. With respect to this, it is likely that downregulated GRIA1 deubiquitination may be involved in the intractable seizures to AMPAR antagonists, and CsA co-treatment would also inhibit deubiquitinases of GRIA1 in non-responders via unknown mechanisms. However, retigabine, an AED and a Kv7 channel opener, alleviates the acute stress-induced GRIA1 downregulation by increasing USP2 expression [61]. Therefore, further studies are needed to elucidate the role of GRIA1 deubiqutination in intractable seizures to AMPAR antagonists.

5. Conclusions

The present study reveals that AMPAR antagonists ameliorated spontaneous seizure activity by affecting the PP2B-mediated ERK1/2-SGK1-NEDD4-2 signaling pathway, which is relevant to the enhanced GRIA1 ubiquitination. In addition, the dysregulation of this pathway was one of the causes of refractory seizures to AMPAR antagonists. Therefore, our findings suggest that PP2B-ERK1/2-SGK1-NEDD4-2 pathway may be one of the potential therapeutic targets for the treatment of intractable TLE.

Supplementary Materials: The following are available online at https://www.mdpi.com/article/10.3390/biomedicines9081069/s1; Figure S1: Representative full-gel images of Western blots in Figure 3; Figure S2: Representative full-gel images of Western blots in Figure 4; Figure S3: Representative full-gel images of Western blots in Figure 5; Figure S4: Representative full-gel images of Western blots in Figure 6; Figure S5: Representative full-gel images of Western blots in Figure 8.

Author Contributions: J.-E.K. and T.-C.K. designed and supervised the project. J.-E.K., D.-S.L., H.P., T.-H.K. and T.-C.K. performed the experiments described in the manuscript. J.-E.K. and T.-C.K. analyzed the data and wrote the manuscript. All authors have read and agreed to the published version of the manuscript.

Funding: This study was supported by a grant from the National Research Foundation of Korea (NRF) grant (No. 2021R1A2C4002003 and No. 2021R1A2B5B01001482).

Institutional Review Board Statement: All experimental protocols were approved by the Animal Care and Use Committee of Hallym University (#Hallym 2018-2, 26 April 2018, #Hallym 2018-21, 8 June 2018 and #Hallym 2021-3, 27 April 2021).

Conflicts of Interest: The authors declare that the research was conducted in the absence of any commercial or financial relationships that could be construed as a potential conflict of interest. The funders had no role in the design of the study; in the collection, analyses, or interpretation of data; in the writing of the manuscript; or in the decision to publish the results.

References

1. Fiest, K.M.; Sauro, K.M.; Wiebe, S.; Patten, S.B.; Kwon, C.S.; Dykeman, J.; Pringsheim, T.; Lorenzetti, D.L.; Jetté, N. Prevalence and incidence of epilepsy: A systematic review and meta-analysis of international studies. *Neurology* **2017**, *88*, 296–303. [CrossRef] [PubMed]
2. Herman, S.T. Epilepsy after brain insult: Targeting epileptogenesis. *Neurology* **2002**, *59*, S21–S26. [CrossRef] [PubMed]
3. Sillanpää, M.; Schmidt, D. Natural history of treated childhood-onset epilepsy: Prospective, long-term population-based study. *Brain* **2006**, *129*, 617–624. [CrossRef] [PubMed]
4. Kim, J.E.; Park, H.; Lee, J.E.; Kim, T.H.; Kang, T.C. PTEN is required for the anti-epileptic effects of AMPA receptor antagonists in chronic epileptic rats. *Int. J. Mol. Sci.* **2020**, *21*, 5643. [CrossRef]
5. Löscher, W. Animal models of epilepsy for the development of antiepileptogenic and disease-modifying drugs. A comparison of the pharmacology of kindling and post-status epilepticus models of temporal lobe epilepsy. *Epilepsy Res.* **2002**, *50*, 105–123. [CrossRef]
6. Egbenya, D.L.; Hussain, S.; Lai, Y.C.; Xia, J.; Anderson, A.E.; Davanger, S. Changes in synaptic AMPA receptor concentration and composition in chronic temporal lobe epilepsy. *Mol. Cell. Neurosci.* **2018**, *92*, 93–103. [CrossRef]
7. Anggono, V.; Huganir, R.L. Regulation of AMPA receptor trafficking and synaptic plasticity. *Curr. Opin. Neurobiol.* **2012**, *22*, 461–469. [CrossRef]
8. Fritsch, B.; Stott, J.J.; Joelle Donofrio, J.; Rogawski, M.A. Treatment of early and late kainic acid-induced status epilepticus with the noncompetitive AMPA receptor antagonist GYKI 52466. *Epilepsia* **2010**, *51*, 108–117. [CrossRef]
9. Mohammad, H.; Sekar, S.; Wei, Z.; Moien-Afshari, F.; Taghibiglou, C. Perampanel but not amantadine prevents behavioral alterations and epileptogenesis in pilocarpine rat model of status epilepticus. *Mol. Neurobiol.* **2019**, *56*, 2508–2523. [CrossRef]
10. Kim, J.E.; Lee, D.S.; Park, H.; Kang, T.C. Src/CK2/PTEN-mediated GluN2B and CREB dephosphorylation regulate the responsiveness to AMPA receptor antagonists in chronic epilepsy rats. *Int. J. Mol. Sci.* **2020**, *21*, 9633. [CrossRef]
11. Zhu, J.; Lee, K.Y.; Jewett, K.A.; Man, H.Y.; Chung, H.J.; Tsai, N.P. Epilepsy-associated gene NEDD4-2 mediates neuronal activity and seizure susceptibility through AMPA receptors. *PLoS Genet.* **2017**, *13*, e1006634. [CrossRef]
12. Ekberg, J.A.; Boase, N.A.; Rychkov, G.; Manning, J.; Poronnik, P.; Kumar, S. Nedd4-2 (NEDD4L) controls intracellular Na(+)-mediated activity of voltage-gated sodium channels in primary cortical neurons. *Biochem. J.* **2014**, *457*, 27–31. [CrossRef]
13. Ekberg, J.; Schuetz, F.; Boase, N.A.; Conroy, S.J.; Manning, J.; Kumar, S.; Poronnik, P.; Adams, D.J. Regulation of the voltage-gated K(+) channels KCNQ2/3 and KCNQ3/5 by ubiquitination. Novel role for Nedd4-2. *J. Biol. Chem.* **2007**, *282*, 12135–12142. [CrossRef]

14. Goel, P.; Manning, J.A.; Kumar, S. NEDD4-2 (NEDD4L): The ubiquitin ligase for multiple membrane proteins. *Gene* **2015**, *557*, 1–10. [CrossRef]
15. Schuetz, F.; Kumar, S.; Poronnik, P.; Adams, D.J. Regulation of the voltage-gated K(+) channels KCNQ2/3 and KCNQ3/5 by serum- and glucocorticoid-regulated kinase-1. *Am. J. Physiol. Cell. Physiol.* **2008**, *295*, C73–C80. [CrossRef]
16. Yu, T.; Calvo, L.; Anta, B.; López-Benito, S.; López-Bellido, R.; Vicente-García, C.; Tessarollo, L.; Rodriguez, R.E.; Arévalo, J.C. In vivo regulation of NGF-mediated functions by Nedd4-2 ubiquitination of TrkA. *J. Neurosci.* **2014**, *34*, 6098–6106. [CrossRef] [PubMed]
17. Kim, J.E.; Lee, D.S.; Kim, M.J.; Kang, T.C. PLPP/CIN-mediated NEDD4-2 S448 dephosphorylation regulates neuronal excitability via GluA1 ubiquitination. *Cell Death Dis.* **2019**, *10*, 545. [CrossRef] [PubMed]
18. Epi4K Consortium; Epilepsy Phenome/Genome Project; Allen, A.S.; Berkovic, S.F.; Cossette, P.; Delanty, N.; Dlugos, D.; Eichler, E.E.; Epstein, M.P.; Glauser, T.; et al. De novo mutations in epileptic encephalopathies. *Nature* **2013**, *501*, 217–221. [PubMed]
19. Dibbens, L.M.; Ekberg, J.; Taylor, I.; Hodgson, B.L.; Conroy, S.J.; Lensink, I.L.; Kumar, S.; Zielinski, M.A.; Harkin, L.A.; Sutherland, G.R.; et al. NEDD4-2 as a potential candidate susceptibility gene for epileptic photosensitivity. *Genes Brain Behav.* **2007**, *6*, 750–755. [CrossRef]
20. Vanli-Yavuz, E.N.; Ozdemir, O.; Demirkan, A.; Catal, S.; Bebek, N.; Ozbek, U.; Baykan, B. Investigation of the possible association of NEDD4-2 (NEDD4L) gene with idiopathic photosensitive epilepsy. *Acta Neurol. Belg.* **2015**, *115*, 241–245. [CrossRef]
21. Kim, J.E.; Lee, D.S.; Kim, T.H.; Park, H.; Kim, M.J.; Kang, T.C. PLPP/CIN-mediated Mdm2 dephosphorylation increases seizure susceptibility via abrogating PSD95 ubiquitination. *Exp. Neurol.* **2020**, *331*, 113383. [CrossRef]
22. Kim, J.E.; Lee, D.S.; Kim, T.H.; Park, H.; Kim, M.J.; Kang, T.C. PLPP/CIN-mediated NF2-serine 10 dephosphorylation regulates F-actin stability and Mdm2 degradation in an activity-dependent manner. *Cell Death Dis.* **2021**, *12*, 37. [CrossRef] [PubMed]
23. Löscher, W.; Potschka, H. Blood-brain barrier active efflux transporters: ATP-binding cassette gene family. *NeuroRx* **2005**, *2*, 86–98. [CrossRef] [PubMed]
24. Vezzani, A.; Balosso, S.; Ravizza, T. Neuroinflammatory pathways as treatment targets and biomarkers in epilepsy. *Nat. Rev. Neurol.* **2019**, *15*, 459–472. [CrossRef]
25. Tang, F.; Hartz, A.M.S.; Bauer, B. Drug-resistant epilepsy: Multiple hypotheses, few answers. *Front. Neurol.* **2017**, *8*, 301. [CrossRef] [PubMed]
26. Kim, J.E.; Lee, D.S.; Park, H.; Kim, T.H.; Kang, T.C. Inhibition of AKT/GSK3β/CREB pathway improves the responsiveness to AMPA receptor antagonists by regulating GRIA1 surface expression in chronic epilepsy rats. *Biomedicines* **2021**, *9*, 425. [CrossRef] [PubMed]
27. Widagdo, J.; Chai, Y.J.; Ridder, M.C.; Chau, Y.Q.; Johnson, R.C.; Sah, P.; Huganir, R.L.; Anggono, V. Activity-Dependent Ubiquitination of GluA1 and GluA2 Regulates AMPA Receptor Intracellular Sorting and Degradation. *Cell Rep.* **2015**, *10*, 783–795. [CrossRef]
28. Lin, A.; Hou, Q.; Jarzylo, L.; Amato, S.; Gilbert, J.; Shang, F.; Man, H.Y. Nedd4-mediated AMPA receptor ubiquitination regulates receptor turnover and trafficking. *J. Neurochem.* **2011**, *119*, 27–39. [CrossRef] [PubMed]
29. Schwarz, L.A.; Hall, B.J.; Patrick, G.N. Activity-dependent ubiquitination of GluA1 mediates a distinct AMPA receptor endocytosis and sorting pathway. *J. Neurosci.* **2010**, *30*, 16718–16729. [CrossRef]
30. Kim, J.E.; Choi, H.C.; Song, H.K.; Kang, T.C. Perampanel affects up-stream regulatory signaling pathways of GluA1 phosphorylation in normal and epileptic rats. *Front. Cell. Neurosci.* **2019**, *13*, 80. [CrossRef] [PubMed]
31. Ko, A.R.; Kang, T.C. Blockade of endothelin B receptor improves the efficacy of levetiracetam in chronic epileptic rats. *Seizure* **2015**, *31*, 133–140. [CrossRef] [PubMed]
32. Racine, R.J. Modification of seizure activity by electrical stimulation. II. Motor seizure. *Electroencephalogr. Clin. Neurophysiol.* **1972**, *32*, 281–294. [CrossRef]
33. Lee, K.Y.; Jewett, K.A.; Chung, H.J.; Tsai, N.P. Loss of fragile X protein FMRP impairs homeostatic synaptic downscaling through tumor suppressor p53 and ubiquitin E3 ligase Nedd4-2. *Hum. Mol. Genet.* **2018**, *27*, 2805–2816. [CrossRef] [PubMed]
34. Wu, L.; Peng, J.; Kong, H.; Yang, P.; He, F.; Deng, X.; Gan, N.; Yin, F. The role of ubiquitin/Nedd4-2 in the pathogenesis of mesial temporal lobe epilepsy. *Physiol. Behav.* **2015**, *143*, 104–112. [CrossRef]
35. Chandran, S.; Li, H.; Dong, W.; Krasinska, K.; Adams, C.; Alexandrova, L.; Chien, A.; Hallows, K.R.; Bhalla, V. Neural precursor cell-expressed developmentally downregulated protein 4-2 (Nedd4-2) regulation by 14-3-3 protein binding at canonical serum and glucocorticoid kinase 1 (SGK1) phosphorylation sites. *J. Biol. Chem.* **2011**, *286*, 37830–37840. [CrossRef]
36. Zhou, R.; Snyder, P.M. Nedd4-2 phosphorylation induces serum and glucocorticoid-regulated kinase (SGK) ubiquitination and degradation. *J. Biol. Chem.* **2005**, *280*, 4518–4523. [CrossRef]
37. Kobayashi, T.; Cohen, P. Activation of serum- and glucocorticoid-regulated protein kinase by agonists that activate phosphatidylinositide 3-kinase is mediated by 3-phosphoinositide-dependent protein kinase-1 (PDK1) and PDK2. *Biochem. J.* **1999**, *339*, 319–328. [CrossRef]
38. Lee, C.T.; Ma, Y.L.; Lee, E.H. Serum- and glucocorticoid-inducible kinase1 enhances contextual fear memory formation through downregulation of the expression of Hes5. *J. Neurochem.* **2007**, *100*, 1531–1542.
39. Lee, C.T.; Tyan, S.W.; Ma, Y.L.; Tsai, M.C.; Yang, Y.C.; Lee, E.H. Serum- and glucocorticoid-inducible kinase (SGK) is a target of the MAPK/ERK signaling pathway that mediates memory formation in rats. *Eur. J. Neurosci.* **2006**, *23*, 1311–1320. [CrossRef]

40. García-Martínez, J.M.; Alessi, D.R. mTOR complex 2 (mTORC2) controls hydrophobic motif phosphorylation and activation of serum- and glucocorticoid-induced protein kinase 1 (SGK1). *Biochem. J.* **2008**, *416*, 375–385. [CrossRef]
41. Lee, I.H.; Dinudom, A.; Sanchez-Perez, A.; Kumar, S.; Cook, D.I. Akt mediates the effect of insulin on epithelial sodium channels by inhibiting Nedd4-2. *J. Biol. Chem.* **2007**, *282*, 29866–29873. [CrossRef]
42. Waskiewicz, A.J.; Cooper, J.A. Mitogen and stress response pathways: MAP kinase cascades and phosphatase regulation in mammals and yeast. *Curr. Opin. Cell Biol.* **1995**, *7*, 798–805. [CrossRef]
43. Gabryel, B.; Pudelko, A.; Adamczyk, J.; Fischer, I.; Malecki, A. Calcineurin and Erk1/2-signaling pathways are involved in the antiapoptotic effect of cyclosporin A on astrocytes exposed to simulated ischemia in vitro. *Naunyn. Schmiedebergs Arch. Pharmacol.* **2006**, *374*, 127–139. [CrossRef] [PubMed]
44. Park, J.; Leong, M.L.; Buse, P.; Maiyar, A.C.; Firestone, G.L.; Hemmings, B.A. Serum and glucocorticoid-inducible kinase (SGK) is a target of the PI 3-kinase-stimulated signaling pathway. *EMBO J.* **1999**, *18*, 3024–3033. [CrossRef] [PubMed]
45. Hashimoto, Y.; King, M.M.; Soderling, T.R. Regulatory interactions of calmodulin-binding proteins: Phosphorylation of calcineurin by autophosphorylated Ca^{2+}/calmodulin-dependent protein kinase II. *Proc. Natl. Acad. Sci. USA* **1988**, *85*, 7001–7005. [CrossRef] [PubMed]
46. MacDonnell, S.M.; Weisser-Thomas, J.; Kubo, H.; Hanscome, M.; Liu, Q.; Jaleel, N.; Berretta, R.; Chen, X.; Brown, J.H.; Sabri, A.K.; et al. CaMKII negatively regulates calcineurin-NFAT signaling in cardiac myocytes. *Circ. Res.* **2009**, *105*, 316–325. [CrossRef]
47. Schwarz, L.A.; Patrick, G.N. Ubiquitin-dependent endocytosis, trafficking and turnover of neuronal membrane proteins. *Mol. Cell. Neurosci.* **2012**, *49*, 387–393. [CrossRef] [PubMed]
48. Hallengren, J.; Chen, P.C.; Wilson, S.M. Neuronal ubiquitin homeostasis. *Cell Biochem. Biophys.* **2013**, *67*, 67–73. [CrossRef] [PubMed]
49. Bruce, M.C.; Kanelis, V.; Fouladkou, F.; Debonneville, A.; Staub, O.; Rotin, D. Regulation of Nedd4-2 self-ubiquitination and stability by a PY motif located within its HECT-domain. *Biochem. J.* **2008**, *415*, 155–163. [CrossRef] [PubMed]
50. García-Tardón, N.; González-González, I.M.; Martínez-Villarreal, J.; Fernández-Sánchez, E.; Giménez, C.; Zafra, F. Protein kinase C (PKC)-promoted endocytosis of glutamate transporter GLT-1 requires ubiquitin ligase Nedd4-2-dependent ubiquitination but not phosphorylation. *J. Biol. Chem.* **2012**, *287*, 19177–19187. [CrossRef]
51. Snyder, P.M.; Olson, D.R.; Kabra, R.; Zhou, R.; Steines, J.C. cAMP and serum and glucocorticoid-inducible kinase (SGK) regulate the epithelial Na^+ channel through convergent phosphorylation of Nedd4-2. *J. Biol. Chem.* **2004**, *279*, 45753–45758. [CrossRef]
52. Wang, L.; Zhou, C.; Zhu, Q.; Luo, J.; Xu, Y.; Huang, Y.; Zhang, X.; Wang, X. Upregulation of serum- and glucocorticoid-induced protein kinase 1 in the brain tissue of human and experimental epilepsy. *Neurochem. Int.* **2010**, *57*, 899–905. [CrossRef]
53. Pérez, M.; Avila, J. The expression of casein kinase 2α' and phosphatase 2A activity. *Biochim. Biophys. Acta* **1999**, *1449*, 150–156. [CrossRef]
54. Pellegrini-Giampietro, D.E.; Gorter, J.A.; Bennett, M.V.; Zukin, R.S. The GluR2 (GluR-B) hypothesis: Ca^{2+}-permeable AMPA receptors in neurological disorders. *Trends Neurosci.* **1997**, *20*, 464–470. [CrossRef]
55. Hell, J.W. How Ca^{2+}-permeable AMPA receptors, the kinase PKA, and the phosphatase PP2B are intertwined in synaptic LTP and LTD. *Sci. Signal.* **2016**, *9*, e2. [CrossRef] [PubMed]
56. Ma, Y.; Sun, X.; Li, J.; Jia, R.; Yuan, F.; Wei, D.; Jiang, W. Melatonin Alleviates the Epilepsy-Associated Impairments in Hippocampal LTP and Spatial Learning Through Rescue of Surface GluR2 Expression at Hippocampal CA1 Synapses. *Neurochem. Res.* **2017**, *42*, 1438–1448. [CrossRef]
57. Lorgen, J.Ø.; Egbenya, D.L.; Hammer, J.; Davanger, S. PICK1 facilitates lasting reduction in GluA2 concentration in the hippocampus during chronic epilepsy. *Epilepsy Res.* **2017**, *137*, 25–32. [CrossRef] [PubMed]
58. Taubøll, E.; Gerdts, R.; Gjerstad, L. Cyclosporin A and brain excitability studied in vitro. *Epilepsia* **1998**, *39*, 687–691. [CrossRef] [PubMed]
59. Handreck, A.; Mall, E.M.; Elger, D.A.; Gey, L.; Gernert, M. Different preparations, doses, and treatment regimens of cyclosporine A cause adverse effects but no robust changes in seizure thresholds in rats. *Epilepsy Res.* **2015**, *112*, 1–17. [CrossRef]
60. Huo, Y.; Khatri, N.; Hou, Q.; Gilbert, J.; Wang, G.; Man, H.Y. The deubiquitinating enzyme USP46 regulates AMPA receptor ubiquitination and trafficking. *J. Neurochem.* **2015**, *134*, 1067–1080. [CrossRef]
61. Li, C.; Zhang, J.; Xu, H.; Chang, M.; Lv, C.; Xue, W.; Song, Z.; Zhang, L.; Zhang, X.; Tian, X. Retigabine ameliorates acute stress-induced impairment of spatial memory retrieval through regulating USP2 signaling pathways in hippocampal CA1 area. *Neuropharmacology* **2018**, *135*, 151–162. [CrossRef] [PubMed]

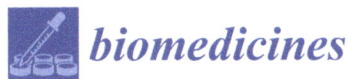

Article

Inhibition of AKT/GSK3β/CREB Pathway Improves the Responsiveness to AMPA Receptor Antagonists by Regulating GRIA1 Surface Expression in Chronic Epilepsy Rats

Ji-Eun Kim, Duk-Shin Lee, Hana Park, Tae-Hyun Kim and Tae-Cheon Kang *

Department of Anatomy and Neurobiology, Institute of Epilepsy Research, College of Medicine, Hallym University, Chuncheon 24252, Korea; jieunkim@hallym.ac.kr (J.-E.K.); dslee84@hallym.ac.kr (D.-S.L.); M19050@hallym.ac.kr (H.P.); hyun1028@hallym.ac.kr (T.-H.K.)
* Correspondence: tckang@hallym.ac.kr; Tel.: +82-33-248-2524; Fax: +82-33-248-2525

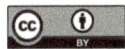

Citation: Kim, J.-E.; Lee, D.-S.; Park, H.; Kim, T.-H.; Kang, T.-C. Inhibition of AKT/GSK3β/CREB Pathway Improves the Responsiveness to AMPA Receptor Antagonists by Regulating GRIA1 Surface Expression in Chronic Epilepsy Rats. *Biomedicines* 2021, 9, 425. https://doi.org/10.3390/biomedicines9040425

Academic Editor: Prosper N'Gouemo

Received: 26 March 2021
Accepted: 13 April 2021
Published: 14 April 2021

Publisher's Note: MDPI stays neutral with regard to jurisdictional claims in published maps and institutional affiliations.

Copyright: © 2021 by the authors. Licensee MDPI, Basel, Switzerland. This article is an open access article distributed under the terms and conditions of the Creative Commons Attribution (CC BY) license (https://creativecommons.org/licenses/by/4.0/).

Abstract: α-Amino-3-hydroxy-5-methylisoxazole-4-propionic acid receptor (AMPAR) has been reported as one of the targets for treatment of epilepsy. Although maladaptive regulation of surface expression of glutamate ionotropic receptor AMPA type subunit 1 (GRIA1) subunit is relevant to the responsiveness to AMPAR antagonists (perampanel and GYKI 52466) in LiCl-pilocarpine-induced chronic epilepsy rats, the underlying mechanisms of refractory seizures to AMPAR antagonists have yet been unclear. In the present study, we found that both AMPAR antagonists restored the up-regulations of GRIA1 surface expression and Src family-mediated glycogen synthase kinase 3β (GSK3β)-Ca^{2+}/cAMP response element-binding protein (CREB) phosphorylations to control levels in responders (whose seizure activities were responsive to AMPAR) but not non-responders (whose seizure activities were uncontrolled by AMPAR antagonists). In addition, 3-chloroacetyl indole (3CAI, an AKT inhibitor) co-treatment attenuated spontaneous seizure activities in non-responders, accompanied by reductions in AKT/GSK3β/CREB phosphorylations and GRIA1 surface expression. Although AMPAR antagonists reduced GRIA2 tyrosine (Y) phosphorylations in responders, they did not affect GRIA2 surface expression and protein interacting with C kinase 1 (PICK1) protein level in both responders and non-responders. Therefore, our findings suggest that dysregulation of AKT/GSK3β/CREB-mediated GRIA1 surface expression may be responsible for refractory seizures in non-responders, and that this pathway may be a potential target to improve the responsiveness to AMPAR antagonists.

Keywords: 3CAI; GRIA1; GRIA2; intractable epilepsy; PICK1; protein kinase C

1. Introduction

Epilepsy is a common clinical neurological disease characterized by spontaneous seizures due to abnormal neuronal discharges. Over decades, the incidence of epilepsy presents an increasing tendency with a reported number of 65 million patients worldwide. About 30% temporal lobe epilepsy (TLE) patients show refractory seizures that are uncontrolled by standard medications with antiepileptic drugs (AEDs). In addition, patients with intractable seizures have a high mortality rate [1,2]. Given the inefficacy of AEDs and the unrelenting nature of intractable epilepsy, therefore, the necessity to explore the underlying mechanisms of generation of refractory seizures is undoubted.

Although the pathogenesis of epilepsy remains to be fully elucidated, hyper-activation of the glutamate receptor is one of the important causes of epilepsy. A massive release of glutamate and the subsequent over-activation of glutamate receptors cause aberrant neuronal hyper-excitability, followed by delayed neuronal death and secondary injury [3,4]. Recently, α-amino-3-hydroxy-5-methylisoxazole-4-propionic acid receptor (AMPAR) has been focused on as one of the major therapeutic targets for treatment of epilepsy [5] since AMPAR antagonists, but not N-methyl-D-aspartate receptor (NMDAR) antagonists, terminate status epilepticus (SE, a prolonged seizure activity) and seizure activity in animal models and preferentially suppress seizure-related long-term consequences [6–8].

AMPAR is one of the ionotropic glutamate receptors, which exists as a homomeric or heteromeric assembly of four subunits (glutamate ionotropic receptor AMPA type subunit (GRIA) 1–4) encoded by different genes [9]. GRIA subunits preferentially dimerize soon after the translocation in the endoplasmic reticulum (ER) and tetramerize prior to ER exit [10]. Activity-dependent phosphorylation/dephosphorylation of intracellular C-terminal sites on the AMPAR subunits GRIA1 and GRIA2 regulate their synaptic trafficking and functional properties [11,12]: Phosphorylation of GRIA1 at serine (S) 831 and/or S845 sites increases both open channel conductance and its surface expression [13,14]. In contrast, GRIA2 S880 phosphorylation facilitates its internalization [15]. Interestingly, GRIA2 subunit regulates the ion-permeable properties of AMPAR. GRIA2-containing AMPAR is permeable to Na^+ and K^+ but not Ca^{2+}. In contrast, GRIA2-lacking AMPAR is highly permeable to Ca^{2+}, which activates a series of intracellular protein kinases or immediate early genes. In the hippocampus of epileptic animals, GRIA2 surface expression is decreased [16,17], while >95% of AMPARs contain the GRIA2 subunit under physiological conditions [18]. Therefore, it is likely that increased membrane GRIA1/GRIA2 ratio may be an important component of the ictogenesis and the seizure-associated consequences by leading to a high Ca^{2+} permeability of AMPAR in the epileptic brain. Indeed, we have reported that membrane GRIA1/GRIA2 ratio is significantly higher in chronic epilepsy rats than that in control animals, indicating the existing preponderance of Ca^{2+}-permeable AMPAR, although both GRIA1 and GRIA2 levels are lower in the hippocampus. In addition, AMPAR antagonists (perampanel and GYKI 52466) decrease membrane GRIA1/GRIA2 ratio by reducing GRIA1, but not GRIA2, surface expression [19,20]. These effects of AMPAR antagonists are relevant to Src family/casein kinase 2 (CK2)/phosphatase and tensin homolog deleted on chromosome ten (PTEN)-mediated Ca^{2+}/cAMP response element-binding protein (CREB) S133 phosphorylation, which are observed in responders (whose seizure activities are responsive to AMPA antagonists), but not non-responders (whose seizure activities are not uncontrolled) [19]. However, the up-stream signaling pathways regulating membrane GRIA1/GRIA2 ratio in the epileptic hippocampus have yet been elusive.

On the other hand, GRIA2 phosphorylations regulate their surface expression through interactions with glutamate receptor interacting protein 1 (GRIP1) and protein interacting with C kinase 1 (PICK1) that contains the postsynaptic density-95/Discs large/zona occludens-1 (PDZ) domain. GRIP1 enhances GRIA2 surface expression, whereas PICK1 facilitates its internalization [21,22]. Src family-mediated GRIA2 phosphorylations on tyrosine (Y) 869, Y873, and Y876 sites destabilize its interaction with GRIP1 and allow more GRIA2–PICK1 binding to promote its internalization [23,24]. In addition, protein kinase C (PKC)-mediated S880 phosphorylation also decreases GRIA2 binding to GRIP1, but not to PICK1, and results in rapid GRIA2 internalization [21]. However, the regulations of the GRIA2 subunit phosphorylations in response to AMPAR antagonists in the epileptic hippocampus are largely unknown. In an effort to understand the pathogenesis of intractable epilepsy, therefore, it will be noteworthy to more specifically investigate the underlying mechanisms of refractory seizures to AMPAR antagonists.

Here, we demonstrated that the anti-convulsive effects of AMPAR antagonists were closely relevant to the regulation of AKT/glycogen synthase kinase 3β (GSK3β)/CREB-mediated GRIA1 surface expression rather than the modulation of PICK1–GRIA2 internalization. In addition, impairment of this signaling pathway resulted in refractory seizures in response to AMPAR antagonists, which were improved by 3-chloroacetyl indole (3CAI, an AKT inhibitor) co-treatment. Therefore, our findings suggest that AKT/GSK3β/CREB pathway may be a potential therapeutic strategy to improve the treatment of intractable TLE in response to AMPAR antagonists.

2. Materials and Methods

2.1. Experimental Animals and Chemicals

Male Sprague–Dawley (SD) rats (7 weeks old) were provided with a commercial diet and water ad libitum under controlled temperature, humidity, and lighting conditions (22 ± 2 °C, $55 \pm 5\%$ and a 12:12 light/dark cycle with lights). Animal protocols were approved by the Institutional Animal Care and Use Committee of Hallym University (Hallym 2018-2, 26 April 2018 and Hallym 2018-21, 8 June 2018). All reagents were purchased from Sigma-Aldrich (St. Louis, MO, USA), except as noted.

2.2. Generation of Chronic Epilepsy Rats

Figure 1 illustrates the design of the drug trial methodology, which was a modified protocol based on Ko and Kang [25]. Animals were intraperitoneally (i.p.) given LiCl (127 mg/kg) 24 h before the pilocarpine treatment. Animals were treated with pilocarpine (30 mg/kg, i.p.) 20 min after atropine methylbromide (5 mg/kg i.p.). Two hours after SE on-set, animals were administered diazepam (Valium; Hoffman la Roche, Neuilly sur-Seine, France; 10 mg/kg, i.p.) and dosage was repeated, as needed. Control animals received saline in place of pilocarpine. Animals were video-monitored 8 h a day for general behavior and occurrence of spontaneous seizures by 4 weeks after SE induction. Behavioral seizure severity was evaluated according to Racine's scale [26]: 1, immobility, eye closure, twitching of vibrissae, sniffing, facial clonus; 2, head nodding associated with more severe facial clonus; 3, clonus of one forelimb; 4, rearing, often accompanied by bilateral forelimb clonus; and 5, rearing with loss of balance and falling accompanied by generalized clonic seizures. We classified chronic epilepsy rats that showed behavioral seizures with seizure score ≥ 3 more than once.

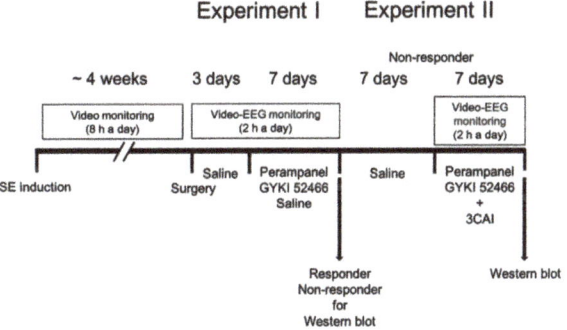

Figure 1. Scheme of the experimental design in the present study.

2.3. Surgery

Control and epilepsy rats were implanted with monopolar stainless steel electrodes (Plastics One, Roanoke, VA, USA) in the right hippocampus (stereotaxic coordinates were -3.8 mm posterior; 2.0 mm lateral; -2.6 mm depth to bregma) under Isoflurane anesthesia (3% induction, 1.5–2% for surgery, and 1.5% maintenance in a 65:35 mixture of $N_2O:O_2$). Animals were also implanted with a brain infusion kit 1 (Alzet, Cupertino, CA, USA) to infuse with 3CAI (an AKT inhibitor, 25 µM) into the right lateral ventricle (1 mm posterior; 1.5 mm lateral; -3.5 mm depth to the bregma, see below). Throughout surgery, core temperature of each rat was maintained at 37–38 °C. Electrode was secured to the exposed skull with dental acrylic.

2.4. Drug Trials, EEG Analysis and Quantification of Behavioral Seizure Activity

2.4.1. Experiment I

After baseline seizure activity was determined over 3 days, perampanel (2-(2-oxo-1-phenyl-5-pyridin-2-yl-1,2-dihydropyridin-3-yl)benzonitrile; 8 mg/kg, i.p, Eisai Korea Inc, Seoul, South Korea), GYKI 52466 (1-(4-aminophenyl)-4-methyl-7,8-methylenedioxy-5H-2,3-benzodiazepine hydrochloride, 10 mg/kg, i.p.) or saline (vehicle) was daily administered at 6:00 p.m. over a 1-week period [19,20,27]. Electroencephalographic (EEG) signals were detected with a DAM 80 differential amplifier (0.1–3000 Hz bandpass; World Precision Instruments, Sarasota, FL, USA) 2 h a day at the same time over a 1-week period. The data were digitized and analyzed using LabChart Pro v7 (ADInstruments, Bella Vista, New South Wales, Australia). Behavioral seizure severity was measured according to Racine's scale [26], as aforementioned. Non-responders were defined as showing no reduction in total seizure frequency in a 7-day period, as compared with the pre-treatment stage. After recording (18 h after the last drug treatment), animals were used for Western blot.

2.4.2. Experiment II

Some non-responders in experiment I were given saline (i.p.) over a 7-day period. Thereafter, animals were daily given perampanel or GYKI 52466 by the aforementioned method. Rats were also connected with Alzet 1007D osmotic pump (Alzet, Cupertino, CA, USA) containing vehicle or 3CAI (25 µM) [28]. The pump was placed in a subcutaneous pocket in the dorsal region. In a pilot study and our previous study [28], this dosage of 3CAI did not show behavioral and neurological defects and could not change the seizure susceptibility and seizure severity in response to pilocarpine. After recording (18 h after the last drug treatment), animals were used for Western blot.

2.5. Western Blot

Animals were sacrificed by decapitation, and their hippocampi were obtained and homogenized in lysis buffer containing protease inhibitor cocktail (Roche Applied Sciences, Branford, CT, USA) and phosphatase inhibitor cocktail (PhosSTOP®, Roche Applied Science, Branford, CT, USA). Thereafter, total protein concentration calibrated using a Micro BCA Protein Assay Kit (Pierce Chemical, Rockford, IL, USA). To analyze membrane GRIA subunit expressions, the bilateral hippocampal tissues (~100 mg) were washed gently with ice-cold PBS and chopped and homogenized for 10 strokes using a Dounce tissue homogenizer. Thereafter, membrane proteins were extracted with a subcellular Protein Fractionation Kit for Tissues (Thermo Scientific Korea, Seoul, South Korea), according to the manufacturer's instructions. Western blot was performed by the standard protocol: Sample proteins (10 µg) were separated on a Bis-Tris sodium dodecyl sulfate-poly-acrylamide gel (SDS-PAGE) and transferred to membranes. Membranes were incubated with 2% bovine serum albumin (BSA) in Tris-buffered saline (TBS; in mM 10 Tris, 150 NaCl, pH 7.5, and 0.05% Tween 20), and then reacted with primary antibodies (Table 1) overnight at 4 °C. After washing, membranes were incubated in a solution containing horseradish peroxidase (HRP)-conjugated secondary antibodies for 1 h at room temperature. Immunoblots were detected and quantified using ImageQuant LAS4000 system (GE Healthcare Korea, Seoul, South Korea). Optical densities of proteins were calculated with the corresponding amount of β-actin or N-cadherin.

Table 1. Primary antibodies used in the present study.

Antigen	Host	Manufacturer (Catalog Number)	Dilution Used
CREB	Rabbit	Novus biologicals (NBP1-90364)	1:500 (WB)
GRIA1	Mouse	Synaptic systems (#182011)	1:1000 (WB)
GRIA2	Rabbit	Sigma (AB1768-I)	1:1000 (WB)
GSK3β	Rabbit	Elapscience (ENT2082)	1:1000 (WB)
N-cadherin	Rabbit	Abcam (ab182030)	1:4000 (WB)
p-CREB S133	Rabbit	Novus biologicals (NB110-55727)	1:5000 (WB)
p-GRIA2 Y869/Y873/Y876	Rabbit	Cell signaling (#3921)	1:1000 (WB)
p-GRIA2 S880	Rabbit	Invitrogen (#PA5-38134)	1:1000 (WB)
p-GSK3β S9	Rabbit	Biorbyt (orb14745)	1:1000 (WB)
p-PKC T497	Rabbit	Abcam (ab76016)	1:1000 (WB)
p-Src family Y416	Rabbit	Cell signaling (#6943)	1:1000 (WB)
p-Src family Y527	Rabbit	Cell signaling (#2105)	1:1000 (WB)
PICK1	Rabbit	Abcam (ab3420)	1:1000 (WB)
PKC	Rabbit	Abcam (ab23511)	1:1000 (WB)
Src family	Rabbit	Cell signaling (#2108)	1:1000 (WB)
β-actin	Mouse	Sigma (#A5316)	1:5000 (WB)

2.6. Data Analysis

Seizure parameters (frequency, duration and Racine scores) were assessed by different investigators who were blind to the classification of animal groups and treatments. Shapiro–Wilk W-test was used to evaluate the values on normality. Mann–Whitney U-test, Wilcoxon signed rank test, Student's *t*-test, and paired Student's *t*-test were applied to determine statistical significance of data. Comparisons among groups were also performed using repeated measures ANOVA, Friedman test, and one-way ANOVA followed by Bonferroni's post hoc comparisons. A *p*-value less than 0.05 was considered to be significant.

3. Results

3.1. Effects of AMPAR Antagonists on Chronic Spontaneous Seizure Activity

In epileptic rats, the total seizure frequency (number of seizures), the total electroencephalographic (EEG) seizure duration, and average seizure severity (behavioral seizure core) were 11.9 ± 2.5, 996.4 ± 121 s, and 3.7 ± 0.5 over 1-week period, respectively ($n = 7$, Figure 2A–C). In responders, perampanel gradually reduced seizure frequency ($\chi^2_{(1)} = 5.5$, $p = 0.019$, Friedman test, $n = 7$), seizure duration ($F_{(1,12)} = 6.6$, $p = 0.025$, repeated measures ANOVA, $n = 7$), and the seizure severity ($\chi^2_{(1)} = 5.3$, $p = 0.021$, Friedman test, $n = 7$) over 1-week period (Figure 2A,B). The total seizure frequency was 6.42 ± 1.5 ($Z = 3.14$, $p = 0.001$ vs. vehicle, Mann–Whitney U-test, $n = 7$), the total seizure duration was 538.3 ± 127 s ($t_{(12)} = 13.43$, $p < 0.001$ vs. vehicle, Student *t*-test, $n = 7$), and the average seizure severity was 1.9 ± 0.2 over 1-week period ($Z = 2.89$, $p = 0.002$ vs. vehicle, Mann–Whitney U-test, $n = 7$; Figure 2C). Six out of thirteen rats in perampanel-treated group were identified as non-responders whose seizure activities were uncontrolled by perampanel (total seizure frequency, 10.8 ± 2.5; total seizure duration, 852.2 ± 150.5 s; average seizure severity, 3.8 ± 0.3; Figure 2B,C).

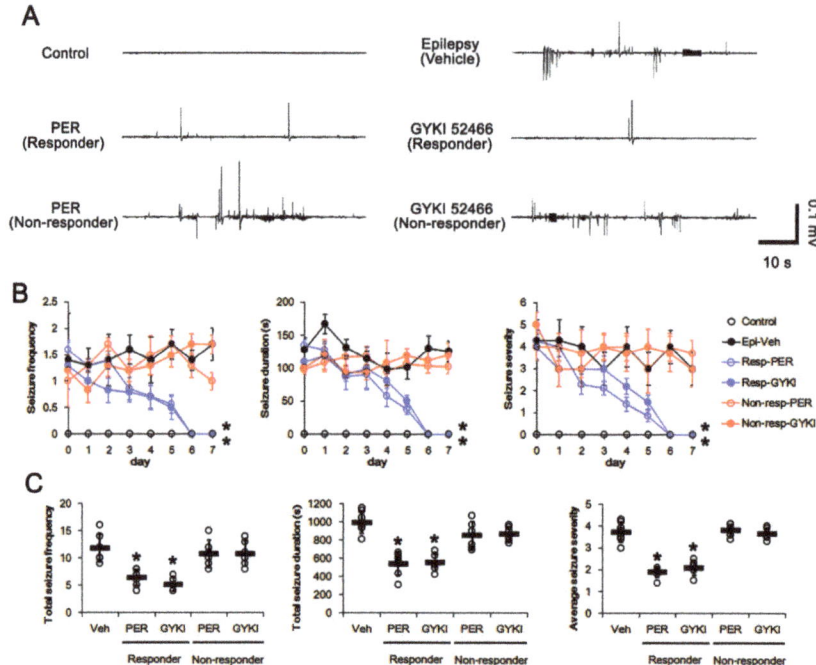

Figure 2. The effects of perampanel (PER) and GYKI 52466 (GYKI) on spontaneous seizure activities in chronic epilepsy rats. Both α-amino-3-hydroxy-5-methylisoxazole-4-propionic acid receptor (AMPAR) antagonists effectively attenuate spontaneous seizure activities in responders. (**A**) Representative electroencephalograms (EEG) in each group at 2 days after treatment. (**B**) Quantitative analyses of the chronological effects of AMPAR antagonists on seizure frequency, seizure duration, and seizure severity (seizure score) over 7-day period. Error bars indicate SD (* $p < 0.05$ vs. vehicle (Veh)-treated animals; Friedman test for seizure frequency and seizure severity; Repeated measures ANOVA for seizure duration). (**C**) Quantitative analyses of seizure frequency, total seizure duration and average behavioral seizure score (seizure severity) in 7-day period. Open circles indicate each individual value. Horizontal bars indicate mean value. Error bars indicate SD (* $p < 0.05$ vs. vehicle (Veh)-treated animals; Mann–Whitney U-test for seizure frequency and seizure severity; Student t-test for seizure duration).

GYKI 52466 also decreased seizure frequency ($\chi^2_{(1)}$ = 6.2, p = 0.013, Friedman test, n = 6), total seizure duration ($F_{(1,11)}$ = 5.9, p = 0.033, repeated measures ANOVA, n = 6), and the seizure severity ($\chi^2_{(1)}$ = 4.8, p = 0.029, Friedman test, n = 6) in responders over 1-week period (Figure 2A,B). In responders to GYKI 52466, the total seizure frequency was 5.2 ± 1.2 (Z = 3.01, p = 0.001 vs. vehicle, Mann–Whitney U-test, n = 6), the total seizure duration was 551.7 ± 92.9 s ($t_{(11)}$ = 10.01, $p < 0.001$ vs. vehicle, Student t-test, n = 6), and the average seizure severity was 2.1 ± 0.3 over 1-week period (Z = 2.86, p = 0.002 vs. vehicle, Mann–Whitney U-test, n = 6; Figure 2C). Six out of twelve rats in GYKI 52466-treated group were identified as non-responders (total seizure frequency, 10.8 ± 2.3; total seizure duration, 870.8 ± 80.5 s; average seizure severity, 3.7 ± 0.3; Figure 2B,C).

3.2. Effects of AMPAR Antagonists on GRIA2 Phosphorylations

The phosphorylations of GRIA2 regulate its surface expression and influence AMPAR functionality [15,21–24]. Therefore, we first explored whether AMPAR antagonists affect GRIA2 protein expression and its phosphorylation levels in the epileptic hippocampus. Consistent with previous studies [16,17], total GRIA2 protein level was 37% lower in the epileptic hippocampus ($t_{(12)}$ = 10.0, $p < 0.001$ vs. control animals, Student t-test; Figure 3A,B and Figure S1), as compared to control animals. Compatible to its protein level, GRIA2 Y869/Y873/Y876 phosphorylation levels were decreased to 0.49-fold of control level in the vehicle-treated epilepsy rats ($t_{(12)} = 14.8$, $p < 0.001$ vs. control animals, Student t-test; Figure 3A,C). GRIA2 Y phosphorylation ratio was 0.79-fold of control level in the vehicle-treated epilepsy rats ($t_{(12)} = 3.8$, $p < 0.001$ vs. control animals, Student t-test; Figure 3A,D).

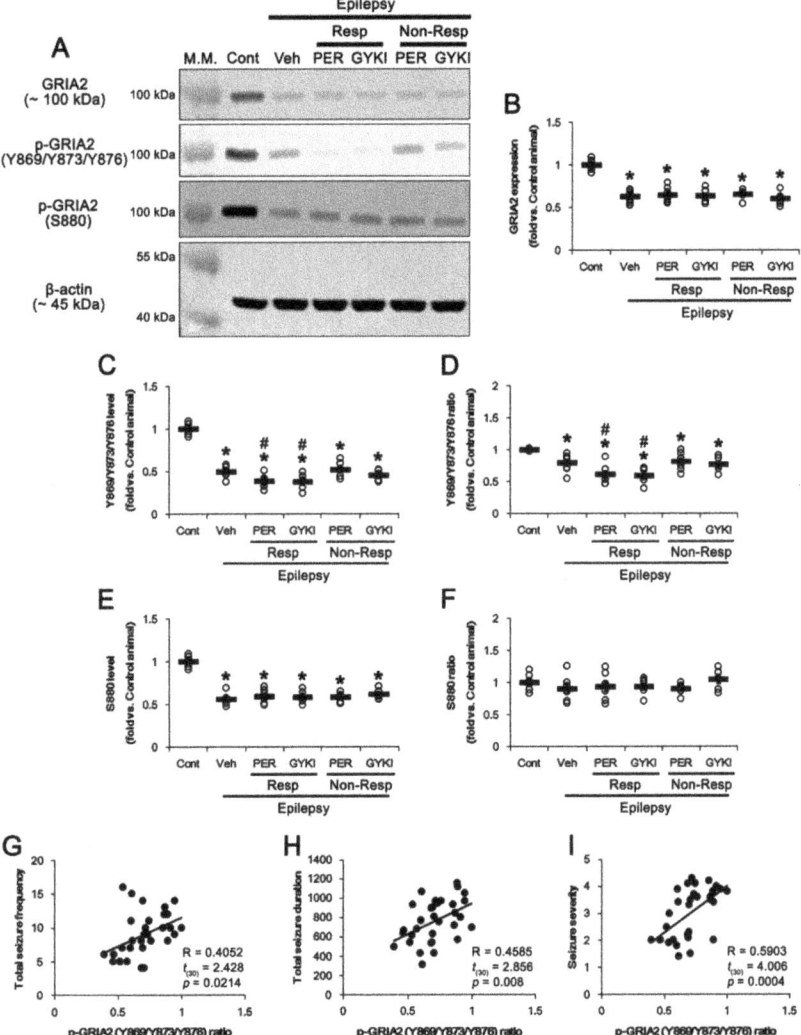

Figure 3. The effects of perampanel (PER) and GYKI 52466 (GYKI) on total glutamate ionotropic receptor AMPA type subunit 2 (GRIA2) expression and its phosphorylations in chronic epilepsy rats. (**A**) Representative images for Western blot of GRIA2 and its phosphorylation levels in the hippocampal tissues. (**B–F**) Quantifications of GRIA2 (**B**), p-GRIA2 Y869/Y873/Y876 (**C**), p-GRIA2 Y869/Y873/Y876/GRIA2 ratio (**D**), p-GRIA2 S880 (**E**), and p-GRIA2 S880/GRIA2 ratio (**F**) in the hippocampal tissues. Open circles indicate each individual value. Horizontal bars indicate mean value. Error bars indicate SEM (*, # $p < 0.05$ vs. control (Cont) and vehicle (Veh)-treated animals, respectively; one-way ANOVA with post hoc Bonferroni's multiple comparison). (**G–I**) Linear regression analyses between p-GRIA2 Y869/Y873/Y876/GRIA2 ratio and total seizure frequency (**G**), total seizure duration (**H**), and seizure severity (**I**) in chronic epilepsy rats.

In responders to perampanel and GYKI 52466, GRIA2 Y869/Y873/Y876 phosphorylation levels were significantly reduced to 0.39- and 0.38-fold of control levels without affecting GRIA2 protein levels, respectively ($F_{(2,17)}$ = 4.8, p = 0.02 vs. vehicle, one-way ANOVA; Figure 3A–C and Figure S1). Thus, its Y phosphorylation ratios were 0.61- and 0.6-fold of control levels, respectively ($F_{(2,17)}$ = 4.1, p = 0.04 vs. vehicle, one-way ANOVA; Figure 3A,D). In non-responders to perampanel and GYKI 52466, GRIA2 protein level and its Y869/Y873/Y876 phosphorylation levels/ratios were unaffected by each compound (Figure 3A–D). Similar to Y869/Y873/Y876 phosphorylation level, GRIA2 S880 phosphorylation level was reduced to 0.56-fold of control level in the vehicle-treated epilepsy rats ($t_{(12)}$ = 12.6, p < 0.001 vs. control animals, Student t-test; Figure 3A,E and Figure S1). Thus, S880 phosphorylation ratio was 0.91-fold of control level in the vehicle-treated epilepsy rats ($t_{(12)}$ = 1.2, p = 0.26 vs. control animals, Student t-test; Figure 3A,F). In responders, GRIA2 S880 phosphorylation level ($F_{(2,17)}$ = 0.4, p = 0.65 vs. vehicle, one-way ANOVA; Figure 3A,E) and its ratio ($F_{(2,17)}$ = 0.08, p = 0.92 vs. vehicle, one-way ANOVA; Figure 3A,F) were unaffected by perampanel and GYKI 52466. In non-responders, both perampanel and GYKI 52466 did not alter GRIA2 S880 phosphorylation level/ratio (Figure 3A,E,F). In addition, we analyzed the correlation between GRIA2 Y phosphorylation ratio and seizure parameters in chronic epilepsy rats. Linear regression analysis showed a direct proportional relationship between GRIA2 Y phosphorylation ratio and total seizure frequency with linear correlation coefficients of 0.4052 ($t_{(30)}$ = 2.428, p = 0.0214; Figure 3G). The GRIA2 Y phosphorylation ratio also showed direct proportional relationships with total seizure duration (linear correlation coefficients, 0.4585; $t_{(30)}$ = 2.856, p = 0.008; Figure 3H) and seizure severity (linear correlation coefficients, 0.5903; $t_{(30)}$ = 4.006, p = 0.0004; Figure 3I). These findings indicate that anti-epileptic effects of AMPAR antagonists may be correlated with GRIA2 Y869/Y873/Y876 phosphorylations.

3.3. Effects of AMPAR Antagonists on PKC and Src Phosphorylations

Src family and PKC phosphorylate GRIA2 at Y869/Y873/Y876 and S880 sites, respectively [21,23,24]. Therefore, we confirmed whether both AMPAR antagonists affect GRIA2 phosphorylations through PKC and/or Src family-mediated signaling pathways.

In epileptic rats, PKC expression and its phosphorylation level were decreased to 0.72- ($t_{(12)}$ = 7.9, p < 0.001 vs. control animals, Student t-test; Figure 4A,B and Figure S2) and 0.68-fold ($t_{(12)}$ = 7.6, p < 0.001 vs. control animals, Student t-test; Figure 4A,C) of control levels, respectively. However, PKC phosphorylation ratio was similar to that in controls ($t_{(12)}$ = 0.97, p = 0.35 vs. control animals, Student t-test; Figure 4A,D). Both perampanel and GYKI 52466 did not affect PKC protein level ($F_{(4,27)}$ = 1.4, p = 0.26 vs. vehicle, one-way ANOVA), PKC phosphorylation ($F_{(4,27)}$ = 1.1, p = 0.36 vs. vehicle, one-way ANOVA), and its phosphorylation ratio ($F_{(4,27)}$ = 0.7, p = 0.58 vs. vehicle, one-way ANOVA) in non-responders as well as responders (Figure 4A–D and Figure S2).

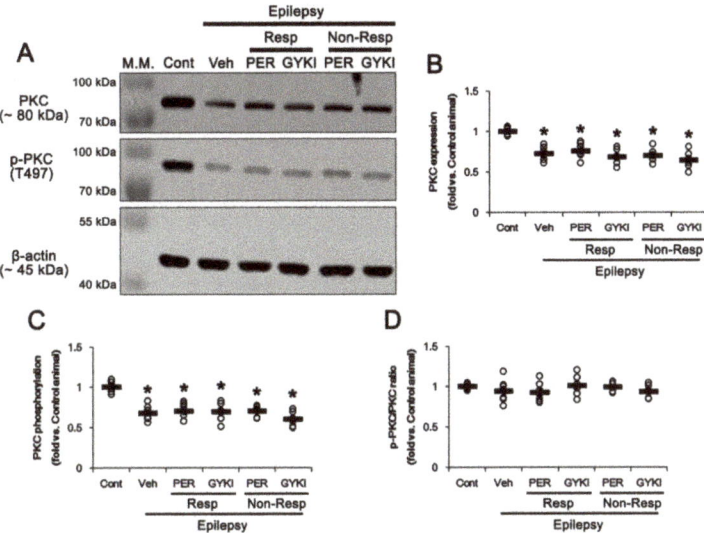

Figure 4. The effects of perampanel (PER) and GYKI 52466 (GYKI) on total protein kinase C (PKC) expression and its threonine (T) 497 phosphorylation in chronic epilepsy rats. (**A**) Representative images for western blot of PKC and its T497 phosphorylation level in the hippocampal tissues. (**B–D**) Quantifications of PKC (**B**), p-PKC T497 (**C**), and p-PKC/PKC ratio (**D**) in the hippocampal tissues. Open circles indicate each individual value. Horizontal bars indicate mean value. Error bars indicate SEM (* $p < 0.05$ vs. control animals; one-way ANOVA with post hoc Bonferroni's multiple comparison).

In chronic epilepsy rats, Src family protein level was similarly observed, as compared to controls. Both AMPAR antagonists did not affect it ($F_{(4,27)} = 0.9$, $p = 0.49$, one-way ANOVA; Figure 5A,B and Figure S3). Src Y416 phosphorylation level was 0.54-fold lower in the epileptic hippocampus than that in controls ($t_{(12)} = 8.6$, $p < 0.001$ vs. control animals, Student t-test; Figure 5A,C) and its phosphorylation ratio was 0.57-fold of control level ($t_{(12)} = 7.4$, $p < 0.001$ vs. control animals, Student t-test; Figure 5A,D). In responders, perampanel and GYKI 52466 decreased Src Y416 phosphorylation level to 0.25- and 0.3-fold of control level, respectively ($F_{(2,17)} = 19.6$, $p < 0.001$ vs. vehicle, one-way ANOVA; Figure 5A,C and Figure S3). Both perampanel and GYKI 52466 reduced Y416 phosphorylation ratios to 0.25- and 0.31-fold of control level, respectively ($F_{(2,17)} = 19.3$, $p < 0.001$ vs. vehicle, one-way ANOVA; Figure 5A,D). In non-responders, both AMPAR antagonists did not affect Y416 phosphorylation level ($F_{(2,16)} = 0.11$, $p = 0.89$ vs. vehicle, one-way ANOVA; Figure 5A,C) and its ratio ($F_{(2,15)} = 0.14$, $p = 0.87$, one-way ANOVA; Figure 5A,D). In the epileptic hippocampus, Src Y527 phosphorylation level was also decreased to 0.65-fold of control level ($t_{(12)} = 10.1$, $p < 0.001$ vs. control animals, one-way ANOVA, Student t-test; Figure 5A,E and Figure S3). Y527 phosphorylation ratio was 0.69-fold of control level ($t_{(12)} = 8.9$, $p < 0.001$, Student t-test; Figure 5A,F). In responders, perampanel and GYKI 52466 recovered Src Y527 phosphorylation level ($F_{(2,17)} = 31.1$, $p < 0.001$ vs. vehicle, one-way ANOVA) and its phosphorylation ratio to control level ($F_{(2,17)} = 16.5$, $p < 0.001$ vs. vehicle, one-way ANOVA), respectively (Figure 5A,E,F). In non-responders, both AMPAR antagonists did not affect Y527 phosphorylation level ($F_{(2,16)} = 0.22$, $p = 0.81$ vs. vehicle, one-way ANOVA; Figure 5A,E) and its ratio ($F_{(2,16)} = 0.3$, $p = 0.74$, one-way ANOVA; Figure 5A,F). Src family activities are reversely modulated by phosphorylation of two distinct tyrosine sites: Y416 autophosphorylation upregulates Src kinase activity. In contrast, Y527 phosphorylation inhibits its activity, although dephosphorylation at this site cannot fully activate it [29,30]. Therefore, these findings indicate that refractory seizure activity to AMPAR antagonists may be relevant to dysregulated Src activity rather than PKC phosphorylation in responders.

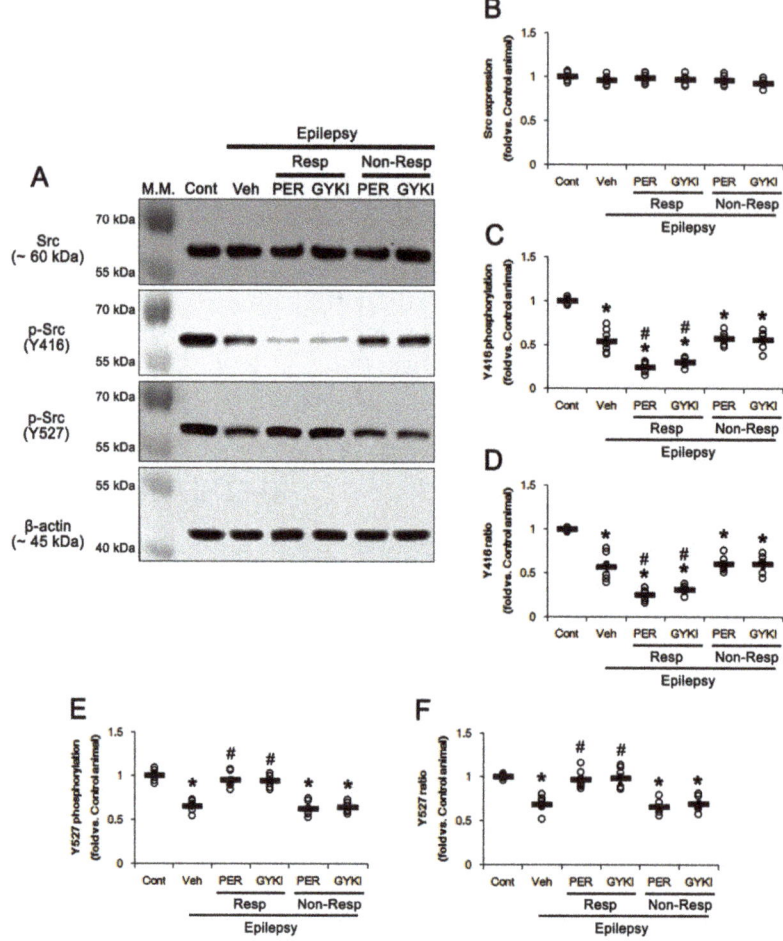

Figure 5. The effects of perampanel (PER) and GYKI 52466 (GYKI) on Src family and its phosphorylations in chronic epilepsy rats. (**A**) Representative images for Western blot of Src family and its phosphorylation levels in the hippocampal tissues. (**B–F**) Quantifications of Src2 (**B**), p-Src Y416 (**C**), p-Src Y416/Src ratio (**D**), p-Src Y527 (**E**), and p-Src Y527/GRIA2 ratio (**F**) in the hippocampal tissues. Open circles indicate each individual value. Horizontal bars indicate mean value. Error bars indicate SEM (*, # $p < 0.05$ vs. control (Cont) and vehicle (Veh)-treated animals, respectively; one-way ANOVA with post hoc Bonferroni's multiple comparison).

3.4. Effects of AMPAR Antagonists on PICK1 Expression

PICK1 negatively regulates GRIA2 surface expression [21,22]. Src family and/or PKC-mediated GRIA2 phosphorylations facilitate GRIA2–PICK1 bindings, which lead to GRIA2 internalization and a relative increase of GRIA2-lacking, Ca^{2+}-permeable AMPARs [21,23,24]. However, both perampanel and GYKI 52466 decrease GRIA1/GRIA2 ratio by reducing GRIA1, but not GRIA2, surface expression [19,20]. Considering GRIA2 phosphorylations, it is likely that altered PICK1 expression may be involved in unaffected GRIA2 surface expression by AMPAR antagonists. To confirm this, we evaluated the effects of perampanel and GYKI 52466 on PICK1 expression in the epileptic hippocampus. In the present study, PICK1 protein level was lower in chronic epilepsy rats than that in controls ($t_{(12)} = 10.4$, $p < 0.001$, Student *t*-test; Figure 6A,B and Figure S4), which was unaffected by AMPAR antagonists ($F_{(4,27)}$ = 0.2, p = 0.93, one-way ANOVA; Figure 6A,B). These findings indicate that reduced PICK1 expression may decrease its binding to phosphorylated GRIA2, which would serve to maintain GRIA2 surface expression as an adaptive response. In addition, it is unlikely that PICK1-mediated GRIA2 internalization may be a contributor to generation of refractory seizures in response to AMPAR antagonists.

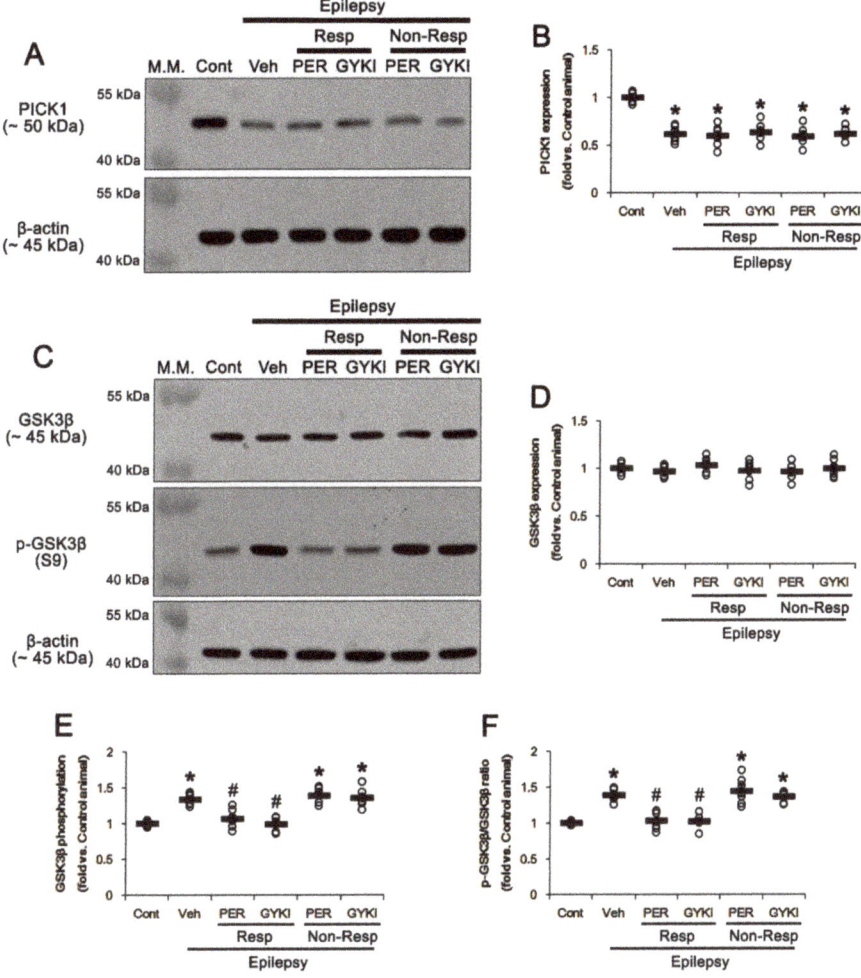

Figure 6. The effects of perampanel (PER) and GYKI 52466 (GYKI) on protein interacting with C kinase 1 (PICK1) expression and glycogen synthase kinase 3β (GSK3β) expression and its phosphorylation in chronic epilepsy rats. (**A,B**) Representative images for Western blot of PICK1 expression (**A**) and quantifications of PICK1 expression (**B**) in the hippocampal tissues. (**C–F**) Representative images for Western blot of GSK3β expression and its phosphorylation (**C**) and quantifications of GSK3β (**D**), p-GSK3β S9 (**E**), and p-GSK3β S9/GSK3β ratio (**F**) in the hippocampal tissues. Open circles indicate each individual value. Horizontal bars indicate mean value. Error bars indicate SEM (*, # p < 0.05 vs. control (Cont) and vehicle (Veh)-treated animals, respectively; one-way ANOVA with post hoc Bonferroni's multiple comparison).

3.5. Effects of AMPAR Antagonists on GSK3β Phosphorylation

GSK3β is a serine/threonine kinase that phosphorylates various substrates and is involved in cellular and synaptic functions. Phosphoinositide 3-kinases (PI3K)/AKT-mediated S9 phosphorylation inhibits its activity, which is negatively regulated by PTEN [31–33]. GSK3β phosphorylates PICK1 and promotes the GRIA2–PICK1 interaction [34]. Furthermore, inactivated (phosphorylated) GSK3β promotes CREB S133 phosphorylation [32] that increases in human patients and animal models of epilepsy and participates in ictogenesis [35,36]. Furthermore, AMPAR antagonists activate PTEN-mediated CREB S133 dephosphorylation [19]. Since CREB is required for the maintenance of the GRIA1 surface expression under physiological conditions [37], it is likely that impaired AKT/GSK3β-mediated CREB S133 phosphorylation would result in refractory seizures in response to AMPAR antagonist.

In the present study, there was no difference in GSK3β protein level between control and the epileptic hippocampus ($t_{(12)}$ = 1.1, p = 0.27, Student *t*-test; Figure 6C,D and Figure S5). Both perampanel and GYKI 52466 did not affect GSK3β protein level in responders and non-responders ($F_{(4,27)}$ = 0.8, p = 0.53, one-way ANOVA; Figure 6C,D and Figure S5). However, GSK3β S9 phosphorylation level was 1.34-fold higher in the epileptic hippocampus than that in controls ($t_{(12)}$ = 10.2, p < 0.001, Student *t*-test; Figure 6C,E and Figure S5) and its phosphorylation ratio was 1.39-fold of control level ($t_{(12)}$ = 12.4, p < 0.001, Student *t*-test; Figure 6C,F). In responders, perampanel and GYKI 52466 restored GSK3β phosphorylation level to control level ($F_{(2,17)}$ = 20.3, p < 0.001, one-way ANOVA; Figure 6C,E and Figure S5). Both AMPAR antagonists also recovered GSK3β phosphorylation ratio to control level ($F_{(2,17)}$ = 27.5, p < 0.001, one-way ANOVA; Figure 6C,F). In non-responders, perampanel and GYKI 52466 did not affect GSK3β phosphorylation level ($F_{(2,16)}$ = 0.5, p = 0.62, one-way ANOVA; Figure 6C,E) and its ratio ($F_{(2,16)}$ = 0.7, p = 0.5, one-way ANOVA; Figure 6C,F). These findings indicate that AMPAR antagonists may liberate GSK3β from S9 phosphorylation-mediated inhibition.

Consistent with our previous study [19], furthermore, CREB protein level in the epileptic hippocampus was 1.25-fold higher than that in controls ($t_{(12)}$ = 7.1, p < 0.001, Student *t*-test; Figure 7A,B and Figure S6), which was unaffected by AMPAR antagonists ($F_{(4,27)}$ = 0.2, p = 0.94, one-way ANOVA; Figure 7A,B). CREB S133 phosphorylation level was 1.51-fold higher in the epileptic hippocampus than that in controls ($t_{(12)}$ = 9.8, p < 0.001, Student *t*-test; Figure 7A,C and Figure S6) and its phosphorylation ratio was 1.41-fold of control level ($t_{(12)}$ = 6.9, p < 0.001, Student *t*-test; Figure 7A,D). In responders, perampanel and GYKI 52466 decreased CREB S133 phosphorylation level to 1.21- and 1.23-fold of control level, respectively ($F_{(2,17)}$ = 9.1, p = 0.002, one-way ANOVA; Figure 7A,C). Both AMPAR antagonists reduced S133 phosphorylation ratios to control level ($F_{(2,17)}$ = 7.7, p = 0.004, one-way ANOVA; Figure 7A,D). In non-responders, perampanel and GYKI 52466 did not affect CREB S133 phosphorylation level ($F_{(2,16)}$ = 0.3, p = 0.75, one-way ANOVA; Figure 7A,C) and its ratio ($F_{(2,16)}$ = 0.1, p = 0.89, one-way ANOVA; Figure 7A,D). These findings indicate that the GSK3β-CREB signaling pathway may be involved in anti-convulsive effects of AMPAR antagonists.

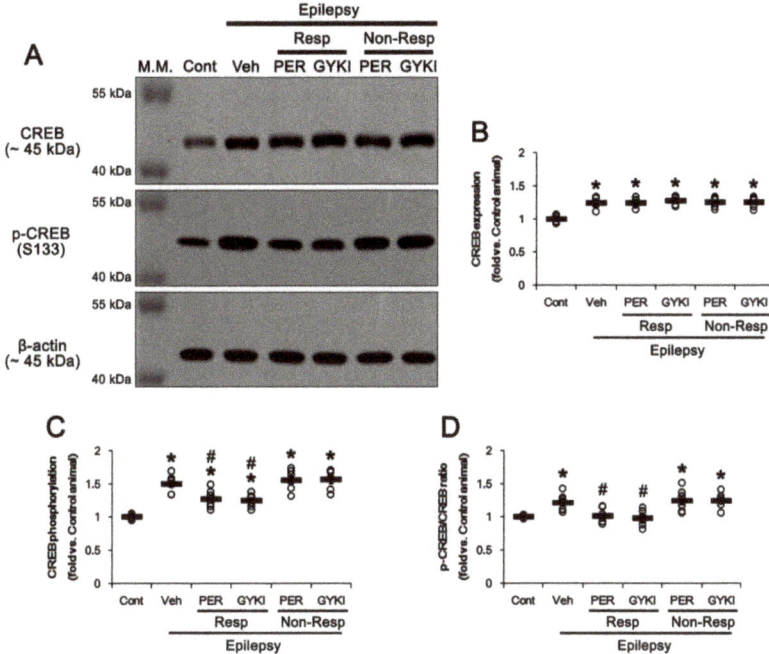

Figure 7. The effects of perampanel (PER) and GYKI 52466 (GYKI) on total Ca^{2+}/cAMP response element-binding protein (CREB) expression and its S133 phosphorylation in chronic epilepsy rats. (**A**) Representative images for Western blot of CREB and its S133 phosphorylation level in the hippocampal tissues. (**B–D**) Quantifications of CREB (**B**), p-CREB S133 (**C**), and p-CREB/CREB ratio (**D**) in the hippocampal tissues. Open circles indicate each individual value. Horizontal bars indicate mean value. Error bars indicate SEM (*,# $p < 0.05$ vs. control (Cont) and vehicle (Veh)-treated animals, respectively; one-way ANOVA with post hoc Bonferroni's multiple comparison).

3.6. Effect of 3CAI Co-Treatment on Refractory Seizures in Non-Responders to AMPAR Antagonists

As mentioned earlier, GSK3β is inhibited by AKT-mediated S9 phosphorylation, which inhibits GRIA2–PICK1 interaction but promotes CREB S133 phosphorylation [31–34]. To confirm the roles of GSK3β signaling pathway in CREB activity and refractory seizures to AMPAR antagonists, 3CAI (an AKT inhibitor) was co-treated with perampanel or GYKI 52466 in non-responders (Figure 1). This is because the direct GSK3β activator is unavailable. In non-responders to perampanel, total seizure frequency was 9.6 ± 2.3, total seizure duration was 815.6 ± 213.7 s, and average seizure severity was 3.6 ± 0.3 over 1-week period ($n = 5$, Figure 8A–C). In non-responders to GYKI 52466, total seizure frequency was 9.2 ± 2.5, total seizure duration was 839 ± 144.1 s, and average seizure severity was 3.6 ± 0.4 over 1-week period ($n = 5$, Figure 8A–C). 3CAI co-treatment gradually decreased seizure frequency ($\chi^2_{(3)} = 8.9$, $p = 0.031$, Friedman test, $n = 5$), total seizure duration ($F_{(3,16)} = 4.8$, $p = 0.014$, repeated measures ANOVA, $n = 5$), and the seizure severity ($\chi^2_{(3)} = 8.3$, mboxemphp = 0.041, Friedman test, $n = 5$) in both perampanel- and GYKI 52466-treated groups over 1-week period (Figure 8A,B). In non-responders to peramanel, 3CAI co-treatment reduced the total seizure frequency to 5.4 ± 1.6 ($Z = 2.02$, $p = 0.04$, Wilcoxon signed rank test, $n = 5$; Figure 8A,C), the total seizure duration to 409.2 ± 131.6 s ($t_{(4)} = 3.12$, $p = 0.04$, paired Student t-test, $n = 5$; Figure 8A,C), and average seizure severity to 1.6 ± 0.4 ($Z = 2.04$, $p = 0.04$, Wilcoxon signed rank test, $n = 5$; Figure 8A,C). In non-responders to GYKI 52466, 3CAI co-treatment also attenuated the seizure frequency to 5.8 ± 1.6 ($Z = 2.03$, $p = 0.04$, Wilcoxon signed rank test, $n = 5$; Figure 8A,C), the total seizure duration to

433.2 ± 100.1 s ($t_{(4)}$ = 2.91, p = 0.04, paired Student t-test, n = 5; Figure 8A,C), and the seizure severity to 2.1 ± 0.7 (Z = 2.06, p = 0.04 vs. vehicle, Wilcoxon signed rank test, n = 5; Figure 8A,C). These findings indicate that PI3K/AKT-mediated GSK3β inhibition may be one of the important signaling pathways for generation of refractory seizures to AMPAR antagonists.

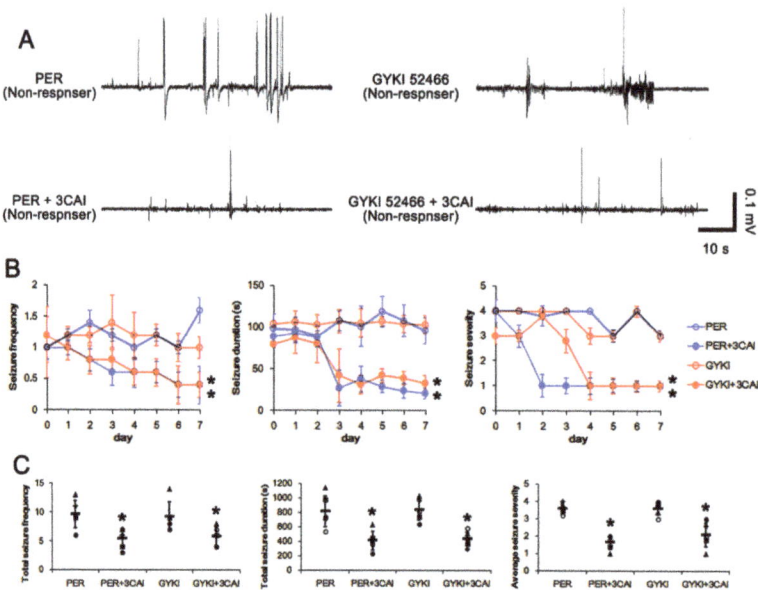

Figure 8. The effects of 3CAI co-treatment with perampanel (PER) and GYKI 52466 (GYKI) on spontaneous seizure activities in non-responders. 3CAI co-treatment effectively improves the anti-epileptic effects of both AMPAR antagonists in non-responders. (**A**) Representative electroencephalograms (EEG) in each group at 2 days after 3CAI co-treatment. (**B**) Quantitative analyses of the chronological effects of 3CAI co-treatment with AMPAR antagonists on seizure frequency, seizure duration, and seizure severity (seizure score) over 7-day period. Error bars indicate SD (* p < 0.05 vs. vehicle (Veh)-treated animals; Friedman test for seizure frequency and seizure severity; Repeated measures ANOVA for seizure duration). (**C**) Quantitative analyses of total seizure frequency, total seizure duration, and average behavioral seizure score (seizure severity) in 7-day period. Symbols indicate each individual value. Horizontal bars indicate mean value. Error bars indicate SD (* p < 0.05 vs. vehicle (Veh)-treated animals; Wilcoxon signed rank test for seizure frequency and seizure severity; paired Student t-test for seizure duration).

3.7. Effect of 3CAI Co-Treatment on PICK1 Expression and Phosphorylations of GSK3β and CREB in Non-Responders

Next, we investigated whether 3CAI co-treatment affects PICK1 expression and phosphorylations of GSK3β and CREB in non-responders to AMPAR antagonists. 3CAI co-treatment did not affect GSK3β protein level in non-responders (Figure 9A,B). However, 3CAI co-treatment reduced GSK3β S9 phosphorylation level to control level in non-responders to perampanel ($t_{(8)}$ = 6.1, p < 0.001, Student t-test) and GYKI 52466 ($t_{(8)}$ = 4.0, p = 0.004, Student t-test; Figure 9A,C and Figure S7). Thus, 3CAI co-treatment restored GSK3β S9 phosphorylation ratio to control level in non-responders to perampanel ($t_{(8)}$ = 4.2, p = 0.003, Student t-test) and GYKI 52466 ($t_{(8)}$ = 3.2, p = 0.01, Student t-test), respectively (Figure 9A,D). Similar to the case of GSK3β, 3CAI co-treatment did not alter CREB protein level in non-responders to perampanel and GYKI 52466 (Figure 9A,E and Figure S7). However, 3CAI co-treatment decreased CREB S133 phosphorylation level in non-responders to perampanel ($t_{(8)}$ = 6.4, p < 0.001, Student t-test) and GYKI 52466 ($t_{(8)}$ = 5.7, p < 0.001,

Student *t*-test), respectively Figure 9A,F and Figure S7). 3CAI co-treatment restored CREB S133 phosphorylation ratio to control level in non-responders to perampanel ($t_{(8)}$ = 5.4, $p < 0.001$, Student *t*-test) and GYKI 52466 ($t_{(8)}$ = 4.9, $p = 0.001$, Student *t*-test), respectively (Figure 9A,G). 3CAI co-treatment did not alter PICK1 protein level in non-responders to perampanel and GYKI 52466 (Figure 9A,H). These findings indicate that the GSK3β activation may improve anti-convulsive effects of AMPAR antagonists in non-responders by regulating CREB activity rather than PICK1 expression.

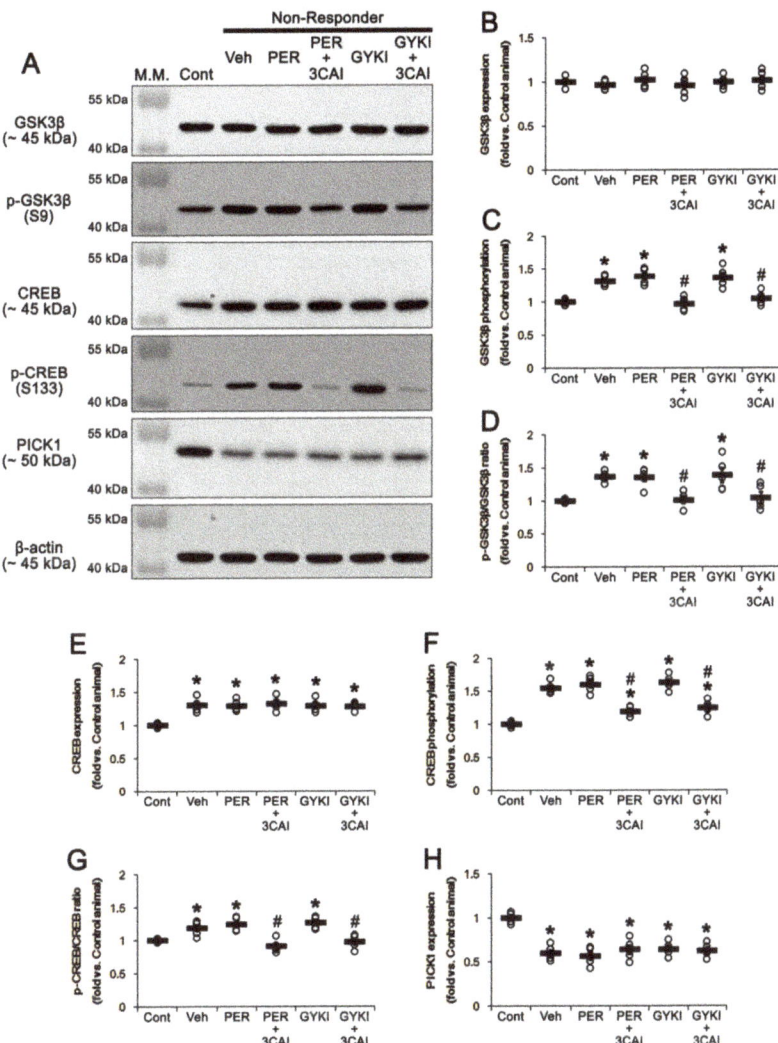

Figure 9. The effects of 3CAI co-treatment with perampanel (PER) and GYKI 52466 (GYKI) on expression levels of GSK3β, CREB, and PICK1 and the phosphorylation levels of GSK3β and CREB in non-responders. (**A**) Representative images for Western blot of total GSK3β, CREB, and PICK1 levels and the phosphorylation levels of GSK3β and CREB. (**B–H**) Quantifications of GSK3β (**B**), p-GSK3β S9 (**C**), p-GSK3β S9/GSK3β ratio (**D**), CREB (**E**), p-CREB S133 (**F**), p-CREB S133/CREB ratio (**G**), and PICK1 (**H**) in the hippocampal tissues. Open circles indicate each individual value. Horizontal bars indicate mean value. Error bars indicate SEM (*, # $p < 0.05$ vs. control (Cont) and vehicle (Veh)-treated animals, respectively; one-way ANOVA with post hoc Bonferroni's multiple comparison).

3.8. Effect of 3CAI Co-Treatment on Surface GRIA Expressions in Non-Responders

Finally, we investigated whether 3CAI co-treatment affects surface GRIA1 and GRIA2 expressions in the hippocampus of non-responders. The present study showed total GRIA1 protein level in the epileptic hippocampus was 0.74-fold of control level ($t_{(8)} = 7.7$, $p < 0.001$ vs. control animals, Student *t*-test; Figure 10A,B), which was further reduced to 0.51- and 0.54-fold of control level in responders by perampanel and GYKI 52466, respectively ($F_{(2,12)} = 24.4$, $p < 0.001$ vs. vehicle, one-way ANOVA; Figure 10A,B). However, both AMPAR antagonists did not influence total GRIA1 protein level in non-responders, which was unaffected by 3CAI co-treatment (Figure 10A,B and Figure S8).

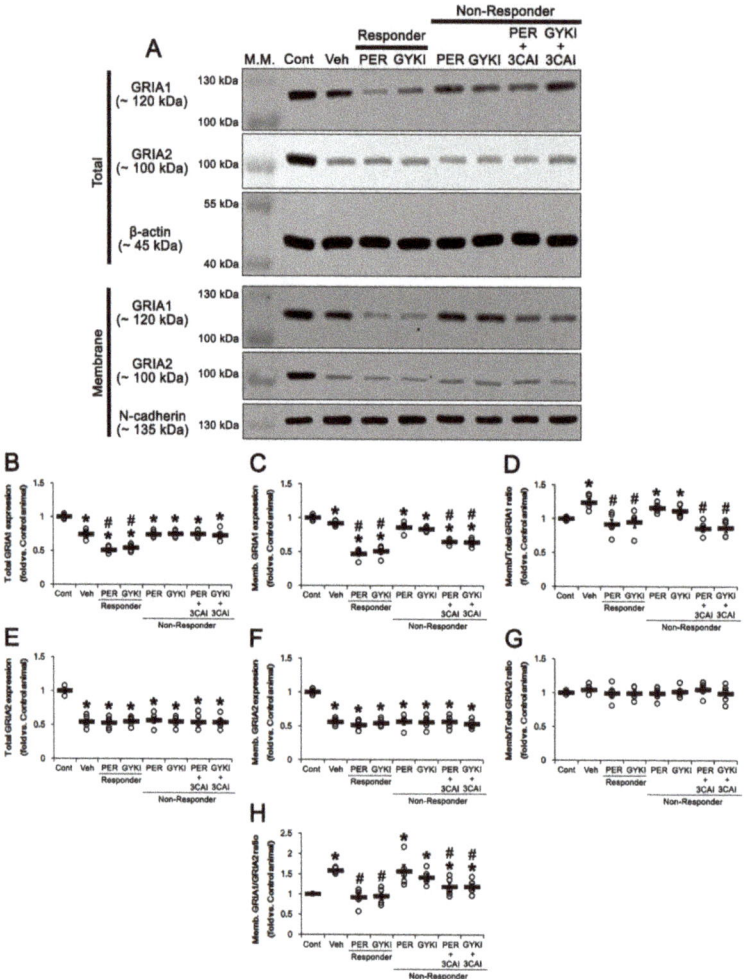

Figure 10. The effects of 3CAI co-treatment with perampanel (PER) and GYKI 52466 (GYKI) on surface expressions of GRIA1 and GRIA2 in chronic epilepsy rats. (**A**) Representative images for Western blot of total and membrane GRIA1 and GRIA2 expression levels. (**B–H**) Quantifications of total GRIA1 expression (**B**), membrane GRIA1 expression (**C**), membrane/total GRIA1 ratio (**D**), total GRIA2 expression (**E**), membrane GRIA2 expression (**F**), membrane/total GRIA2 ratio (**G**), and membrane GRIA1/GRIA2 ratio in the hippocampal tissues. Open circles indicate each individual value. Horizontal bars indicate mean value. Error bars indicate SEM (*, # $p < 0.05$ vs. control (Cont) and vehicle (Veh)-treated animals, respectively; one-way ANOVA with post hoc Bonferroni's multiple comparison).

Membrane GRIA1 expression in the epileptic hippocampus was 0.89-fold of control level ($t_{(8)}$ = 4.1, p = 0.004 vs. control animals, Student t-test; Figure 10A,C). Thus, membrane/total GRIA1 ratio in the epileptic hippocampus was increased to 1.23-fold of control level ($t_{(8)}$ = 3.4, p = 0.01 vs. control animals, Student t-test; Figure 10A,D and Figure S8). Perampanel and GYKI 52466 decreased membrane GRIA1 expression to 0.47- and 0.51-fold of control level in responders, respectively ($F_{(2,12)}$ = 51.5, p < 0.001 vs. vehicle, one-way ANOVA; Figure 10A,C). Both AMPAR antagonists restored membrane/total GRIA1 ratio to control level in responders ($F_{(2,12)}$ = 5.2, p = 0.02 vs. vehicle, one-way ANOVA; Figure 10A,D). Although both AMPAR antagonists did not affect membrane GRIA1 expression in non-responders, 3CAI co-treatment reduced it to 0.65- and 0.64-fold of control level in non-responders to perampanel ($t_{(8)}$ = 5.7, p < 0.001, Student t-test) and GYKI 52466 ($t_{(8)}$ = 6.4, p < 0.001, Student t-test), respectively (Figure 10A,C and Figure S8). 3CAI co-treatment also diminished membrane/total GRIA1 ratio to control level in non-responders to perampanel ($t_{(8)}$ = 5.4, p < 0.001, Student t-test) and GYKI 52466 ($t_{(8)}$ = 4.1, p = 0.003, Student t-test), respectively (Figure 10A,D). Both AMPAR antagonists and 3CAI co-treatment did not affect total GRIA2 protein level, membrane GRIA2 expression, and membrane/total GRIA2 ratio in both responders and non-responders (Figure 10A,E–G and Figure S8).

Membrane GRIA1/GRIA2 ratio in the epileptic hippocampus was 1.6-fold of control level ($t_{(8)}$ = 18.8, p < 0.001 vs. control animals, Student t-test; Figure 10A,H and Figure S8). Both AMPAR antagonists restored membrane GRIA1/GRIA2 ratio to control level in responders ($F_{(2,12)}$ = 23.1, p < 0.001 vs. vehicle, one-way ANOVA) but not non-responders (Figure 10A,H). 3CAI co-treatment decreased membrane GRIA1/GRIA2 ratio to 1.12- and 1.23-fold of control level in non-responders to perampanel ($t_{(8)}$ = 2.9, p = 0.02, Student t-test) and GYKI 52466 ($t_{(8)}$ = 3.2, p = 0.01, Student t-test), respectively (Figure 10A,H and Figure S8). These findings indicate that 3CAI may increase the responsiveness to AMPAR antagonists in non-responders by reducing surface GRIA1 expression.

4. Discussion

The principal findings of the present study were that AMPAR antagonists ameliorated spontaneous seizure activity by regulating surface expression of GRIA1 but not GRIA2. In addition, impaired AKT/GSK3β-mediated CREB S133 activation was involved in refractory seizures in response to AMPAR antagonists, which suggests that the regulation of these pathways may be a potential therapeutic strategy to improve the medication of intractable TLE.

Since the activation and desensitization kinetics of AMPAR are much faster than those of NMDAR [38], AMPAR antagonists have been focused to prevent ictogenesis and steadily progressive seizure-related brain pathologic plasticity in the epileptic brain [5]. Indeed, AMPAR antagonists terminate SE and seizure activity that are uncontrolled by NMDAR antagonists [6–8]. Among them, only perampanel is marketed for the treatment of focal epilepsy, which is a novel non-competitive AMPAR antagonist without affecting the NMDAR or kainate receptors [5], although its effects on signaling pathways remain to be elucidated. In the present study, both perampanel and GYKI 52466 ameliorated spontaneous seizure activity in 54% and 50% of animals (responders) in each group, concomitant with the reduced membrane expression of GRIA1 but not GRIA2. Furthermore, both AMPAR antagonists restored upregulated membrane/total GRIA1 ratio and membrane GRIA1/GRIA2 ratio to control levels. These effects of AMPAR antagonists were relevant to inhibition of AKT/GSK3β/CREB signaling pathway in responders. Because both AMPAR subunits are also located in endomembrane systems, such as the Golgi complex, endosomes, and ER [39,40], the GRIA1 and GRIA2 concentrations in membrane fraction may not directly represent the "pure surface expressions" in the present study. Considering that AMPAR trafficking is tightly regulated from the synthesis in ER to surface expression [41,42] and CREB regulates surface GRIA1 expression [37], however, the decreases in membrane/total GRIA1 ratio and membrane GRIA1/GRIA2 ratio indicate the diminished surface GRIA expression [19,20].

CREB activity (phosphorylation) is increased in human patients and animal models of epilepsy [35,36]. CREB phosphorylation is regulated by the activation of multiple signaling cascades, including GSK3β, PKC, protein kinase A (PKA), and Ca^{2+}-calmodulin-dependent protein kinase II (CAMKII) [32,33,43,44]. In the present study, we found that GSK3β S9 (but not PKC) and CREB S133 phosphorylations were higher in the epileptic hippocampus than those in normal one, which were abolished by both AMPAR antagonists in responders, but not non-responders. Since the increased GSK3β-mediated CREB S133 phosphorylation participates in ictogenesis in human patients and animal models of epilepsy [32,35,36], these findings indicate that AMPAR antagonists may negatively regulate surface GRIA expression via GSK3β/CREB signaling pathway in responders.

PI3K/AKT-mediated GSK3β phosphorylation inhibits its activity, which is conversely regulated by PTEN [31,33]. Recently, we have reported that PTEN expression is decreased in the epileptic hippocampus, concomitant with the reduced Src/CK2-mediated phosphorylations [19]. Regarding phosphorylation-mediated inhibition of PTEN activity [45], we have postulated that the reduced PTEN phosphorylation (the increased activity) may be an adaptive response to the decreased expression in the epileptic hippocampus, while this alteration may be insufficient to suppress spontaneous seizure activities. This is because AMPAR antagonists further diminish PTEN phosphorylation only in responders, accompanied by increasing its expression, which is abrogated by dipotassium bisperoxovanadium(pic) dihydrate (BpV(pic), a PTEN inhibitor) [19,20]. In the present study, 3CAI-induced AKT inhibition improved the responsiveness to AMPAR antagonists in non-responders through GSK3β-mediated CREB regulation. Furthermore, 3CAI reduced surface GRIA1 expression in non-responders to AMPAR antagonists. Therefore, it is likely that the regulation of the PTEN/AKT/GSK3β/CREB pathway be essentially required for the anti-epileptic effects of AMPAR antagonists. Indeed, the hippocampi of animal models and the surgically resected hippocampal tissues from drug-resistant TLE patients show upregulated AKT activity (phosphorylation) [46–48]. Similar to the present data, furthermore, topiramate (TPM, an AED) modulates AMPAR-mediated AKT/GSK3β/CREB signaling pathway [49]. Therefore, our findings suggest that maladaptive regulation of AKT/GSK3β/CREB pathway may be one of the important causes in pharmacoresistant seizures in response to AMPAR antagonists.

PICK1 contributes to a shift in the AMPAR composition to GRIA2-lacking (Ca^{2+}-permeable) by facilitating GRIA2 internalization [21,23,24]. In the present study, GRIA2 and PICK1 expression levels in the epileptic hippocampus were lower than those in the control (normal) hippocampus. These findings are consistent with a previous study demonstrating downregulation of GRIA2 and PICK1 expression in kainic acid-induced chronic epilepsy rats [17]. The present study also demonstrates that both AMPAR antagonists effectively reduced GRIA2 Y phosphorylations in responders, but not in non-responders, without affecting its S880 phosphorylation. Furthermore, GRIA2 Y phosphorylations showed direct proportional relationships with seizure parameters. Phosphorylations regulate surface GRIA2 expression through interactions with GRIP1 and PICK1: PKC-mediated S880 phosphorylation reinforces its internalization by inhibiting GRIP1–GRIA2 bindings [15,21]. In contrast, Src family-mediated Y phosphorylations facilitate PICK1–GRIA2 interaction to promote GRIA2 internalization [23,24]. Consistent with our previous studies [19,50], both AMPAR antagonists reduced Src family, but not PKC, activity. Considering the roles of GRIA2 phosphorylations in its interactions with GRIP1/PICK1 [15,21,23,24], it is plausible that both AMPAR antagonists would attenuate seizure activity by inhibiting PICK1-mediated GRIA2 internalization. However, AMPAR antagonists cannot influence surface GRIA2 expression [20]. In addition, the present data show that AMPAR antagonists did not influence the reduced PICK1 expression in the hippocampi of both responders and non-responders, which was unaffected by 3CAI co-treatment in non-responders, although PICK1 is a substrate of AKT/GSK3β pathway [34]. Therefore, it is likely that the reduced GRIA2 Y phosphorylations may reflect the decreased Src family activity induced by AMPAR antagonists rather than the inhibition of GRIA2-lacking AMPAR assembly.

Furthermore, it is hypothesized that reduced PICK1 expression in the hippocampus would be involved in ictogenesis in chronic epilepsy rats via other pathways rather than the regulation of surface GRIA2 expression since PICK1 interacts with type III metabotropic glutamate receptor (mGlu7R) in the presynaptic active zone and regulates glutamate release [50]. Indeed, mGlu7R deletion and a polypeptide interfering PICK1 and mGlu7R show typical epileptic seizures [51,52]. Therefore, our findings indicate that PICK1-mediated regulation of surface GRIA2 expression may not be involved in the anti-epileptic effects and responsiveness of AMPAR antagonists, although both perampanel and GYKI 52466 inhibited Src-mediated GRIA2 Y phosphorylations.

On the other hand, SE and spontaneous seizure activity lead to vasogenic edema formation (serum extravasation) induced by brain–blood barrier (BBB) disruption, which deteriorates seizure activity [53–55]. During recovery of vasogenic edema, multidrug efflux transporter expressions, such as p-glycoprotein (p-GP), breast cancer resistance protein (BCRP), and multidrug resistance protein-4 (MRP4), are increased in the hippocampus, which reduce AED concentrations in the brain and cause pharmacoresistant epilepsy [53]. Since we did not compare the pharmacokinetics of AMPAR antagonists between responders and non-responders in the present study, the possibility could not be excluded that the decreased responsiveness of AMPAR antagonists in non-responders would be a consequence from the lower concentration of these compounds induced by over-expression or hyperactivation of drug efflux transporters. In addition, AKT is one of the common down-stream molecules during seizure-induced BBB leakage. Indeed, 3CAI effectively attenuates SE-induced vasogenic edema formation, although it does not show anti-epileptic effects [28]. Thus, it is likely that 3CAI would also increase the efficacies of AMPAR antagonist by inhibiting AKT-mediated serum leakage or upregulation of multidrug efflux transporter. On the other hand, CREB activation plays a protective role against BBB disruption [56,57]. Considering the inhibitory effect of 3CAI on AKT/GSK3β/CREB signaling pathway in the present study, however, it is unlikely that 3CAI may be involved in the CREB-mediated regulation of vascular permeability. Further studies are needed to elucidate whether 3CAI enhances the responsiveness to AMPAR antagonists by inhibiting serum extravasation and/or multidrug efflux systems.

5. Conclusions

The present study revealed that AMPAR antagonists ameliorated spontaneous seizure activity by affecting the Src-mediated AKT/GSK3β/CREB signaling pathway, which was relevant to the regulation of surface expression of GRIA1 rather than GRIA2. In addition, the dysregulation of this pathway was one of the causes of refractory seizures to AMPAR antagonists. Therefore, our findings suggest that the Src/AKT/GSK3β/CREB pathway may be one of the potential therapeutic targets for the treatment of intractable TLE.

Supplementary Materials: The following are available online at https://www.mdpi.com/article/10.3390/biomedicines9040425/s1, Figure S1: Representative full-gel images of Western blots in Figure 3A, Figure S2: Representative full-gel images of Western blots in Figure 4A, Figure S3: Representative full-gel images of Western blots in Figure 5A, Figure S4: Representative full-gel images of Western blots in Figure 6A, Figure S5: Representative full-gel images of Western blots in Figure 6B, Figure S6: Representative full-gel images of Western blots in Figure 7A, Figure S7: Representative full-gel images of Western blots in Figure 9A, Figure S8: Representative full-gel images of Western blots in Figure 10A.

Author Contributions: T.-C.K. designed and supervised the project. J.-E.K., D.-S.L., H.P., T.-H.K., and T.-C.K. performed the experiments described in the manuscript. J.-E.K. and T.-C.K. analyzed the data and wrote the manuscript. All authors have read and agreed to the published version of the manuscript.

Funding: This study was supported by a grant of National Research Foundation of Korea (NRF) grant (No. 2021R1A2B5B01001482).

Institutional Review Board Statement: All experimental protocols were approved by the Animal Care and Use Committee of Hallym University (#Hallym 2018-2, 26 April 2018 and #Hallym 2018-21, 8 June 2018).

Conflicts of Interest: The authors declared that the research was conducted in the absence of any commercial or financial relationships that could be construed as a potential conflict of interest. The funders had no role in the design of the study; in the collection, analyses, or interpretation of data; in the writing of the manuscript, or in the decision to publish the results.

References

1. Aylward, R.L. Epilepsy: A review of reports, guidelines, recommendations and models for the provision of care for patients with epilepsy. *Clin. Med.* **2008**, *8*, 433–438. [CrossRef]
2. Mohanraj, R.; Norrie, J.; Stephen, L.J.; Kelly, K.; Hitiris, N.; Brodie, M.J. Mortality in adults with newly diagnosed and chronic epilepsy: A retrospective comparative study. *Lancet Neurol.* **2006**, *5*, 481–487. [CrossRef]
3. Blair, R.E.; Deshpande, L.S.; Sombati, S.; Elphick, M.R.; Martin, B.R.; DeLorenzo, R.J. Prolonged exposure to WIN55,212-2 causes downregulation of the CB1 receptor and the development of tolerance to its anticonvulsant effects in the hippocampal neuronal culture model of acquired epilepsy. *Neuropharmacology* **2009**, *57*, 208–218. [CrossRef]
4. Blair, R.E.; Sombati, S.; Churn, S.B.; Delorenzo, R.J. Epileptogenesis causes an N-methyl-d-aspartate receptor/Ca2+-dependent decrease in Ca2+/calmodulin-dependent protein kinase II activity in a hippocampal neuronal culture model of spontaneous recurrent epileptiform discharges. *Eur. J. Pharmacol.* **2008**, *588*, 64–71. [CrossRef]
5. Roberta, C.; Francesco, F. Targeting ionotropic glutamate receptors in the treatment of epilepsy. *Curr. Neuropharmacol.* **2020**. [CrossRef] [PubMed]
6. Fritsch, B.; Stott, J.J.; Joelle Donofrio, J.; Rogawski, M.A. Treatment of early and late kainic acid-induced status epilepticus with the noncompetitive AMPA receptor antagonist GYKI 52466. *Epilepsia* **2010**, *51*, 108–117. [CrossRef] [PubMed]
7. Niquet, J.; Baldwin, R.; Norman, K.; Suchomelova, L.; Lumley, L.; Wasterlain, C.G. Simultaneous triple therapy for the treatment of status epilepticus. *Neurobiol. Dis.* **2017**, *104*, 41–49. [CrossRef] [PubMed]
8. Mohammad, H.; Sekar, S.; Wei, Z.; Moien-Afshari, F.; Taghibiglou, C. Perampanel but not amantadine prevents behavioral alterations and epileptogenesis in pilocarpine rat model of status epilepticus. *Mol. Neurobiol.* **2019**, *56*, 2508–2523. [CrossRef] [PubMed]
9. Essin, K.; Nistri, A.; Magazanik, L. Evaluation of GluR2 subunit involvement in AMPA receptor function of neonatal rat hypoglossal motoneurons. *Eur. J. Neurosci.* **2002**, *15*, 1899–1906. [CrossRef] [PubMed]
10. Greger, I.H.; Khatri, L.; Ziff, E.B. RNA editing at arg607 controls AMPA receptor exit from the endoplasmic reticulum. *Neuron* **2002**, *34*, 759–772. [CrossRef]
11. Barria, A.; Derkach, V.; Soderling, T. Identification of the Ca2+/calmodulin-dependent protein kinase II regulatory phosphorylation site in the alpha-amino-3-hydroxyl-5-methyl-4-isoxazole-propionate-type glutamate receptor. *J. Biol. Chem.* **1997**, *272*, 32727–32730. [CrossRef] [PubMed]
12. Seidenman, K.J.; Steinberg, J.P.; Huganir, R.; Malinow, R. Glutamate receptor subunit 2 Serine 880 phosphorylation modulates synaptic transmission and mediates plasticity in CA1 pyramidal cells. *J. Neurosci.* **2003**, *23*, 9220–9228. [CrossRef]
13. Lee, H.K.; Barbarosie, M.; Kameyama, K.; Bear, M.F.; Huganir, R.L. Regulation of distinct AMPA receptor phosphorylation sites during bidirectional synaptic plasticity. *Nature* **2000**, *405*, 955–959. [CrossRef] [PubMed]
14. Malinow, R.; Malenka, R.C. AMPA receptor trafficking and synaptic plasticity. *Annu. Rev. Neurosci.* **2002**, *25*, 103–126. [CrossRef] [PubMed]
15. Wyszynski, M.; Valtschanoff, J.G.; Naisbitt, S.; Dunah, A.W.; Kim, E.; Standaert, D.G.; Weinberg, R.; Sheng, M. Association of AMPA receptors with a subset of glutamate receptor-interacting protein in vivo. *J. Neurosci.* **1999**, *19*, 6528–6537. [CrossRef] [PubMed]
16. Ma, Y.; Sun, X.; Li, J.; Jia, R.; Yuan, F.; Wei, D.; Jiang, W. Melatonin alleviates the epilepsy-associated impairments in hippocampal LTP and spatial learning through rescue of surface GluR2 expression at hippocampal CA1 synapses. *Neurochem. Res.* **2017**, *42*, 1438–1448. [CrossRef]
17. Lorgen, J.Ø.; Egbenya, D.L.; Hammer, J.; Davanger, S. PICK1 facilitates lasting reduction in GluA2 concentration in the hippocampus during chronic epilepsy. *Epilepsy Res.* **2017**, *137*, 25–32. [CrossRef]
18. Pellegrini-Giampietro, D.E.; Gorter, J.A.; Bennett, M.V.; Zukin, R.S. The GluR2 (GluR-B) hypothesis: Ca(2+)-permeable AMPA receptors in neurological disorders. *Trends Neurosci.* **1997**, *20*, 464–470. [CrossRef]
19. Kim, J.E.; Lee, D.S.; Park, H.; Kang, T.C. Src/CK2/PTEN-mediated GluN2B and CREB dephosphorylations regulate the responsiveness to AMPA receptor antagonists in chronic epilepsy Rats. *Int. J. Mol. Sci.* **2020**, *21*, 9633. [CrossRef] [PubMed]
20. Kim, J.E.; Park, H.; Lee, J.E.; Kim, T.H.; Kang, T.C. PTEN is required for the anti-epileptic effects of AMPA receptor antagonists in chronic epileptic rats. *Int. J. Mol. Sci.* **2020**, *21*, 5643. [CrossRef] [PubMed]
21. Chung, H.J.; Xia, J.; Scannevin, R.H.; Zhang, X.; Huganir, R.L. Phosphorylation of the AMPA receptor subunit GluR2 differentially regulates its interaction with PDZ domain-containing proteins. *J. Neurosci.* **2000**, *20*, 7258–7267. [CrossRef] [PubMed]
22. Kim, C.H.; Chung, H.J.; Lee, H.K.; Huganir, R.L. Interaction of the AMPA receptor subunit GluR2/3 with PDZ domains regulates hippocampal long-term depression. *Proc. Natl. Acad. Sci. USA* **2001**, *98*, 11725–11730. [CrossRef] [PubMed]

23. Ahmadian, G.; Ju, W.; Liu, L.; Wyszynski, M.; Lee, S.H.; Dunah, A.W.; Taghibiglou, C.; Wang, Y.; Lu, J.; Wong, T.P.; et al. Tyrosine phosphorylation of GluR2 is required for insulin-stimulated AMPA receptor endocytosis and LTD. *EMBO J.* **2004**, *23*, 1040–1050. [CrossRef]
24. Hayashi, T.; Huganir, R.L. Tyrosine phosphorylation and regulation of the AMPA receptor by SRC family tyrosine kinases. *J. Neurosci.* **2004**, *24*, 6152–6160. [CrossRef] [PubMed]
25. Ko, A.R.; Kang, T.C. Blockade of endothelin B receptor improves the efficacy of levetiracetam in chronic epileptic rats. *Seizure* **2015**, *31*, 133–140. [CrossRef] [PubMed]
26. Racine, R.J. Modification of seizure activity by electrical stimulation. II. Motor seizure. *Electroencephalogr. Clin. Neurophysiol.* **1972**, *32*, 281–294. [CrossRef]
27. Kim, J.E.; Choi, H.C.; Song, H.K.; Kang, T.C. Perampanel affects up-stream regulatory signaling pathways of GluA1 phosphorylation in normal and epileptic rats. *Front. Cell. Neurosci.* **2019**, *13*, 80. [CrossRef]
28. Kim, J.E.; Park, H.; Lee, J.E.; Kang, T.C. Blockade of 67-kDa laminin receptor facilitates AQP4 down-regulation and BBB disruption via ERK1/2-and p38 MAPK-mediated PI3K/AKT activations. *Cells* **2020**, *9*, 1670. [CrossRef]
29. Roskoski, R., Jr. Src kinase regulation by phosphorylation and dephosphorylation. *Biochem. Biophys. Res. Commun.* **2005**, *331*, 1–14. [CrossRef]
30. Roskoski, R., Jr. Src protein-tyrosine kinase structure and regulation. *Biochem. Biophys. Res. Commun.* **2004**, *324*, 1155–1164. [CrossRef]
31. Takashima, A. Drug development targeting the glycogen synthase kinase-3beta (GSK-3beta)-mediated signal transduction pathway: Role of GSK-3beta in adult brain. *J. Pharmacol. Sci.* **2009**, *109*, 174–178. [CrossRef] [PubMed]
32. Grimes, C.A.; Jope, R.S. CREB DNA binding activity is inhibited by glycogen synthase kinase-3 beta and facilitated by lithium. *J. Neurochem.* **2001**, *78*, 1219–1232. [CrossRef] [PubMed]
33. Grimes, C.A.; Jope, R.S. The multifaceted roles of glycogen synthase kinase 3beta in cellular signaling. *Prog. Neurobiol.* **2001**, *65*, 391–426. [CrossRef]
34. Yagishita, S.; Murayama, M.; Ebihara, T.; Maruyama, K.; Takashima, A. Glycogen synthase kinase 3β-mediated phosphorylation in the most C-terminal region of protein interacting with C kinase 1 (PICK1) regulates the binding of PICK1 to glutamate receptor subunit GluA2. *J. Biol. Chem.* **2015**, *290*, 29438–29448. [CrossRef] [PubMed]
35. Becker, A.J.; Chen, J.; Zien, A.; Sochivko, D.; Normann, S.; Schramm, J.; Elger, C.E.; Wiestler, O.D.; Blümcke, I. Correlated stage- and subfield-associated hippocampal gene expression patterns in experimental and human temporal lobe epilepsy. *Eur. J. Neurosci.* **2003**, *18*, 2792–2802. [CrossRef]
36. Zhu, X.; Dubey, D.; Bermudez, C.; Porter, B.E. Suppressing cAMP response element-binding protein transcription shortens the duration of status epilepticus and decreases the number of spontaneous seizures in the pilocarpine model of epilepsy. *Epilepsia* **2015**, *56*, 1870–1878. [CrossRef]
37. Middei, S.; Houeland, G.; Cavallucci, V.; Ammassari-Teule, M.; D'Amelio, M.; Marie, H. CREB is necessary for synaptic maintenance and learning-induced changes of the AMPA receptor GluA1 subunit. *Hippocampus* **2013**, *23*, 488–499. [CrossRef]
38. Paoletti, P. Molecular basis of NMDA receptor functional diversity. *Eur. J. Neurosci.* **2011**, *33*, 1351–1365. [CrossRef]
39. Parkinson, G.T.; Hanley, J.G. Mechanisms of AMPA Receptor Endosomal Sorting. *Front. Mol. Neurosci.* **2018**, *11*, 440. [CrossRef]
40. Moretto, E.; Passafaro, M. Recent Findings on AMPA Receptor Recycling. *Front. Cell. Neurosci.* **2018**, *12*, 286. [CrossRef]
41. Greger, I.H.; Esteban, J.A. AMPA receptor biogenesis and trafficking. *Curr. Opin. Neurobiol.* **2007**, *17*, 289–297. [CrossRef]
42. Zhu, J.J. Mechanisms of synaptic plasticity: From membrane to intracellular AMPAR trafficking. *Mol. Interv.* **2003**, *3*, 15–18. [CrossRef] [PubMed]
43. Brindle, P.K.; Montminy, M.R. The CREB family of transcription activators. *Curr. Opin. Genet. Dev.* **1992**, *2*, 199–204. [CrossRef]
44. Sassone-Corsi, P. Transcription factors responsive to cAMP. *Annu. Rev. Cell Dev. Biol.* **1995**, *11*, 355–377. [CrossRef] [PubMed]
45. Moult, P.R.; Cross, A.; Santos, S.D.; Carvalho, A.L.; Lindsay, Y.; Connolly, C.N.; Irving, A.J.; Leslie, N.R.; Harvey, J. Leptin regulates AMPA receptor trafficking via PTEN inhibition. *J. Neurosci.* **2010**, *30*, 4088–4101. [CrossRef] [PubMed]
46. Shacka, J.J.; Lu, J.; Xie, Z.L.; Uchiyama, Y.; Roth, K.A.; Zhang, J. Kainic acid induces early and transient autophagic stress in mouse hippocampus. *Neurosci. Lett.* **2007**, *414*, 57–60. [CrossRef]
47. Zhu, F.; Kai, J.; Chen, L.; Wu, M.; Dong, J.; Wang, Q.; Zeng, L.H. Akt Inhibitor perifosine prevents epileptogenesis in a rat model of temporal lobe epilepsy. *Neurosci. Bull.* **2018**, *34*, 283–290. [CrossRef]
48. Talos, D.M.; Jacobs, L.M.; Gourmaud, S.; Coto, C.A.; Sun, H.; Lim, K.C.; Lucas, T.H.; Davis, K.A.; Martinez-Lage, M.; Jensen, F.E. Mechanistic target of rapamycin complex 1 and 2 in human temporal lobe epilepsy. *Ann. Neurol.* **2018**, *83*, 311–327. [CrossRef]
49. Shalaby, H.N.; El-Tanbouly, D.M.; Zaki, H.F. Topiramate mitigates 3-nitropropionic acid-induced striatal neurotoxicity via modulation of AMPA receptors. *Food Chem. Toxicol.* **2018**, *118*, 227–234. [CrossRef]
50. Rothstein, J.D.; Martin, L.; Levey, A.I.; Dykes-Hoberg, M.; Jin, L.; Wu, D.; Nash, N.; Kuncl, R.W. Localization of neuronal and glial glutamate transporters. *Neuron* **1994**, *13*, 713–725. [CrossRef]
51. Arstikaitis, P.; Gauthier-Campbell, C. BARS at the synapse: PICK-1 lipid binding domain regulates targeting, trafficking, and synaptic plasticity. *J. Neurosci.* **2006**, *26*, 6909–6910. [CrossRef] [PubMed]
52. Bertaso, F.; Zhang, C.; Scheschonka, A.; de Bock, F.; Fontanaud, P.; Marin, P.; Huganir, R.L.; Betz, H.; Bockaert, J.; Fagni, L.; et al. PICK1 uncoupling from mGluR7a causes absence-like seizures. *Nat. Neurosci.* **2008**, *11*, 940–948. [CrossRef] [PubMed]

53. Kim, Y.J.; Kim, J.E.; Choi, H.C.; Song, H.K.; Kang, T.C. Cellular and regional specific changes in multidrug efflux transporter expression during recovery of vasogenic edema in the rat hippocampus and piriform cortex. *BMB Rep.* **2015**, *48*, 348–353. [CrossRef] [PubMed]
54. Kim, J.E.; Kang, T.C. TRPC3- and ET_B receptor-mediated PI3K/AKT activation induces vasogenic edema formation following status epilepticus. *Brain Res.* **2017**, *1672*, 58–64. [CrossRef] [PubMed]
55. Broekaart, D.W.M.; Anink, J.J.; Baayen, J.C.; Idema, S.; de Vries, H.E.; Aronica, E.; Gorter, J.A.; van Vliet, E.A. Activation of the innate immune system is evident throughout epileptogenesis and is associated with blood-brain barrier dysfunction and seizure progression. *Epilepsia* **2018**, *59*, 1931–1944. [CrossRef]
56. Ruan, W.; Li, J.; Xu, Y.; Wang, Y.; Zhao, F.; Yang, X.; Jiang, H.; Zhang, L.; Saavedra, J.M.; Shi, L.; et al. MALAT1 up-regulator polydatin protects brain microvascular integrity and ameliorates stroke through C/EBPβ/MALAT1/CREB/PGC-1α/PPARγ pathway. *Cell. Mol. Neurobiol.* **2019**, *39*, 265–286. [CrossRef]
57. Wu, X.; Fu, S.; Liu, Y.; Luo, H.; Li, F.; Wang, Y.; Gao, M.; Cheng, Y.; Xie, Z. NDP-MSH binding melanocortin-1 receptor ameliorates neuroinflammation and BBB disruption through CREB/Nr4a1/NF-κB pathway after intracerebral hemorrhage in mice. *J. Neuroinflamm.* **2019**, *16*, 192. [CrossRef]

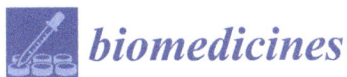

Article

Peripheral Infection after Traumatic Brain Injury Augments Excitability in the Perilesional Cortex and Dentate Gyrus

Ying Wang [1,2], Pedro Andrade [1] and Asla Pitkänen [1,*]

[1] A. I. Virtanen Institute for Molecular Sciences, University of Eastern Finland, P.O. Box 1627, FI-70211 Kuopio, Finland; wangying@dmu.edu.cn (Y.W.); pedro.andrade@uef.fi (P.A.)
[2] Department of Neurology, The First Affiliated Hospital of Dalian Medical University, Dalian 116001, China
* Correspondence: asla.pitkanen@uef.fi; Tel.: +358-50-517-2091; Fax: +358-17-16-3030

Abstract: Peripheral infections occur in up to 28% of patients with traumatic brain injury (TBI), which is a major etiology for structural epilepsies. We hypothesized that infection occurring after TBI acts as a "second hit" and facilitates post-traumatic epileptogenesis. Adult male Sprague–Dawley rats were subjected to lateral fluid-percussion injury or sham-operation. At 8 weeks post-injury, rats were treated with lipopolysaccharide (LPS, 5 mg/kg) to mimic Gram-negative peripheral infection. T2-weighted magnetic resonance imaging was used to detect the cortical lesion type (small focal inflammatory [TBI$_{FI}$] vs. large cavity-forming [TBI$_{CF}$]). Spontaneous seizures were detected with video-electroencephalography, and seizure susceptibility was determined by the pentylenetetrazole (PTZ) test. Post-PTZ neuronal activation was assessed using c-Fos immunohistochemistry. LPS treatment increased the percentage of rats with PTZ-induced seizures among animals with TBI$_{FI}$ lesions ($p < 0.05$). It also increased the cumulative duration of PTZ-induced seizures ($p < 0.01$), particularly in the TBI$_{FI}$ group ($p < 0.05$). The number of c-Fos immunopositive cells was higher in the perilesional cortex of injured animals compared with sham-operated animals ($p < 0.05$), particularly in the TBI-LPS group ($p < 0.05$). LPS treatment increased the percentage of injured rats with bilateral c-Fos staining in the dentate gyrus ($p < 0.05$), particularly in the TBI$_{FI}$ group ($p < 0.05$). Our findings demonstrate that peripheral infection after TBI increases PTZ-induced seizure susceptibility and neuronal activation in the perilesional cortex and bilaterally in the dentate gyrus, particularly in animals with prolonged perilesional T2 enhancement. Our data suggest that treatment of infections and reduction of post-injury neuro-inflammation are important components of the treatment regimen aiming at preventing epileptogenesis after TBI.

Keywords: c-Fos; early gene activation; epileptogenesis; lipopolysaccharide; pentylenetetrazole; post-traumatic epilepsy; seizure susceptibility; traumatic brain injury

Citation: Wang, Y.; Andrade, P.; Pitkänen, A. Peripheral Infection after Traumatic Brain Injury Augments Excitability in the Perilesional Cortex and Dentate Gyrus. *Biomedicines* **2021**, *9*, 1946. https://doi.org/10.3390/biomedicines9121946

Academic Editor: Bruno Meloni

Received: 23 November 2021
Accepted: 17 December 2021
Published: 19 December 2021

Publisher's Note: MDPI stays neutral with regard to jurisdictional claims in published maps and institutional affiliations.

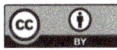

Copyright: © 2021 by the authors. Licensee MDPI, Basel, Switzerland. This article is an open access article distributed under the terms and conditions of the Creative Commons Attribution (CC BY) license (https://creativecommons.org/licenses/by/4.0/).

1. Introduction

Approximately 2.5 million people in both Europe (www.center-tbi.eu/ accessed on 23 November 2021) and the United States (www.cdc.gov/traumaticbraininjury accessed on 22 November 2021) experience traumatic brain injury (TBI) each year. The risk of epileptogenesis increases according to the severity of the TBI: approximately 2- to 4-fold after mild, 8-fold after moderate, and 16-fold after severe TBI [1–3]. Up to 53% of patients with penetrating TBI develop epilepsy [4,5]. TBI causes 10% to 20% of symptomatic epilepsy and 5% of all types of epilepsy [6,7]. Despite the large number of epidemiologic studies reporting risk factors for epileptogenesis after TBI [8], the factors and events occurring over the lifetime of a given subject that lead to post-traumatic epilepsy (PTE) remain largely unknown.

The evolution of post-traumatic epileptogenesis overlaps with the progression of secondary brain damage, which can continue for days to weeks to months after TBI and includes neuroinflammation, oxidative stress, excitation-inhibition imbalance, and blood–brain barrier damage, as well as synaptic and network plasticity alterations [9]. Some of these molecular and cellular changes contribute to post-traumatic epileptogenesis, whereas others can support spontaneous recovery [10]. To date, the effects of additional events modulating secondary damage during the post-TBI aftermath have received little attention, even though their prevention and/or treatment could present an important avenue for mitigating post-traumatic epileptogenesis.

The concept of "microglia priming," in which "the brain is primed by chronic central nervous system (CNS) diseases to show exaggerated responses to a subsequent hit, which induces an inflammatory response, whether systemic or central in origin," was introduced by Combrinck et al. [11]. Activation of innate inflammatory pathways is an elementary component of the secondary injury in both experimental and human TBI [12]. In animal models, the inflammatory response is most robust during the 1 to 3 weeks post-TBI, but microglia can remain activated in the brain for months [13]. A positron emission tomography (PET) imaging study in humans with TBI using [11C] (R)PK11195 demonstrated that microglial activation can last up to 17 years, and is associated with cognitive decline [14].

Bacterial infections represent important post-TBI secondary hits as they commonly occur but seem innocuous because they are treatable by existing medications. Up to 50% of severe TBI patients have been suggested to suffer from infections during their hospital stay, and infection-related mortality can be as high as 28% [15–20]. Infections are most common in patients with the lowest Glasgow Coma Scale scores, that is, in patients with the highest risk of epileptogenesis [18]. To date, no evidence for a clear association between TBI-related infections and PTE has been reported, which may relate to relatively small study populations and short follow-up. Weisbrod and coworkers reported that up to 29% of patients who suffered penetrating TBI in combat due to gunshots or blast had systemic infections, and 25% had meningitis during acute hospitalization; up to 39% developed epilepsy in a 2-year follow-up [21]. In another study, Saadat and coworkers found a poor outcome if the military perforating injury was associated with CNS infection. CNS infections co-occurred with epilepsy, but the association between epilepsy and infections was not specifically analyzed [22]. A recent study demonstrated that elevated systemic levels of lipopolysaccharide (LPS), a component of the outer membrane of Gram-negative bacteria, due to the breakdown of the gastrointestinal barrier was associated with PTE in a rat lateral fluid-percussion injury (FPI) model [23]. Despite the important clinical ramifications, little is known about whether or not the re-activation of inflammation by peripheral infection in an adult TBI-primed brain facilitates epileptogenesis.

The present study was designed to test the hypothesis that LPS-induced peripheral infection at a chronic time-point after TBI in rats will serve as a "second hit," thereby increasing neuronal excitability in the perilesional cortex and hippocampus and facilitating post-traumatic epileptogenesis.

2. Materials and Methods

The study design is summarized in Figure 1.

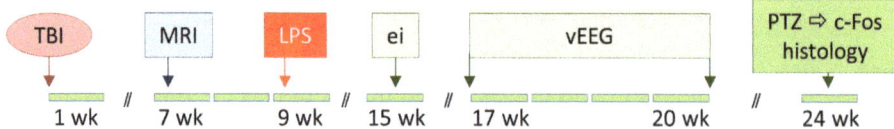

Figure 1. Study design. Traumatic brain injury (TBI) was induced by lateral fluid-percussion injury (FPI). Lesion endophenotype (focal inflammatory [TBI$_{FI}$] vs. cavity-forming [TBI$_{CF}$]) was assessed with T2-weighted magnetic resonance imaging (MRI) at 6 weeks after TBI. At 8 weeks post-TBI, rats received a single injection of lipopolysaccharide (LPS; 5 mg/kg, i.p.) or vehicle. Epidural skull electrodes (ei) were implanted at 14 weeks following TBI. Thereafter, 4-week-long video-electroencephalogram (vEEG) monitoring was performed starting at 16 weeks after TBI to detect spontaneous seizures. The pentylenetetrazole (PTZ) seizure-susceptibility test was performed under vEEG at 23 weeks post-TBI (i.e., 15 weeks after LPS injection). Finally, rats were perfused for histology at 2 h after PTZ administration (~6 months post-TBI). Sham-operated controls underwent all of the same procedures except the induction of TBI.

2.1. Animals

A total of 46 adult (10-week-old) male Sprague–Dawley rats (300–350 g, Harlan Netherlands B.V., Udine, Italy) were used. Throughout the experiments, animals were housed in individual cages in a controlled environment (temperature 22 ± 1 °C; humidity 50 ± 10%; 12 h light/12 h dark cycle). Food and water were available ad libitum. All animal procedures were approved by the Animal Ethics Committee of the Provincial Government of Southern Finland and carried out in accordance with the European Council Directive (2010/63/EU).

2.2. Induction of TBI by Lateral FPI

Traumatic brain injury (TBI) was triggered by lateral FPI, as described previously [24]. Briefly, animals (n = 26) were anesthetized with a cocktail (6 mL/kg, i.p.) containing sodium pentobarbital (58 mg/kg), magnesium sulfate (127.2 mg/kg), propylene glycol (42.8%), and absolute ethanol (11.6%). A craniectomy (Ø 5 mm) was performed over the left parieto-temporal cortex between lambda and bregma (anterior edge 2.0 mm posterior to bregma; lateral edge adjacent to the left lateral ridge). The bone was carefully removed without disruption of the underlying dura. A female Luer-Lock connector was positioned into the craniotomy hole, its edges carefully sealed with Vetbond tissue adhesive (3M, St. Paul, MN, USA), and the cap filled with sterile saline and fixed to the skull with dental acrylate (Selectaplus powder #10009210; Selectaplus liquid CN #D10009102, DeguDent, Germany). About 90 min after administration of anesthesia cocktail, when the toe reflex reappeared, the rat was attached to the fluid-percussion device (AmScien Instruments, Richmond, VA, USA). Lateral FPI was induced by a transient (21–23 ms) fluid pulse impact against the exposed dura. The pendulum height was adjusted to produce severe injury [~3.0 atm; expected <72 h mortality 25%; [4]]. Sham-injured animals (n = 7) also underwent anesthesia and craniectomy procedures without exposure to lateral FPI. Naive animals (n = 5) were not subjected to anesthesia, craniectomy, or injury.

2.3. Magnetic Resonance Imaging (MRI)

Our previous MRI and histologic studies indicated inter-animal heterogeneity in the progression of cortical lesion pathology after lateral FPI-induced TBI [5,25–27]. To stratify the rats into different treatment groups based on the main lesion endophenotype [focal inflammatory (TBI$_{FI}$) vs. cavity-forming (TBI$_{CF}$)], rats underwent MRI at 6 weeks post-TBI. MRI was conducted under isoflurane anesthesia (1.5% isoflurane, O_2/N_2 30/70% as carrier gas) at 9.4 T horizontal magnet (Varian Inc., Palo Alto, CA, USA) interfaced to Bruker Pharmascan console (Bruker Biospin, Ettlingen, Germany) using actively decoupled volume transmitter and quadrature surface receiver coils. Anatomical T2-weighted images were acquired using rapid acquisition with relaxation enhancement (RARE) sequence (TE 40 ms, TR 4000 ms, flip 90°, 25 slices, thickness 1 mm, a field of view 30 × 30 mm, 256 × 256 matrix, 2 averages, RARE factor 8) and T2 maps were acquired using multi-slice multi-echo (MSME) sequence (TR 5000 ms, TE 12, 24, 36, 48, 60, 72, 84, 96, 108, 120 ms, 10–15 slices to cover the lesion area, thickness 1 mm, interleaved collection, 256 × 128 matrix).

Anatomical T-weighted images were acquired at 7 T Bruker Pharmascan MRI scanner using fast spin-echo pulse sequence (TR 4000 ms, effective TE 40 ms, 25 slices, slice thickness 1 mm). In T2-weighted MRI, 10–15 slices that covered the entire rostrocaudal extent of the lesion were analyzed. Imaging was conducted using a 9.4 T horizontal magnet (Varian Inc., Palo Alto, CA, USA) interfaced to a Direct Drive console (Varian Inc.) as previously described by Immonen et al. [5]. According to the distribution and extent of signal intensity in T2-weighted MRI, 15 rats with TBI had developed the TBI$_{FI}$ endophenotype and 11 had developed the TBI$_{CF}$ endophenotype of cortical lesion by the time of the MRI.

2.4. Lipopolysaccharide (LPS) Injection

To model peripheral infection occurring during the post-TBI recovery phase caused by Gram-negative bacteria activating TLR4-mediated signaling [28], rats with the TBI$_{FI}$

or TBI$_{CF}$ endophenotype were randomized into the vehicle or LPS treatment groups. At 8 weeks post-TBI, animals received a single intraperitoneal injection of LPS (serotype 055:B5, Sigma-Aldrich; 5 mg/kg) or vehicle (0.9% NaCl, 2.5 mL/kg). Naïve and sham-operated animals were injected with vehicle only. This resulted in 6 different groups: Naïve-Veh (n = 5), Sham-Veh (n = 7), TBI$_{FI}$-Veh (n = 7), TBI$_{FI}$-LPS (n = 8), TBI$_{CF}$-Veh (n = 5), TBI$_{CF}$-LPS (n = 6).

2.5. Electrode Implantation for Electroencephalogram (EEG) Monitoring

To monitor the spontaneous and pentylenetetrazole (PTZ)-induced epileptiform activity, 4 stainless steel epidural screw electrodes, 1 reference electrode, and 1 ground electrode were inserted into the skull (Ø 1 mm, Plastics One, Inc., Roanoke, VA, USA) on weeks 15 after TBI as described by Kharatishvili et al. [29]. Video-EEG monitoring was initiated after a 7-d recovery period. A lost headset was re-implanted once if the skull was intact and not infected, and monitoring was continued.

2.6. Video-EEG Monitoring and Analysis of Occurrence of Spontaneous Seizures

A 4-weeks continuous (24/7) video-EEG (vEEG) monitoring was started on weeks 17 post-TBI to detect epileptiform activity as described in detail by [30].

Digital EEG files were scanned on the computer screen and manually analyzed by a blinded investigator. A spontaneous electroencephalographic seizure was defined as a high amplitude (more than twice baseline) rhythmic discharge that clearly represented a new pattern of tracing (repetitive spikes, spike-and-wave discharges, and slow waves) and lasted >5 s. Epileptic events occurring with an interval of less than 5 s without the EEG returning to baseline were defined as belonging to the same seizure. In addition, the occurrence of epileptiform discharges (EDs), defined as rhythmic transients ($\geq$1 s, but <5 s) containing spikes and uniform sharp waves, was analyzed.

If an electrographic seizure was observed, its behavioral severity was assessed from the corresponding video recording according to a modified Racine's scale [31]. As described previously by Rodgers et al. [32], we also noted the occurrence of spike-and-wave discharges in both the sham-operated and injured rats, but they were not counted as TBI-related seizures.

2.7. Pentylenetetrazole (PTZ) Seizure Susceptibility Test

Seizure susceptibility was assessed at 23 weeks post-TBI (i.e., 3 weeks after completing the continuous vEEG monitoring). Animals were placed in a transparent plexiglass cage (47 cm × 29 cm × 50 cm) and connected to the vEEG system 24 h before the test. After a baseline vEEG recording, animals were injected with a subconvulsive dose of PTZ (25 mg/kg, i.p., Sigma-Aldrich, YA-Kemia Oy, Finland) and continuously vEEG monitored for 120 min. As outcome parameters, we assessed (1) latency to the first spike (s), (2) latency to the first ED (s), (3) occurrence of electrographic seizures (yes/no), (4) latency to the first electrographic seizure (s), (5) duration of an electrographic seizure (s), and (6) number and severity of induced behavioral seizures [31].

2.8. Histology

Processing of brain tissue. At 120 min after PTZ injection, animals were disconnected from the vEEG, deeply anesthetized (as described before), and perfused intracardially with 4% paraformaldehyde in 0.1 M sodium phosphate buffer (PB), pH 7.4. Brains were post-fixed in 4% paraformaldehyde in 0.1 M PB, cryoprotected in 20% glycerol in 0.02 M potassium phosphate-buffered saline (KPBS, pH 7.4), frozen on dry ice, and stored at −70 °C until further processed.

c-Fos immunohistochemistry. A series of free-floating sections (1-in-10 series, 25 μm) was rinsed, and then, treated with 1% H_2O_2 in 0.02 M KPBS at room temperature (RT) for 15 min to remove endogenous peroxidase. Then, sections were incubated for 72 h at 4 °C in a primary antibody solution containing rabbit-polyclonal antibody raised against c-Fos (1:20 000, sc-253, Santa Cruz Biotechnology), 1% NGS, and 0.5% TX-100 in 0.02 M KPBS. After 3 washes in 2% NGS in 0.02 M KPBS, sections were incubated at RT for 1 h in a secondary antibody solution containing biotinylated goat anti-rabbit IgG (1:200, BA-1000, Vector Laboratories, Burlingame, CA, USA) with 1% NGS and 0.5% TX-100 in 0.02 M KPBS. After 3 washes, sections were incubated in avidin–biotin solution (1:200, PK-4000, Vector Laboratories) in 0.02 M KPBS for 45 min at RT. Then, sections were recycled into the secondary antibody solution (45 min at RT), washed 3 times, and recycled into avidin–biotin solution (30 min at RT). After 3 washes (0.02 M KPBS, 10 min each), the sections were incubated in a solution containing 0.1% 3′,3′-diaminobenzidine (DAB, Pierce Chemicals, Rockford, IL, USA) and 0.08 % H_2O_2 in 0.02 M KPBS for visualization of the staining. Then, the sections were mounted on gelatin-coated microscope slides, dried overnight at 37 °C and the reaction product was intensified with osmium (OsO_4; #19170; Electron Microscopy Sciences, Hatfield, PA, USA) and thiocarbohydrate (TCH; #21900; Electron Microscopy Sciences) according to by Lewis et al. [33]. Finally, slides were covered using DePex as a mounting medium.

2.9. Assessment of the Density of c-Fos Immunoreactive Neurons in the Perilesional and Corresponding Contralateral Cortex

To assess the pattern of PTZ-induced neuronal activation in the brain undergoing epileptogenesis after TBI, we measured the distribution and density of c-Fos labeling in the cerebral cortex from digital photomicrographs of immunostained sections using Image J software (version 1.46r, http://rsb.info.nih.gov/ij/ accessed on 22 November 2021). For the analysis, we selected 2 sections from each rat: 1 from the most rostral and another from the most caudal level of the cortical lesion. A series of contiguous images was then captured from each section at 5× magnification, and a single montage image of the whole section was generated using a Zeiss Imager M2 microscope equipped with a Zeiss Axiocam 506 color camera operated by ZEN software. Four regions of interest (ROIs) were drawn in each section: a 1 mm wide cortical area bordering the lesion core medially (medial perilesional cortex) and laterally (lateral perilesional cortex), and the corresponding areas in the contralateral cortex. Each cortical area was further subdivided into the area containing layers II-IV and layers V-VI. This resulted in the following 4 ROIs: medial perilesional supragranular layers (including internal granular layer IV), medial perilesional infragranular layers, lateral perilesional supragranular layers, and lateral perilesional infragranular layers. Accordingly, the corresponding contralateral cortex was also divided into 4 areas, resulting in a total of 8 ROIs per section. Next, the RGB color images were converted into gray-scale images. Then, gray-scale images were thresholded manually to match with the c-Fos positivity in the immunostained section. Then, the (a) total area of the ROI (total number 8) and (b) area of c-Fos positivity in a thresholded image were calculated. The c-Fos expression-% (c-Fos-%) in each ROI was calculated as (c-Fos positive area/ROI area) × 100%.

2.10. Statistical Analysis

Statistical analysis was performed using SPSS for Windows (version 19.0) and Graph-Pad Prism5. The non-parametric Kruskal–Wallis test was used to assess differences in the parameters of the PTZ test (latency to the first electrographic seizure, latency to the first spike, latency to the first ED, seizure duration, and behavioral score) and the density of c-Fos expression between treatment groups. *Post hoc* analysis was performed using the Mann–Whitney U test. The Wilcoxon test was applied to test the differences in c-Fos expression between different brain areas (ipsilateral vs. contralateral, rostral vs. caudal, medial vs. lateral, supragranular layers vs. infragranular layers) within the same animal. The chi-square (χ^2) test was applied to analyze differences in the occurrence of PTZ-induced seizures and increased c-Fos expression in the dentate gyrus between experimental groups. The non-parametric Spearman rank correlation test was used to analyze correlations between c-Fos expression density and the total seizure duration or the maximum behavioral score in the PTZ test. Data are presented as mean ± standard deviation or as mean ± standard error of the mean. Statistical significance was set at $p < 0.05$.

3. Results

3.1. Impact Pressure, Occurrence of Post-Impact Seizure-Like Behavior, Apnea Time, and Mortality

Impact pressure. The impact pressure used to induce lateral FPI was 3.23 ± 0.09 atm (range 2.91–3.39 atm). There was no difference between the rats that developed TBI_{FI} (3.21 ± 0.07) or TBI_{CF} (3.23 ± 0.11) endophenotypes at 6 weeks post-TBI ($p = 0.096$).

Apnea. The post-impact time in apnea was 20 ± 14 s (range 5–60 s). There was no difference between the TBI_{FI} (23 ± 16) and TBI_{CF} (17 ± 11) endophenotypes ($p = 0.3709$).

Acute and follow-up mortality. Acute post-impact mortality (<72 h) was 21% (7/33 rats with TBI), indicating moderate severity of the TBI [24,34,35]. Follow-up mortality (>72 h post-injury) was 31% (8/26) and typically occurred during the anesthesia-related to electrode implantation or unknown causes. In sham-operated animals, acute mortality was 0% (0/7) and follow-up mortality 28% (2/7; during electrode implantation-related anesthesia).

3.2. MRI Indicated Equal Distribution of TBI_{FI} and TBI_{CF} Endophenotypes at 6 Weeks Post-TBI

Consistent with our previous follow-up studies [5,26,27], MRI analysis of cortical pathology at 6 weeks post-TBI ($n = 26$) indicated 2 major structural cortical lesion endophenotypes. One endophenotype was characterized by a focal cortical lesion surrounded by an enhanced T2 signal, reporting on ongoing perilesional inflammation, and is referred to here as "focal inflammatory endophenotype" (TBI_{FI}) (Figure 2A). The second endophenotype presented as a large cortical cavity accompanied by an enlarged ipsilateral lateral ventricle and very narrow or no perilesional inflammation, referred to here as a "cavity-forming endophenotype" (TBI_{CF}) (Figure 2B). At 6 weeks post-TBI, 58% (15/26) of the TBI rats had developed a TBI_{FI} endophenotype, and 42% (11/26) developed a TBI_{CF} endophenotype. Consequently, the 26 surviving rats of both endophenotypes were randomized into the LPS or vehicle treatment groups, resulting in 4 experimental groups: TBI_{FI}-Veh (7), TBI_{FI}-LPS (8), TBI_{CF}-Veh (5), and TBI_{CF}-LPS (6).

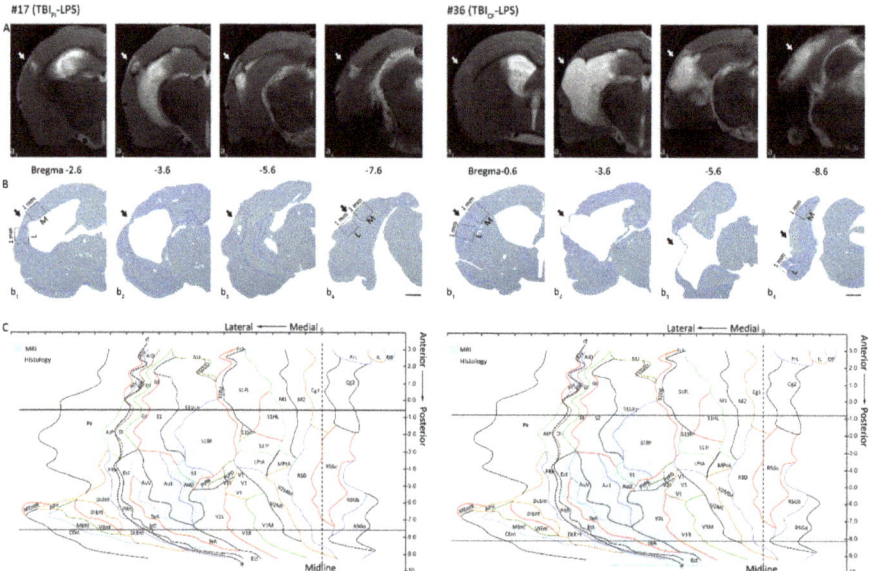

Figure 2. Cortical lesion endophenotypes. Representative unfolded MRI and histologic cortical maps of 2 rats with lateral

fluid-percussion-induced traumatic brain injury (TBI), showing the extent and location of the cortical lesion in the focal-inflammatory (rat #17 from the TBI$_{FI}$-LPS group; left panels) and cavity-forming (rat #36 from the TBI$_{CF}$-LPS group; right panels) endophenotypes. The horizontal lines indicate the 2 rostrocaudal levels, from which the immunostained sections were sampled for analysis of c-Fos expression. (**A**) Four representative coronal T$_2$-weighted MRI slices (a$_1$ most rostral, a$_4$ most caudal) used for the unfolding of the lesion in MRI images at 6 weeks post-TBI. White arrows indicate the lesion. (**B**) Four thionin-stained sections (23 weeks post-TBI) corresponding to levels of MRI slices in panel (**A**). Dashed 1 mm wide squares in b$_1$ (rostral) and b$_4$ (caudal), extending throughout layers I-VI indicate the areas used for the quantitative analysis of c-Fos-immunoreactivity (ir) in the medial (m) and lateral (l) perilesional cortex. (**C**) Unfolded MRI (blue) and histologic (pink) cortical lesion overlaid on the unfolded template prepared as previously described [26]. Abbreviations: CF, cavity-forming; FI, focal inflammatory; ir, immunoreactivity; L, lateral; LPS, lipopolysaccharide; M, medial; MRI, magnetic resonance imaging; TBI, traumatic brain injury. Scale bar = 1 mm.

3.3. Spontaneous Seizures and Epileptiform Discharges

In the 4-weeks vEEG monitoring that started on weeks 17 post-TBI (i.e., 8 weeks after LPS injection) 1 rat in the TBI$_{FI}$-Veh group (#22) expressed 1 spontaneous seizure (Racine score 1) lasting for 117 s (Figure 3A). Another rat in the TBI$_{FI}$-Veh group (#43) had a spontaneous seizure during the overnight vEEG recording preceding the PTZ test. The seizure lasted 185 s and had a Racine score of 5. In both animals, the seizures occurred during the transition from N3 sleep to REM (Figure 3A). No handling-related seizures were observed.

One of the 5 rats in the TBI$_{FI}$-LPS group expressed EDs (Figure 3B, no spontaneous seizures were observed). All except 3 sham and TBI rats (1 in TBI$_{FI}$-Veh, 1 in TBI$_{FI}$-LPS, and 1 in TBI$_{CF}$-LPS group) showed spike-and-wave discharges (SWDs, Figure 3C).

3.4. Peripheral Infection at 8 Weeks Post-TBI Increased Seizure Susceptibility in the PTZ Test

The effect of TBI with or without LPS treatment on seizure susceptibility was tested using the PTZ-test at 4 weeks after completing the 4-weeks vEEG monitoring, i.e., 23 weeks after TBI and 15 weeks after LPS injection. Data are summarized in Table 1.

Occurrence of PTZ-induced seizures. PTZ-induced seizures occurred more often in the TBI-LPS group than in the sham-injured group (80% vs. 20%, $p < 0.05$, χ^2-test). Seizure occurrence did not differ between the TBI-LPS and TBI-Veh groups (80% vs. 46%, $p > 0.05$, χ^2-test) (Table 1).

When the 2 endophenotypes were analyzed separately, PTZ-induced seizures within 1 h after PTZ injection occurred more often in the TBI$_{FI}$-LPS group than in the TBI$_{FI}$-Veh group (100% vs. 43%, $p < 0.05$, χ^2-test). Occurrence of induced seizures in the TBI$_{CF}$-LPS group, however, did not differ from that in the TBI$_{CF}$-Veh group (60% vs. 50%, $p > 0.05$, χ^2-test). In addition, there was no difference between the TBI$_{FI}$-LPS and TBI$_{CF}$-LPS groups (100% vs. 60%) or between the TBI$_{FI}$-Veh and TBI$_{CF}$-Veh groups (43% vs. 50%) (Figure 4A).

Number of PTZ-induced seizures. The mean number of PTZ-induced seizures did not differ between the TBI-LPS and TBI-Veh groups (1.8 ± 1.0 vs. 1 ± 0, $p > 0.05$). In addition, no differences were detected between the endophenotypes (data not shown).

Latency to the first electrographic seizure. Only 1 of the sham-operated rats developed a seizure after PTZ injection (latency 1 628 s). The latency to the first electrographic seizure in the TBI-LPS group tended to be shorter than that in the TBI-Veh group (331 ± 258 s vs. 604 ± 345 s, $p > 0.05$) (Table 1). Even though the different pathologic endophenotypes did not differ from each other, the latency to the first PTZ-induced seizures seemed the shortest in the TBI$_{CF}$-LPS group (206 ± 133 s) (Figure 4B).

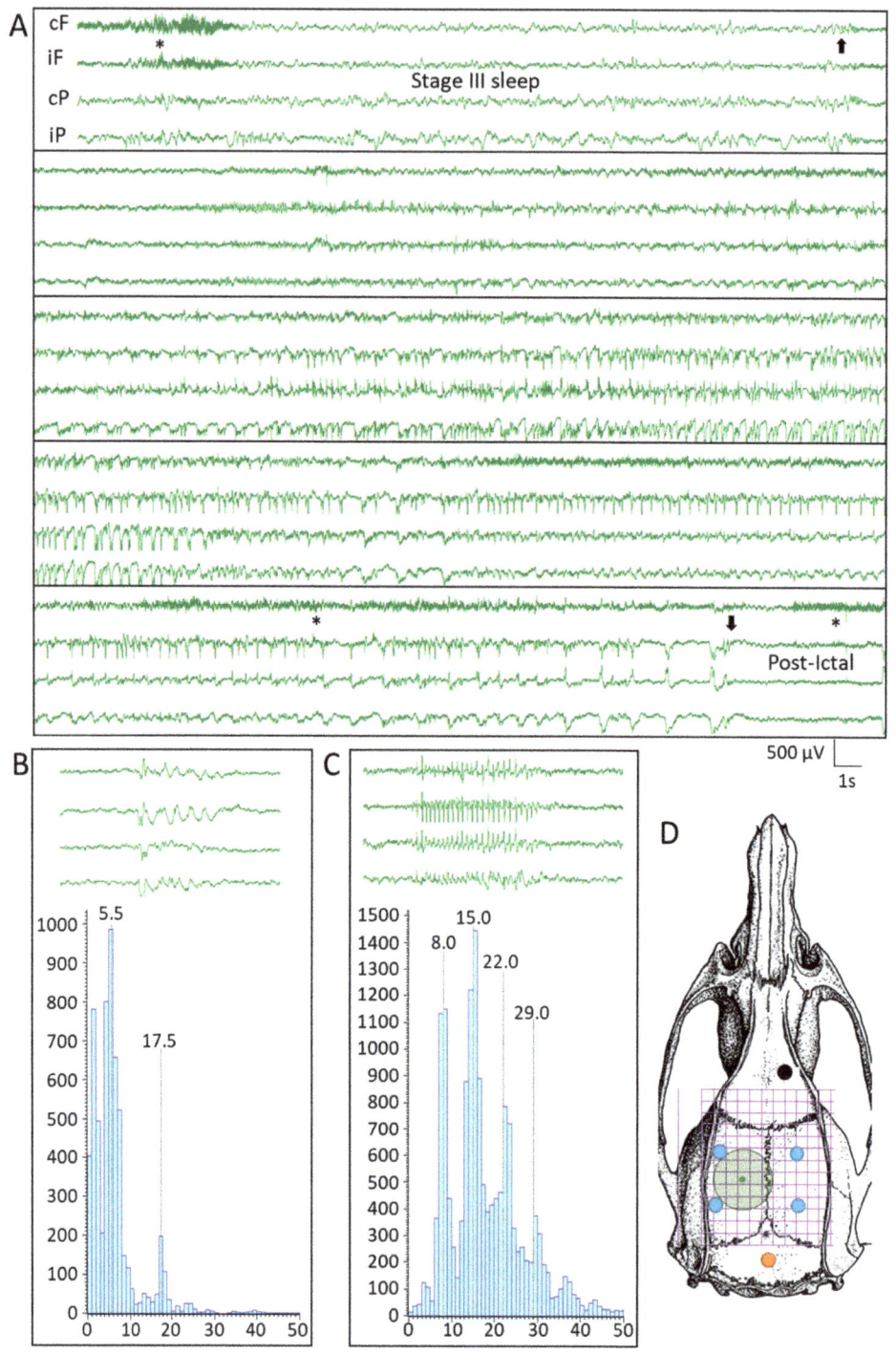

Figure 3. Video-electroencephalogram (vEEG) analysis. (**A**) A spontaneous seizure in a rat (#22) from the TBI$_{FI}$-Veh group

that occurred during the transition from stage III sleep to rapid eye movement sleep (REM). Black arrows indicate the beginning and end of the seizure. Asterisks refer to arousals. The duration of the electrographic seizure was 117 s, and the behavioral Racine score was 3 [31]. The X-Y scale in the right lower corner indicates the voltage and duration or electrographic patterns and applies to panels A-C. Stars indicate muscle artifacts. (**B**) An example of the epileptiform discharge (ED) lasting 1.2 s in a rat (#39) from the TBI$_{FI}$-LPS group. Note the peak in relative power at 5.5 Hz. (**C**) An example of a spike-and-wave discharge (SWD) in a rat (#40) in the TBI$_{FI}$-Veh group. Note the peak in relative power at 8 Hz and subsequent harmonics. SWDs were also found in the sham-operated group and were considered to be age-related oscillations in Sprague–Dawley rats]. (**D**) Green circle indicates the craniotomy. Positions of the 4 epidural recording electrodes (Ø 1 mm, blue circles), a reference electrode (black), and ground electrode (orange). Abbreviations: cF, contralateral frontal; cP, contralateral posterior; ED, epileptiform discharge; FI, focal inflammatory; iF, ipsilateral frontal; iP, ipsilateral posterior; LPS, lipopolysaccharide; REM, rapid eye movement sleep; SWD, spike-and-wave discharge; TBI, traumatic brain injury; Veh, vehicle.

Table 1. Electroencephalograhic (EEG) events in the pentylenetetrazol (PTZ) seizure susceptibility test at 23 weeks after traumatic brain injury (TBI) and 15 weeks after lipopolysaccharide (LPS) administration in the whole animal group.

Parameter	Sham (1/5)	TBI + Veh (5/11)	TBI + LPS (8/10)
latency to the first spike (s)	287 ± 230	730 ± 765	374 ± 401
latency to the first ED (s)	288 ± 229	775 ± 802	400 ± 399
occurrence of PTZ-induced seizures	20%	46%	80%
latency to the first electrographic seizure (s)	1 628	604 ± 345	331 ± 258
mean seizure duration per rat (s)	24	35 ± 19	114 ± 53 *
mean cumulative seizure duration per rat (s)	24	35 ± 19	163 ± 90 **
mean behavioral seizure score per rat	3	3.2 ± 2.0	4.0 ± 1.0

Abbreviations: ED, epileptiform discharge;TBI, traumatic brain injury; Veh, vehicle. Data are shown as mean ± standard deviation of the mean. Statistical significances: * $p < 0.05$; ** $p < 0.01$ (Mann–Whitney U test compared to the TBI-Veh group).

Cumulative duration of PTZ-induced electrographic seizures. Cumulative seizure duration was longer in TBI-LPS rats (163 ± 90 s, range 77–338 s, median 168 s) than in TBI-Veh rats (35 ± 19 s, range 10–52 s, median 46 s, $p < 0.01$) (Figure 4C). In particular, the cumulative seizure duration in the TBI$_{FI}$-LPS group (193 ± 103 s, range 77–338 s, median 196 s) was prolonged compared with that in the TBI$_{FI}$-Veh group (40 ± 18 s, range 20–52 s, median 49 s, $p < 0.05$) (Figure 4D). It should be noted that rats in the TBI$_{CF}$-LPS group also tended to have a prolonged cumulative seizure duration compared with the TBI$_{CF}$-Veh group. As only 2 rats in the TBI$_{CF}$-Veh group had PTZ-induced seizures, however, the difference was not significant (Figure 4D).

Behavioral severity of PTZ-induced seizures. The mean seizure behavioral score was 4.0 ± 1.0 (range 3–5, median 4) in the TBI-LPS group, 3.2 ± 2.0 (range 0–5, median 3) in the TBI-Veh group, and 3 in the sham group (only 1 seizure) (Table 1). No differences were detected between groups or endophenotypes (data not shown).

Latency to the first spike. The latency to the first spike after PTZ treatment tended to be reduced in the TBI-LPS group compared with the TBI-Veh group (Table 1). The difference did not reach statistical significance, however, regardless of whether the 2 endophenotypes were analyzed together or separately (data not shown).

Latency to the first ED. Similarly, the latency to the first ED after PTZ administration tended to be shorter in the TBI-LPS group compared with the TBI-Veh group (Table 1). The difference did not reach statistical significance, however, regardless of whether the 2 endophenotypes were analyzed together or separately (data not shown).

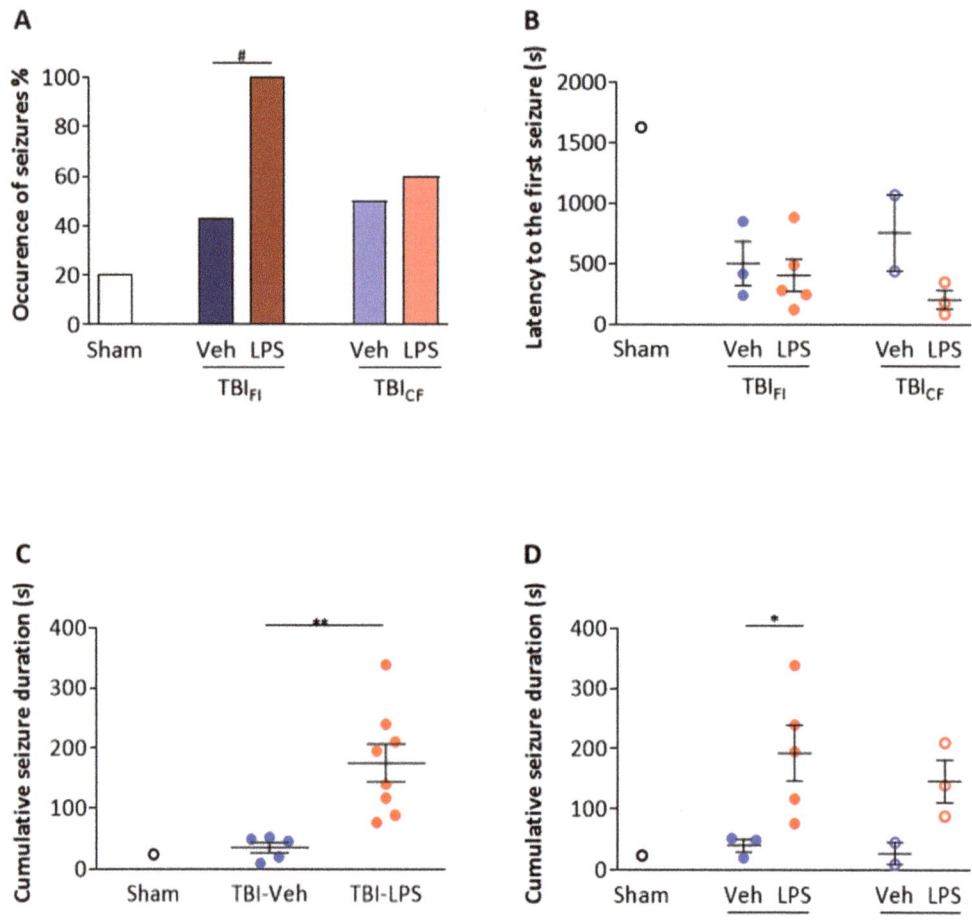

Figure 4. Effect of lesion endophenotype on PTZ seizure susceptibility test. (**A**) Occurrence of PTZ-induced seizures was increased by the "second hit" in the TBI$_{FI}$ endophenotype (TBI$_{FI}$-LPS 100% vs. TBI$_{FI}$-Veh 43%). (**B**) Latency to the first electrographic seizure was not affected by the endophenotype of the cortical lesion. Please note that only a subpopulation of animals developed PTZ-induced seizures (e.g., only 1 rat showed a seizure after PTZ administration in the sham-operated group). (**C**) TBI-LPS rats showed a longer cumulative seizure duration (163 ± 90 s, range 77–338 s, median 168 s) compared with TBI-Veh rats (35 ± 19 s, range 10–52 s, median 46 s). (**D**) Further analysis revealed that the difference resulted from the prolonged cumulative seizure duration in the TBI$_{FI}$ endophenotype. Data are presented as mean ± standard error of the mean (SEM) (panels (**B**,**C**)). Statistical significances: # $p < 0.05$ (χ^2-test); * $p < 0.05$, ** $p < 0.01$ (Mann–Whitney U test). Abbreviations: CF, cavity-forming; FI, focal inflammatory; LPS, lipopolysaccharide; PTZ, pentylenetetrazole; TBI, traumatic brain injury; Veh, vehicle.

3.5. Peripheral Infection at 8 Weeks Post-TBI Enhanced PTZ-Induced c-Fos Expression in the Perilesional Cortex and Dentate Gyrus

We focused our analysis of c-Fos activation on the perilesional cortex and hippocampus, which are known to be involved in PTE-related excitability in the lateral FPI model [27,29,36]. Our initial visual analysis of immunostained preparations revealed differences in PTZ-induced nuclear c-Fos expression (a) along with the rostrocaudal extent of the cortical lesion, (b) between the supragranular and infragranular cortical layers, (c) between the TBI$_{FI}$ and TBI$_{CF}$ endophenotypes (both cortical and hippocampal c-Fos expression), (d) between LPS-

and vehicle-treated injured animals, and (e) between rats with or without induced seizures in the PTZ test.

3.6. Topography of PTZ-Induced c-Fos Expression along the Rostrocaudal Extent of Cortical Lesion

To assess the topography of PTZ-induced c-Fos activation, we divided the lesioned cortex into the medial and lateral perilesional cortex, which were analyzed both rostrally and caudally. As shown in detail below, the c-Fos activation in the TBI-Veh group was greater in the lateral perilesional cortex (area closer to the rhinal fissure) compared with the medial perilesional cortex (closer to midline; $p < 0.05$, Supplementary Figures S1–S4). In addition, the rostral areas were more activated than the caudal areas after TBI (Figure 5 and significances therein). In sham-operated animals, no medial-lateral or rostral-caudal gradients were observed.

Rostral perilesional cortex. In the Sham-Veh group, the density of c-Fos expression was comparable between the ipsilateral (side of craniotomy) and contralateral rostral cortex (AP from -0.96 to -1.80 from the bregma; the levels correspond to rostral levels of the cortical lesion in TBI rats).

Ipsilateral perilesional c-Fos expression was greater in the TBI-Veh group than in the Sham-Veh group ($p < 0.01$). Ipsilateral labeling was also higher than that contralaterally ($p < 0.001$) (Figure 5A).

In the TBI-LPS group, c-Fos expression was increased both ipsilaterally and contralaterally compared with the Sham-Veh group (both $p < 0.001$). Contralateral labeling was also higher than that in the TBI-Veh group ($p < 0.01$). Such as in the TBI-Veh group, the labeling was higher ipsilaterally than contralaterally. ($p < 0.05$) (Figure 5A).

Caudal perilesional cortex. In the Sham-Veh group, the density of c-Fos expression was comparable between the ipsilateral and contralateral caudal cortex (AP -5.88 to -6.24 from bregma; the levels correspond to caudal levels of the cortical lesion in TBI rats).

The density of ipsilateral c-Fos labeling was greater in the TBI-Veh group than in the Sham-Veh group ($p < 0.05$). Ipsilateral labeling was also higher than that contralaterally ($p < 0.001$) (Figure 5B).

Ipsilateral c-Fos expression was greater in the TBI-LPS group than in the Sham-Veh group ($p < 0.001$). Ipsilateral labeling was also higher than that in the TBI-Veh group ($p < 0.05$). Such as in the TBI-Veh group, the labeling was higher ipsilaterally than contralaterally ($p < 0.01$) (Figure 5B).

Rostral vs. caudal perilesional cortex. In the TBI-Veh group, ipsilateral perilesional c-Fos expression was greater rostrally than caudally ($p < 0.05$). In the TBI-LPS group, both ipsilateral and contralateral c-Fos expression was greater rostrally than caudally (both $p < 0.05$) (Figure 5).

3.7. Laminar Analysis of PTZ-Induced c-Fos Expression

Next, we assessed c-Fos expression in layers II-IV (supragranular layers) and layers V-VI (infragranular layers) in the rostral perilesional cortex, in which we found the highest c-Fos expression levels. As shown in Supplementary Figure S2, most of the c-Fos expression was in layers II-IV (medial and lateral perilesional cortex combined). The levels were highest in animals that expressed seizures in the PTZ-test, whether or not they had been treated with vehicle or LPS. Compared with the contralateral side, there was a clear asymmetry in the TBI-Veh group ($p < 0.001$). In the TBI-LPS group, however, c-Fos expression in the superficial layers was increased bilaterally.

In addition, in the caudal perilesional cortex, the most robust activation was observed in layers II-IV (data not shown).

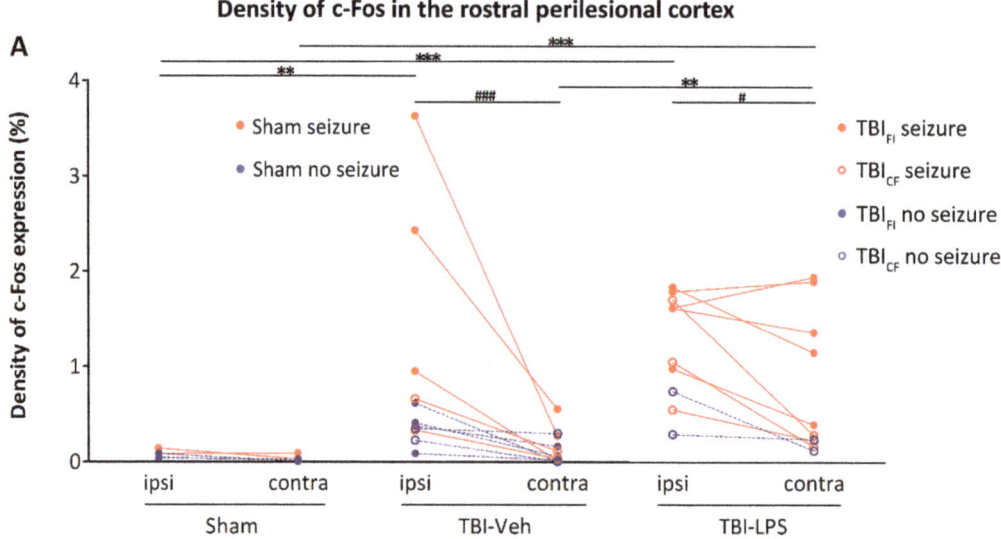

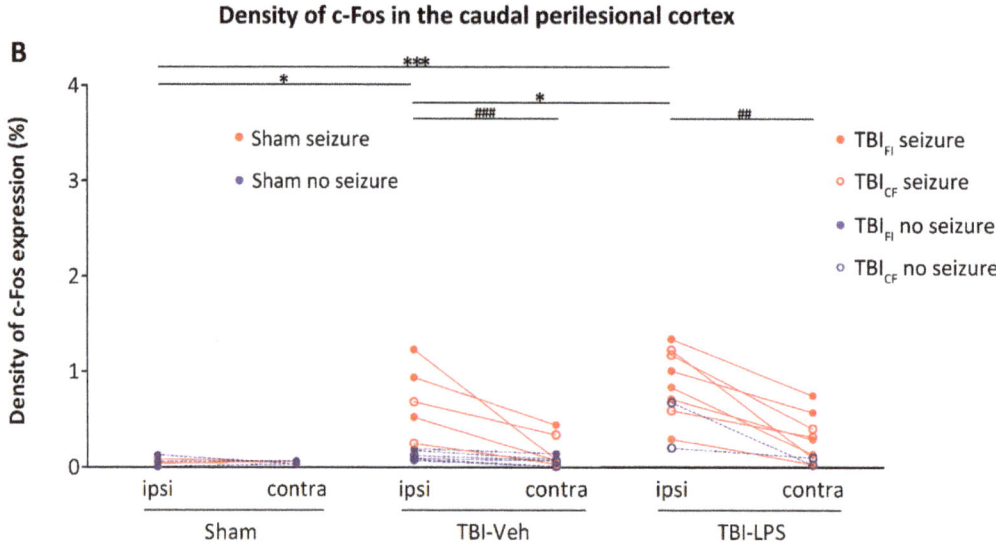

Figure 5. c-Fos expression in the rostral and caudal perilesional cortex. (**A**) *Rostral perilesional cortex.* In the Sham-Veh group, the density of c-Fos expression was comparable between the ipsilateral and contralateral perilesional cortex rostrally. In the TBI-Veh group, c-Fos expression was increased ipsilaterally compared with the Sham-Veh group. In the TBI-LPS group, the density of c-Fos expression was higher both ipsilaterally and contralaterally than in the Sham-Veh group. Contralateral labeling was also higher than that in the TBI-Veh group. Inter-hemispheric analysis showed higher c-Fos labeling ipsilaterally

than contralaterally in both the TBI-Veh and TBI-LPS groups. (**B**) *Caudal perilesional cortex*. In the Sham-Veh group, the density of c-Fos expression was comparable between the ipsilateral and contralateral perilesional cortex caudally. The c-Fos labeling density was higher ipsilaterally in the TBI-Veh group than in the Sham-Veh group. In the TBI-LPS group, c-Fos expression was increased ipsilaterally compared with the Sham-Veh and TBI-Veh groups. Interhemispheric analysis revealed more c-Fos activation ipsilaterally than contralaterally in both the TBI-Veh and TBI-LPS groups. Comparison of c-Fos expression between the rostral and caudal perilesional cortex showed that c-Fos expression in the ipsilateral perilesional cortex was higher rostrally than caudally in the TBI-Veh group ($p < 0.05$, Wilcoxon). In the TBI-LPS group, rostral c-Fos expression was increased bilaterally compared with the caudal c-Fos expression ($p < 0.05$, Wilcoxon). Abbreviations: CF, cavity-forming; contra, contralateral; FI, focal inflammatory; ipsi, ipsilateral; LPS, lipopolysaccharide; TBI, traumatic brain injury; Veh, vehicle. Statistical significances: # $p < 0.05$, ## $p < 0.01$, ### $p < 0.001$ (Wilcoxon); * $p < 0.05$, ** $p < 0.01$, *** $p < 0.001$ (Mann–Whitney U test).

3.8. Effect of Lesion Endophenotype on the Pattern of c-Fos Expression

As the cumulative duration of PTZ-induced seizures was longer in the TBI$_{FI}$ rats than in the TBI$_{CF}$ rats, the highest activation of c-Fos expression was observed in rats with the post-TBI$_{FI}$ endophenotype, whether or not they were treated with LPS (Figure 5, red lines with closed circles). Figures 6 and 7 show representative photomicrographs PTZ-induced c-Fos activation of the rat with TBI$_{FI}$ and Figures 8 and 9 with TBI$_{CF}$ endophenotype.

3.9. Effect of the Occurrence of PTZ-Induced Seizures on the Pattern of c-Fos Expression

Perilesional cortex. As only a subgroup of animals expressed electrographic seizures after PTZ administration, we next compared the activation patterns between animals with or without PTZ-induced seizures.

As summarized in Figure 5, in both the TBI-Veh and TBI-LPS groups, the highest densities of c-Fos activation were observed in rats with PTZ-induced seizures both rostrally and caudally (Figure 5, red circles and lines). Moreover, the activation was more robust ipsilaterally than contralaterally except in the TBI-LPS group, in which the rostral activation was high bilaterally (Figure 5 and significances therein). It should be noted that the injured rats without PTZ-induced seizures also tended to have higher c-Fos expression ipsilaterally than contralaterally (Figure 5).

Next, we assessed whether the density of c-Fos expression was associated with the maximal behavioral seizure score. In the TBI-Veh group, the higher the behavioral score, the greater the c-Fos expression in the ipsilateral rostral perilesional cortex (r = 0.9487, $p < 0.05$) (Figure 10). In the TBI-LPS group, the higher the behavioral seizure score, the higher the c-Fos expression in the contralateral cortex (r = 0.7638, $p < 0.05$) (Figure 10). No associations were detected between the cumulative seizure duration and c-Fos activation in the TBI-Veh and TBI-LPS groups (Figure 10).

In the TBI-Veh group, 9 of 11 rats had a behavioral seizure score < 4 or no seizure in the PTZ-test. Interestingly, 1 of the rats showed increased c-Fos activation in the dentate gyrus. This rat expressed a spontaneous seizure lasting 185 s approximately 23 h before the PTZ injection (in baseline vEEG). Of the 11 rats in the TBI-Veh group, 2 scored 4–5 seizures after PTZ administration, and both of these rats had increased c-Fos activation in the dentate gyrus.

In the TBI-LPS group, 3 of 10 animals had a behavioral seizure score < 4 or no seizure in the PTZ-test. One of these rats (seizure score 3) showed increased c-Fos activation in the dentate gyrus. Of the 10 rats, 7 developed seizures that reached stage 4–5 within 2 h after PTZ administration, and all of these rats had increased c-Fos activation in the dentate gyrus. Consequently, the c-Fos expression increase in the dentate gyrus was higher in the TBI-LPS group (8/10 rats) than in the TBI-Veh group (3/11 rats, $p < 0.05$, χ^2-test) or the sham group (0/5 rats, $p < 0.01$, χ^2-test) (Figure 11).

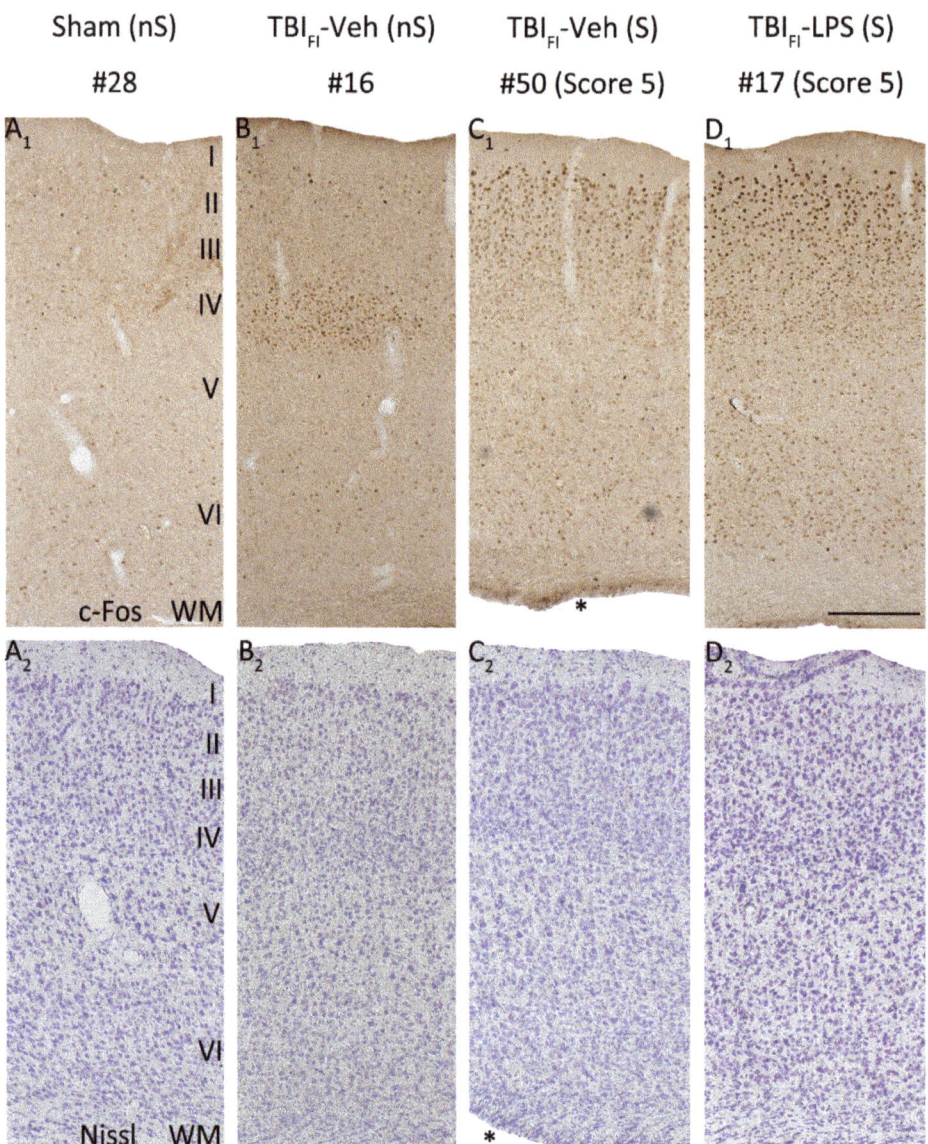

Figure 6. LPS enhances the seizure-induced c-Fos expression and changes its pattern in the rostromedial perilesional cortex. Representative high-magnification photomicrographs showing c-Fos immunolabeling (A_1–D_1) and thionin staining (A_2–D_2) in the rostromedial perilesional cortex (somatosensory cortex, see Figure 3C) of a vehicle-treated sham-operated rat and a vehicle or LPS-treated injured rat with a TBI_{FI} endophenotype at 2 h after PTZ injection (15 weeks after LPS injection and 23 weeks post-TBI). (A_1,A_2) A rat from the Sham-Veh group without PTZ-induced seizure (#28). Note the very low c-Fos expression level throughout the cortical layers. (B_1,B_2) A rat from the TBI_{FI}-Veh group without a PTZ-induced seizure (#16). Note the intense c-Fos labeling in layer IV apparently reporting on the TBI-induced chronic excitability. (C_1,C_2) A rat from the TBI_{FI}-Veh group with a PTZ-induced seizure (#50, Racine score 5 seizure). Note the intense c-Fos labeling in layers II-III. (D_1,D_2) A rat from the TBI_{FI}-LPS group with a PTZ-induced seizure (#17, Racine score 5 seizure) with intense c-Fos labeling in layers II-III and scattered immunopositive cells in deeper layers. Note that the occurrence of PTZ-induced seizures changed the overall pattern of perilesional c-Fos expression in TBI animals (with or without LPS). In addition to

labeling in layer IV, layers I-III were activated (e.g., (**D₁**) vs. (**B₁**)). A rat in the TBI$_{FI}$-Veh group with PTZ-induced seizure (**C₁**) showed higher c-Fos activation than a rat without a seizure ((**C₁**) vs. (**B₁**)), particularly in the supragranular layers. An LPS-treated rat with a TBI$_{FI}$ endophenotype and a PTZ-induced seizure had robustly enhanced c-Fos expression in all cortical layers (**D₁**) compared with a vehicle-treated seizing TBI rat (**C₁**). Abbreviations: FI, focal inflammatory; FPI, fluid-percussion injury; LPS, lipopolysaccharide; nS, no seizure; PTZ, pentylenetetrazole; S, seizure; TBI, traumatic brain injury; Veh, vehicle; WM, white matter. Scale bars = 200 μm. * Enlarged ipsilateral lateral ventricle.

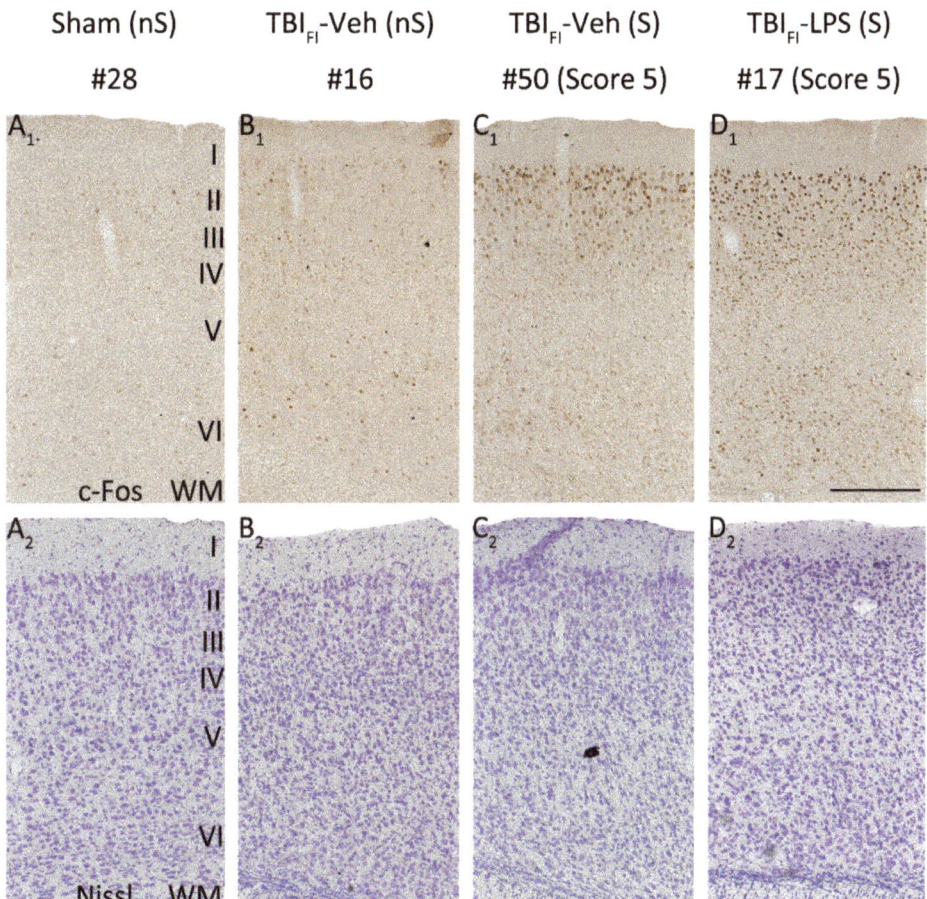

Figure 7. LPS enhances the seizure-induced c-Fos expression and changes its pattern in the caudomedial perilesional cortex. Representative high magnification photomicrographs showing c-Fos immunochemistry (**A₁–D₁**) and Nissl staining (**A₂–D₂**) in the caudomedial perilesional cortex in rats from the Sham-Veh and TBI$_{FI}$ endophenotype groups at 2 h after PTZ injection (23 weeks post-FPI and 15 weeks after LPS injection). (**A₁,A₂**) Example of a rat from the Sham-Veh group without PTZ-induced seizure (#28). (**B₁,B₂**) Example of a rat from the TBI$_{FI}$-Veh group without a PTZ-induced seizure (#16). (**C₁,C₂**) Example of a rat from TBI$_{FI}$-Veh group with a PTZ-induced seizure (#50, seizure Racine score 5). (**D₁,D₂**) Example of a rat from TBI$_{FI}$-LPS group with a PTZ-induced seizure (#17, seizure Racine score 5). Note that in rats without a PTZ-induced seizure, TBI increased PTZ-induced c-Fos expression ((**B₁**) vs. (**A₁**)). In the TBI$_{FI}$-Veh group, a rat with a PTZ-induced seizure (**C₁**) exhibited higher c-Fos activation compared to a rat without a seizure (**B₁**), particularly in the supragranular layers. In the TBI$_{FI}$ endophenotype with PTZ-induced seizure, LPS treatment at a chronic time-point after TBI further enhanced c-Fos expression (**D₁**) compared with vehicle treatment (**C₁**) in all layers. Abbreviations: FI, focal inflammatory; FPI, fluid-percussion injury; LPS, lipopolysaccharide; nS, no seizure; PTZ, pentylenetetrazole; S, seizure; TBI, traumatic brain injury; Veh, vehicle; WM, white matter. Scale bars = 200 μm.

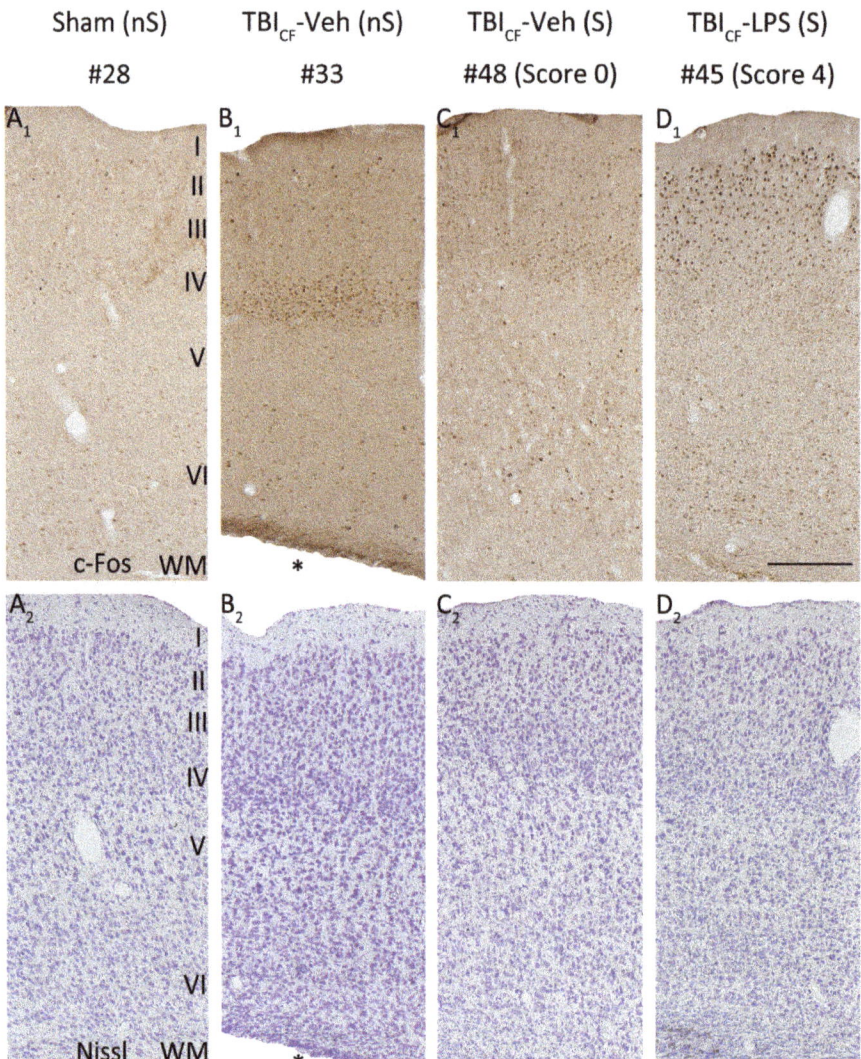

Figure 8. Pattern of c-Fos expression in the rostromedial perilesional cortex. Representative high magnification photomicrographs showing c-Fos immunochemistry (A_1–D_1) and Nissl staining (A_2–D_2) in the rostromedial perilesional cortex in rats from the Sham-Veh group and TBI$_{CF}$ endophenotype at 2 h after PTZ injection (23 weeks post-FPI and 15 weeks after LPS injection). (A_1,A_2) Example of a rat from the Sham-Veh group without a PTZ-induced seizure (#28). (B_1,B_2) Example of a rat from the TBI$_{CF}$-Veh group without a PTZ-induced seizure (#33). (C_1,C_2) Example of a rat from the TBI$_{CF}$-Veh group with a PTZ-induced seizure (#48, seizure Racine score 0, only electroencephalographic seizure). (D_1,D_2) Example of a rat from the TBI$_{CF}$-LPS group with a PTZ-induced seizure (#45, seizure Racine score 4). Note that in rats without a PTZ-induced seizure, TBI increased PTZ-induced c-Fos expression, particularly in layer IV ((B_1) vs. (A_1)). In the TBI$_{CF}$-Veh group, a rat with a PTZ-induced seizure (C_1) revealed higher c-Fos activation compared to a rat without a seizure (B_1), particularly in the supragranular layers. In the TBI$_{CF}$ endophenotype with a PTZ-induced seizure, LPS treatment at a chronic time-point after TBI further enhanced c-Fos expression (D_1) compared with vehicle treatment (C_1) in all layers. Abbreviations: CF, cavity-forming; FPI, fluid-percussion injury; LPS, lipopolysaccharide; nS, no seizure; PTZ, pentylenetetrazole; S, seizure; TBI, traumatic brain injury; Veh, vehicle; WM, white matter. Scale bars = 200 µm. * Enlarged ipsilateral lateral ventricle.

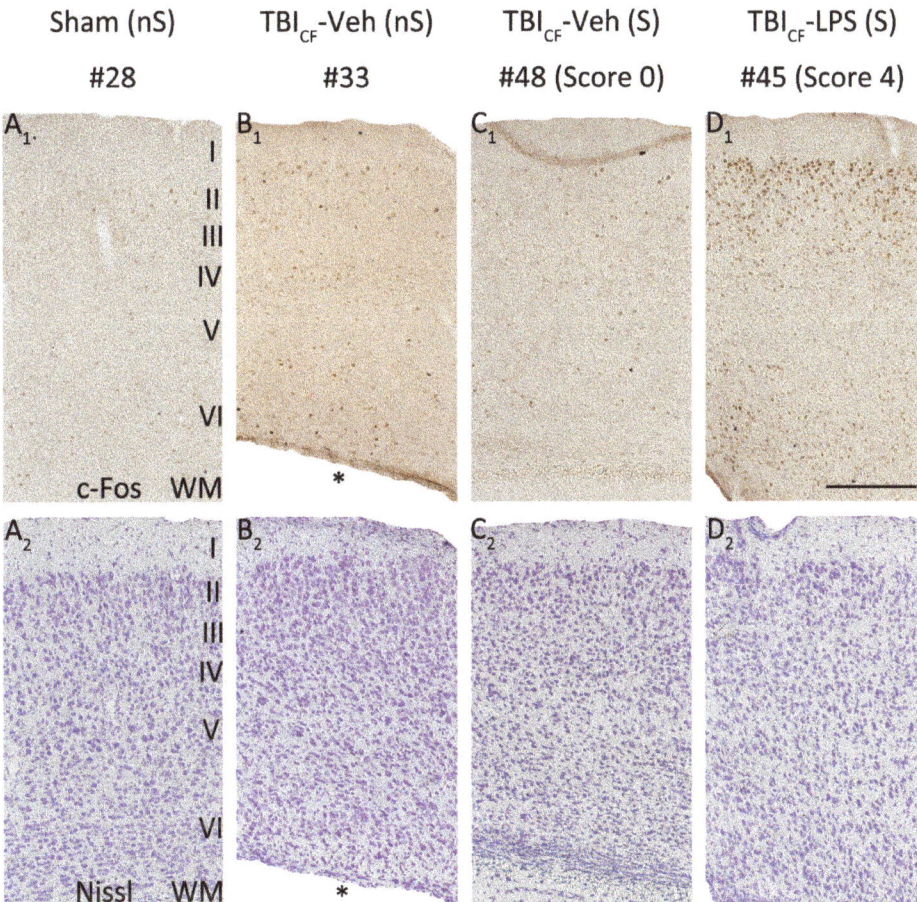

Figure 9. Pattern of c-Fos expression in the caudomedial perilesional cortex. Representative high magnification photomicrographs showing c-Fos immunochemistry (A_1–D_1) and Nissl staining (A_2–D_2) in the caudomedial perilesional cortex in rats from Sham-Veh group and TBI_{CF} endophenotype at 2 h after PTZ injection (23 weeks post-FPI and 15 weeks after LPS injection). (A_1,A_2) Example of a rat from the Sham-Veh group without a PTZ-induced seizure (#28). (B_1,B_2) Example of a rat from the TBI_{CF}-Veh group without a PTZ-induced seizure (#33). (C_1,C_2) Example of a rat from the TBI_{CF}-Veh group with a PTZ-induced seizure (#48, seizure Racine score 0, only electroencephalographic seizure). (D_1,D_2) Example of a rat from the TBI_{CF}-LPS group with a PTZ-induced seizure (#45, seizure Racine score 4). Note that in rats without a PTZ-induced seizure, TBI increased PTZ-induced c-Fos expression ((B_1) vs. (A_1)). In the TBI_{CF}-Veh group, no difference was detected between rats with a PTZ-induced seizure (C_1) and those without a seizure (B_1). In the TBI_{CF} endophenotype with a PTZ-induced seizure, LPS treatment at a chronic time-point after TBI further enhanced c-Fos expression (D_1) compared with vehicle treatment (C_1) in all layers. Abbreviations: CF, cavity-forming; FPI, fluid-percussion injury; LPS, lipopolysaccharide; nS, no seizure; PTZ, pentylenetetrazole; S, seizure; TBI, traumatic brain injury; Veh, vehicle; WM, white matter. Scale bars = 200 µm. * Enlarged ipsilateral lateral ventricle.

Dentate gyrus. Szyndler et al. [37] reported increased c-Fos immunoreactivity in the dentate gyrus in rats that showed a stage 5 generalized tonic-clonic seizure after PTZ induction (35 mg/kg, i.p., repeated administration). Due to the increased seizure susceptibility of TBI rats to PTZ-induced seizures, we administered PTZ at a dose of 25 mg/kg. Consequently, none of the sham-operated animals developed stage 4–5 behavioral seizures, and none of them showed c-Fos activation in the dentate gyrus.

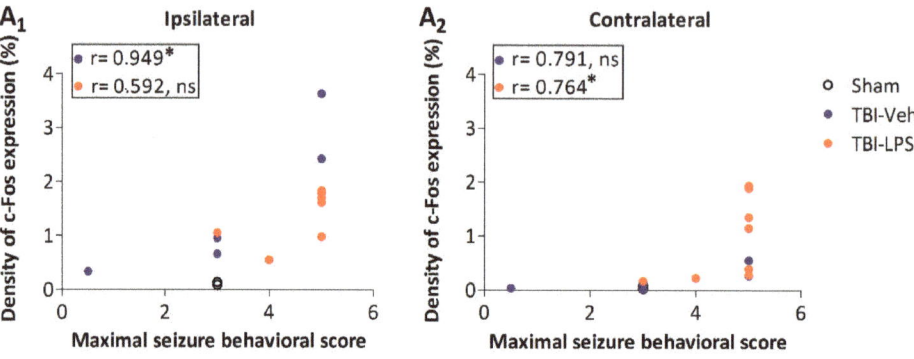

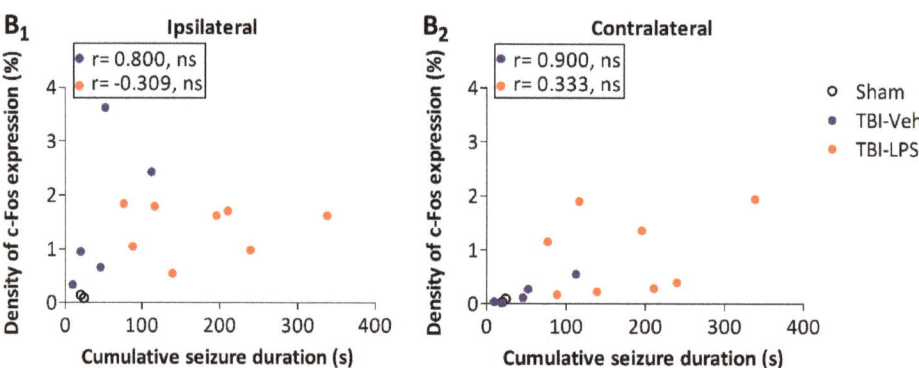

Figure 10. c-Fos expression and seizure susceptibility. Correlations between the density of rostral perilesional c-Fos expression and seizure susceptibility (maximal behavioral seizure score, cumulative seizure duration) in the PTZ-test. (A_1) Ipsilaterally, the higher the density of c-Fos expression, the higher the maximal behavioral seizure score in the TBI-Veh group (r = 0.949, $p < 0.05$). (A_2) Contralaterally, the higher the c-Fos expression, the higher the maximal behavioral score in the TBI-LPS group (r = 0.764, $p < 0.05$). No correlations between the density of c-Fos expression and the cumulative seizure duration were detected (B_1) ipsilaterally or (B_2) contralaterally in the TBI-Veh or TBI-LPS groups. Abbreviations: LPS, lipopolysaccharide; ns, non-significant; r, correlation coefficient; TBI, traumatic brain injury; Veh, vehicle. Statistical significances: * $p < 0.05$ (r, Spearman's rho correlations).

In the TBI_{FI} endophenotype, activation of the dentate gyrus was more common in the TBI_{FI}-LPS group than the TBI_{FI}-Veh group (100% vs. 43%, $p < 0.05$, χ^2-test) or the sham group (100% vs. 0%, $p < 0.01$, χ^2-test) (Figure 12). In the TBI_{CF} endophenotype, c-Fos activation in the dentate gyrus did not differ between the vehicle- and LPS-treated animals (0% vs. 60%, $p > 0.05$) (Figure 11).

In all animals, the increase in c-Fos expression was bilateral along the septotemporal axis of the dentate gyrus.

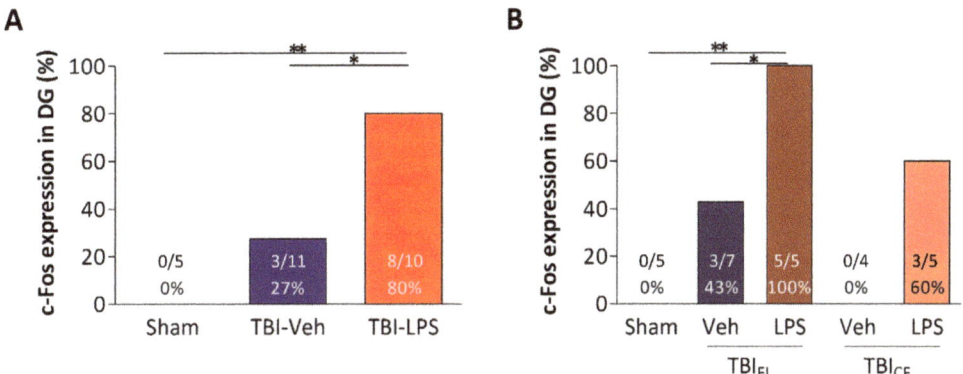

Figure 11. c-Fos expression in the dentate gyrus (DG). (**A**) Percentage of animals with increased c-Fos expression in the dentate gyrus was higher in the TBI-LPS than in the TBI-Veh and Sham-Veh groups. (**B**) All rats in the TBI$_{FI}$-LPS group more commonly showed increased c-Fos activation in the dentate gyrus than rats in the TBI$_{FI}$-Veh and Sham-Veh groups. Abbreviations: CF, cavity-forming; DG, dentate gyrus; FI, focal inflammatory; LPS, lipopolysaccharide; TBI, traumatic brain injury; Veh, vehicle. Statistical significances: * $p < 0.05$, ** $p < 0.01$ (χ^2-test).

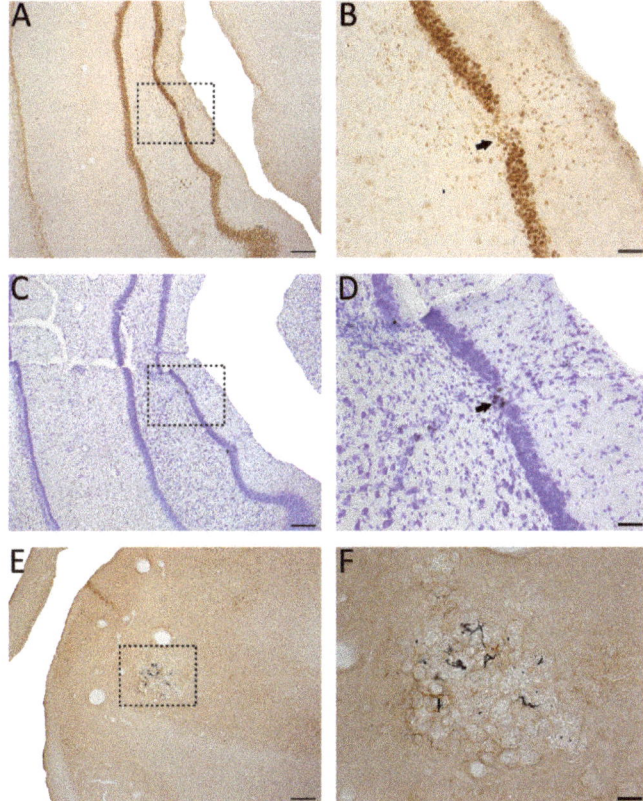

Figure 12. Pattern of c-Fos expression in the dentate gyrus. Representative photomicrographs showing mild granule cell damage and dispersion in the dentate gyrus (**A–D**) and calcifications in the ipsilateral

thalamus (**E,F**) in a rat (#38, Racine score 5) in the TBI$_{FI}$-Veh group with an induced seizure at 2 h after PTZ injection. A c-Fos immunostained (**A**) and a Nissl-stained section (**C**). A higher-magnification photomicrographs of c-Fos immunohistochemistry (**B**) and Nissl staining (**D**) taken from the region indicated with a dashed box in panel (**A,C**), respectively. Note the granule cell loss indicated by a closed arrow with iron deposits (dark dots) and dispersed granule cells in the molecular layer. (**E**) Thalamic calcification (dashed box). (**F**) A higher magnification photomicrograph was taken from the region indicated with a dashed box in panel (**E**). Abbreviations: FI, focal inflammatory; FPI, fluid-percussion injury; PTZ, pentylenetetrazole; TBI, traumatic brain injury; Veh, vehicle. Scale bar = 200 μm (panel (**A,C,E**)); 50 μm (panel (**B,D,F**)).

4. Discussion

The aim of the present study was to identify factors that facilitate epileptogenesis after TBI. We hypothesized that LPS treatment at 8 weeks after TBI, mimicking Gram-negative peripheral infection at a chronic post-injury time-point, will increase neuronal excitability and facilitate post-traumatic epileptogenesis. We had three major findings. First, LPS injection at 8 weeks post-TBI increased seizure susceptibility, particularly in rats with the TBI$_{FI}$ endophenotype. Second, LPS augmented PTZ-induced c-Fos expression, a marker of neuronal activation in the injured ipsilateral cortex. Third, LPS enhanced PTZ-induced c-Fos bilateral expression in the dentate gyrus, particularly in the TBI$_{FI}$ endophenotype.

4.1. Occurrence of Late Spontaneous Seizures

Previous studies demonstrated that approximately 10% of rats with lateral FPI have epilepsy at 3 months, 25% at 6–7 months, and 40% to 50% at 12 months post-injury [29]. Consistent with previous studies, approximately 10% of rats with TBI had electrographic seizures when vEEG-monitored during the fifth post-injury month. Consequently, we used PTZ-induced seizure susceptibility rather than the occurrence of spontaneous seizures as an outcome measure when assessing epileptogenesis in different treatment groups.

4.2. Peripheral Infection at a Chronic Time-Point Post-TBI Increased Seizure Susceptibility

Several studies revealed that peripheral inflammation in normal immature and/or mature rodents induced by LPS increases seizure susceptibility to convulsants, hyperthermic exposure, or kindling [38–44]. Our 6-month follow-up study extended previous observations by showing that LPS injection at 2 months after TBI, modeling peripheral Gram-negative infection in subjects with brain injury, enhanced seizure susceptibility in the PTZ test. This is consistent with earlier studies showing that post-injury immune challenge can worsen the functional post-TBI outcome. For example, LPS administration at 30 days post-TBI exacerbated cognitive impairment and induced depression-like behavior, both of which were associated with microglial reactivation and an exaggerated production of pro-inflammatory cytokines IL1-β and TNFα [45,46].

Such as in humans, brain injury caused by TBI in adult rodents presents differently between animals, even when the impact force is comparable [47]. In addition, the progression of injury varies: smaller lesions with a perilesional inflammatory rim in approximately 50% of rats and fast-progressing cortical lesions with an extensive loss of cortical tissue and large ventricle size in another 50% [47,48]. The inter-animal variability confirmed in the present study allowed us to compare the effect of a second hit induced by LPS treatment according to the lesion type. Interestingly, rats with smaller focal lesions and a perilesional inflammatory rim developed a greater response to PTZ test than animals with large cortical lesions. This correlates with our previous functional MRI study, indicating perilesional focal seizure onset following PTZ-administration in rats with a TBI$_{FI}$ endophenotype on the basis of the blood-oxygen-level-dependent (BOLD) response [27]. Overall, these data suggest a greater presence, and consequently, a more extensive focal reactivation of the immune cells by a "second hit" in rats with the TBI$_{FI}$ endophenotype.

4.3. TBI-Induced Perilesional Cortical Neuronal c-Fos Expression Was Augmented by LPS Treatment

Expression of c-Fos immunoreactivity is widely used as a biologic marker of neuronal activation following various stimuli. Both seizure and injury effects are reported. After PTZ administration, the increase in the brain c-Fos expression peaks at 2 h [49]. Here, we analyzed c-Fos expression to map the PTZ-induced spatial distribution and density of neuronal activation in the perilesional cortex and hippocampus in injured and sham-operated rat brain with or without exposure to LPS treatment at 2 h after convulsant exposure. As expected, we found a clear injury effect on excitability as the neuronal c-Fos activation to the convulsant challenge was substantially greater in rats with TBI as compared to sham-operated experimental controls. In addition, we found an infection effect on c-Fos levels: in non-infected animals, the augmented c-Fos expression was ipsilateral, whereas in LPS-treated animals, not only was the ipsilateral activation greater, but the contralateral cortex was also activated. Laminar analysis of c-Fos activation revealed greater activation in layers II-IV than in layers V-VI in both the TBI-Veh and TBI-LPS groups, indicating the contribution of the supragranular layers to the ictogenic network.

Our observations of the injury effect on c-Fos expression are consistent with previous studies in various TBI models. Following penetrating brain injury, induction of *c-fos* mRNA and protein is focal and restricted to the ipsilateral hemisphere [50]. In controlled cortical impact injury and lateral FPI models, *c-fos* mRNA expression increases in the ipsilateral cortex [51,52]. In addition to injury type, impact severity affects the distribution of c-Fos activation. [52]. Raghupathi et al. reported that mild TBI triggered by lateral FPI induced *c-fos* mRNA in the injured hemisphere, while moderate injury-induced *c-fos* mRNA bilaterally [53].

The functional significance of *c-fos* induction after TBI remains to be investigated. However, the protein product of *c-fos* forms a heterodimer with c-JUN, which binds to the AP-1 DNA site and regulates the function of multiple targets, encoding enzymes, receptors, growth factors or structural proteins, and can contribute to the remodeling of neuronal circuits within the lesioned area, eventually leading to PTE [54].

4.4. TBI-Induced Neuronal c-Fos Expression in the Dentate Gyrus Was Augmented by LPS Treatment

Such as in the cerebral cortex, an injury effect on c-Fos expression in the dentate gyrus has been described both in lateral FPI and cortical contusion injury models [51,52]. Some studies also demonstrated an injury-induced increase in c-Fos expression in the dentate gyrus only when stage 5 generalized tonic-clonic seizures occurred in the PTZ-kindling model [37].

Our data reproduced both the injury and seizure effects on dentate gyrus c-Fos expression in the lateral FPI model. These data add to previous findings by showing that post-injury peripheral infection augmented the dentate gyrus neuronal c-Fos activation. In 2 of 11 rats in the TBI-Veh group and in 7 of 10 rats in the TBI-LPS group with stage 4–5 seizures, increased c-Fos expression was observed in the dentate gyrus. Interestingly, 1 animal in TBI-Veh group also showed enhanced dentate c-Fos expression even though no seizure developed after PTZ injection. This particular rat, however, had experienced a stage 5 spontaneous seizure at 23 h before PTZ injection. Elevated c-Fos expression was also observed in 1 rat in the TBI$_{CF}$-LPS group that developed a stage 3 seizure in the PTZ test. Thus, 80% of rats in the TBI-LPS group and 27% in the TBI-Veh group exhibited neuronal activation in the dentate gyrus, showing augmentation of the dentate gyrus response to convulsant challenge in rats with post-TBI infection. In particular, rats with the TBI$_{FI}$ cortical lesion endophenotype showed robust bilateral dentate gyrus activation to PTZ challenge.

5. Conclusions

In conclusion, our data provide the first evidence that peripheral infection at a chronic post-TBI time-point enhances neuronal excitability in the perilesional cortex and bilaterally in the dentate gyrus, particularly in animals with prolonged focal cortical T2 enhancement around the lesion core. Our results emphasize the need for careful diagnosis and treatment of peripheral infection after TBI as a component of antiepileptogenesis treatment strategies.

Supplementary Materials: The following are available online https://www.mdpi.com/article/10.3390/biomedicines9121946/s1. Figure S1: c-Fos expression in the rostromedial and rostrolateral perilesional cortex and corresponding contralateral cortex. Figure S2: Density of c-Fos expression in layers II-IV (supragranular layers) and layers V-VI (infragranular layers) in the rostral perilesional cortex. Figure S3: Representative higher magnification photomicrographs showing c-Fos immunochemistry and Nissl staining in the rostromedial contralateral cortex. Figure S4: Representative high magnification photomicrographs showing c-Fos immunochemistry and Nissl staining in the caudomedial contralateral cortex.

Author Contributions: Conceptualization, A.P., Y.W., P.A.; methodology, A.P., Y.W., P.A.; software, not applicable; validation, not applicable; formal analysis, Y.W., P.A.; investigation, not applicable; resources, A.P.; data curation, not applicable; writing—original draft preparation, Y.W., P.A., A.P.; writing—review and editing, A.P.; visualization, Y.W., P.A.; supervision, A.P.; project administration, A.P.; funding acquisition, A.P.; All authors have read and agreed to the published version of the manuscript.

Funding: This research was funded by the Medical Research Council of the Academy of Finland (Grants 272249, 273909, 2285733-9), The Sigrid Juselius Foundation and by the European Union's Seventh Framework Programme (FP7/2007-2013) under grant agreement n°602102 (EPITARGET).

Institutional Review Board Statement: All animal procedures were approved by the Animal Ethics Committee of the Provincial Government of Southern Finland (ESAVI/5146/04.10.07/2014) and carried out in accordance with the European Council Directive (2010/63/EU).

Informed Consent Statement: Not applicable.

Acknowledgments: We thank Jarmo Hartikainen and Merja Lukkari for their excellent technical assistance and Biomedical Imaging Unit, A. I. Virtanen Institute for MR imaging.

Conflicts of Interest: No conflicts of interest.

References

1. Annegers, J.F.; Hauser, W.A.; Coan, S.P.; Rocca, W.A. A Population-Based Study of Seizures after Traumatic Brain Injuries. *N. Engl. J. Med.* **1998**, *338*, 20–24. [CrossRef] [PubMed]
2. Haltiner, A.M.; Temkin, N.R.; Dikmen, S.S. Risk of seizure recurrence after the first late posttraumatic seizure. *Arch. Phys. Med. Rehabil.* **1997**, *78*, 835–840. [CrossRef]
3. Pitkänen, A.; Immonen, R. Epilepsy Related to Traumatic Brain Injury. *Neurotherapeutics* **2014**, *11*, 286–296. [CrossRef]
4. Pitkänen, A.; McIntosh, T.K. Animal Models of Post-Traumatic Epilepsy. *J. Neurotrauma* **2006**, *23*, 241–261. [CrossRef] [PubMed]
5. Immonen, R.J.; Kharatishvili, I.; Niskanen, J.-P.; Gröhn, H.; Pitkänen, A.; Gröhn, O.H. Distinct MRI pattern in lesional and perilesional area after traumatic brain injury in rat—11 months follow-up. *Exp. Neurol.* **2009**, *215*, 29–40. [CrossRef] [PubMed]
6. Herman, S.T. Epilepsy after brain insult: Targeting epileptogenesis. *Neurology* **2002**, *59*, S21–S26. [CrossRef]
7. Frey, L.C. Epidemiology of Posttraumatic Epilepsy: A Critical Review. *Epilepsia* **2003**, *44*, 11–17. [CrossRef]
8. Pitkänen, A.; Bolkvadze, T.; Immonen, R. Anti-epileptogenesis in rodent post-traumatic epilepsy models. *Neurosci. Lett.* **2011**, *497*, 163–171. [CrossRef]
9. Pitkänen, A.; Ndode-Ekane, X.E.; Lapinlampi, N.; Puhakka, N. Epilepsy biomarkers—Toward etiology and pathology specificity. *Neurobiol. Dis.* **2019**, *123*, 42–58. [CrossRef]
10. McGinn, M.J.; Povlishock, J.T. Cellular and molecular mechanisms of injury and spontaneous recovery. *Handb. Clin. Neurol.* **2015**, *127*, 67–87. [CrossRef]
11. Combrinck, M.; Perry, V.; Cunningham, C. Peripheral infection evokes exaggerated sickness behaviour in pre-clinical murine prion disease. *Neuroscience* **2002**, *112*, 7–11. [CrossRef]
12. Terrone, G.; Balosso, S.; Pauletti, A.; Ravizza, T.; Vezzani, A. Inflammation and reactive oxygen species as disease modifiers in epilepsy. *Neuropharmacology* **2019**, *167*, 107742. [CrossRef]

13. Van Vliet, E.A.; Ndode-Ekane, X.E.; Lehto, L.J.; Gorter, J.A.; Andrade, P.; Aronica, E.; Gröhn, O.; Pitkänen, A. Long-lasting blood-brain barrier dysfunction and neuroinflammation after traumatic brain injury. *Neurobiol. Dis.* **2020**, *145*, 105080. [CrossRef] [PubMed]
14. Mrcp, A.F.R.; Brooks, D.J.; Greenwood, R.J.; Bose, S.K.; Turkheimer, F.E.; Kinnunen, K.M.; Gentleman, S.; Heckemann, R.A.; Gunanayagam, K.; Gelosa, G.; et al. Inflammation after trauma: Microglial activation and traumatic brain injury. *Ann. Neurol.* **2011**, *70*, 374–383. [CrossRef]
15. Helling, T.S.; Evans, L.L.; Fowler, D.L.; Hays, L.V.; Kennedy, F.R. Infectious Complications in Patients with Severe Head Injury. *J. Trauma Inj. Infect. Crit. Care* **1988**, *28*, 1575–1577. [CrossRef]
16. Dziedzic, T.; Slowik, A.; Szczudlik, A. Nosocomial infections and immunity: Lesson from brain-injured patients. *Crit. Care* **2004**, *8*, 266–270. [CrossRef] [PubMed]
17. Harrison-Felix, C.; Whiteneck, G.; DeVivo, M.J.; Hammond, F.M.; Jha, A. Causes of Death Following 1 Year Postinjury Among Individuals with Traumatic Brain Injury. *J. Head Trauma Rehabil.* **2006**, *21*, 22–33. [CrossRef]
18. Kourbeti, I.; Vakis, A.; Papadakis, J.; Karabetsos, D.; Bertsias, G.; Filippou, M.; Ioannou, A.; Neophytou, C.; Anastasaki, M.; Samonis, G. Infections in traumatic brain injury patients. *Clin. Microbiol. Infect.* **2012**, *18*, 359–364. [CrossRef] [PubMed]
19. Dhillon, N.K.; Tseng, J.; Barmparas, G.; Harada, M.Y.; Ko, A.; Smith, E.J.; Thomsen, G.M.; Ley, E.J. Impact of early positive cultures in the elderly with traumatic brain injury. *J. Surg. Res.* **2018**, *224*, 140–145. [CrossRef] [PubMed]
20. Sharma, R.; Shultz, S.R.; Robinson, M.; Belli, A.; Hibbs, M.L.; O'Brien, T.; Semple, B.D. Infections after a traumatic brain injury: The complex interplay between the immune and neurological systems. *Brain Behav. Immun.* **2019**, *79*, 63–74. [CrossRef]
21. Weisbrod, A.B.; Rodriguez, C.; Bell, R.; Neal, C.; Armonda, R.; Dorlac, W.; Schreiber, M.; Dunne, J.R. Long-term outcomes of combat casualties sustaining penetrating traumatic brain injury. *J. Trauma Acute Care Surg.* **2012**, *73*, 1525–1530. [CrossRef]
22. Saadat, S.; Akbari, H.; Khorramirouz, R.; Mofid, R.; Rahimi-Movaghar, V. Determinants of mortality in patients with traumatic brain injury. *Ulus. Travma Acil. Cerrahi. Derg.* **2012**, *18*, 219–224. [CrossRef]
23. Mazarati, A.; Medel-Matus, J.; Shin, D.; Jacobs, J.P.; Sankar, R. Disruption of intestinal barrier and endotoxemia after traumatic brain injury: Implications for post-traumatic epilepsy. *Epilepsia* **2021**, *62*, 1472–1481. [CrossRef] [PubMed]
24. McIntosh, T.; Vink, R.; Noble, L.; Yamakami, I.; Fernyak, S.; Soares, H.; Faden, A. Traumatic brain injury in the rat: Characterization of a lateral fluid-percussion model. *Neuroscience* **1989**, *28*, 233–244. [CrossRef]
25. Kharatishvili, I.; Sierra, A.; Immonen, R.J.; Gröhn, O.H.; Pitkänen, A. Quantitative T2 mapping as a potential marker for the initial assessment of the severity of damage after traumatic brain injury in rat. *Exp. Neurol.* **2009**, *217*, 154–164. [CrossRef] [PubMed]
26. Ndode-Ekane, X.E.; Kharatishvili, I.; Pitkänen, A. Unfolded Maps for Quantitative Analysis of Cortical Lesion Location and Extent after Traumatic Brain Injury. *J. Neurotrauma* **2017**, *34*, 459–474. [CrossRef] [PubMed]
27. Huttunen, J.K.; Airaksinen, A.M.; Barba, C.; Colicchio, G.; Niskanen, J.-P.; Shatillo, A.; Lopez, A.S.; Ndode-Ekane, X.E.; Pitkanen, A.; Gröhn, O.H. Detection of Hyperexcitability by Functional Magnetic Resonance Imaging after Experimental Traumatic Brain Injury. *J. Neurotrauma* **2018**, *35*, 2708–2717. [CrossRef]
28. Park, B.S.; Lee, J.-O. Recognition of lipopolysaccharide pattern by TLR4 complexes. *Exp. Mol. Med.* **2013**, *45*, e66. [CrossRef]
29. Kharatishvili, I.; Nissinen, J.; McIntosh, T.; Pitkänen, A. A model of posttraumatic epilepsy induced by lateral fluid-percussion brain injury in rats. *Neuroscience* **2006**, *140*, 685–697. [CrossRef]
30. Nissinen, J.; Halonen, T.; Koivisto, E.; Pitkänen, A. A new model of chronic temporal lobe epilepsy induced by electrical stimulation of the amygdala in rat. *Epilepsy Res.* **1999**, *38*, 177–205. [CrossRef]
31. Racine, R.J. Modification of seizure activity by electrical stimulation: II. Motor seizure. *Electroencephalogr. Clin. Neurophysiol.* **1972**, *32*, 281–294. [CrossRef]
32. Rodgers, K.; Dudek, F.E.; Barth, D.S. Progressive, Seizure-Like, Spike-Wave Discharges Are Common in Both Injured and Uninjured Sprague-Dawley Rats: Implications for the Fluid Percussion Injury Model of Post-Traumatic Epilepsy. *J. Neurosci.* **2015**, *35*, 9194–9204. [CrossRef] [PubMed]
33. Lewis, D.; Campbell, M.J.; Morrison, J.H. An immunohistochemical characterization of somatostatin-28 and somatostatin-281-12 in monkey prefrontal cortex. *J. Comp. Neurol.* **1986**, *248*, 1–18. [CrossRef] [PubMed]
34. Thompson, H.J.; Lifshitz, J.; Marklund, N.; Grady, M.S.; Graham, D.I.; Hovda, D.A.; McIntosh, T.K. Lateral Fluid Percussion Brain Injury: A 15-Year Review and Evaluation. *J. Neurotrauma* **2005**, *22*, 42–75. [CrossRef] [PubMed]
35. Dubreuil, C.I.; Marklund, N.; Deschamps, K.; McIntosh, T.K.; McKerracher, L. Activation of Rho after traumatic brain injury and seizure in rats. *Exp. Neurol.* **2006**, *198*, 361–369. [CrossRef]
36. Reid, A.Y.; Bragin, A.; Giza, C.C.; Staba, R.J.; Engel, J. The progression of electrophysiologic abnormalities during epileptogenesis after experimental traumatic brain injury. *Epilepsia* **2016**, *57*, 1558–1567. [CrossRef]
37. Szyndler, J.; Maciejak, P.; Turzyńska, D.; Sobolewska, A.; Taracha, E.; Skórzewska, A.; Lehner, M.; Bidziński, A.; Hamed, A.; Wisłowska-Stanek, A.; et al. Mapping of c-Fos expression in the rat brain during the evolution of pentylenetetrazol-kindled seizures. *Epilepsy Behav.* **2009**, *16*, 216–224. [CrossRef]
38. Sayyah, M.; Javad-Pour, M.; Ghazi-Khansari, M. The bacterial endotoxin lipopolysaccharide enhances seizure susceptibility in mice: Involvement of proinflammatory factors: Nitric oxide and prostaglandins. *Neuroscience* **2003**, *122*, 1073–1080. [CrossRef]
39. Galic, M.A.; Riazi, K.; Heida, J.G.; Mouihate, A.; Fournier, N.M.; Spencer, S.; Kalynchuk, L.E.; Teskey, G.C.; Pittman, Q. Postnatal Inflammation Increases Seizure Susceptibility in Adult Rats. *J. Neurosci.* **2008**, *28*, 6904–6913. [CrossRef]

40. Riazi, K.; Galic, M.A.; Kuzmiski, B.; Ho, W.; Sharkey, K.; Pittman, Q.J. Microglial activation and TNF production mediate altered CNS excitability following peripheral inflammation. *Proc. Natl. Acad. Sci. USA* **2008**, *105*, 17151–17156. [CrossRef]
41. Auvin, S.; Shin, D.; Mazarati, A.; Sankar, R. Inflammation induced by LPS enhances epileptogenesis in immature rat and may be partially reversed by IL1RA. *Epilepsia* **2010**, *51*, 34–38. [CrossRef]
42. Riazi, K.; Galic, M.A.; Pittman, Q.J. Contributions of peripheral inflammation to seizure susceptibility: Cytokines and brain excitability. *Epilepsy Res.* **2010**, *89*, 34–42. [CrossRef]
43. Eun, B.; Abraham, J.; Mlsna, L.; Kim, M.J.; Koh, S. Lipopolysaccharide potentiates hyperthermia-induced seizures. *Brain Behav.* **2015**, *5*, e00348. [CrossRef]
44. Ho, Y.-H.; Lin, Y.-T.; Wu, C.-W.J.; Chao, Y.-M.; Chang, A.Y.W.; Chan, J.Y.H. Peripheral inflammation increases seizure susceptibility via the induction of neuroinflammation and oxidative stress in the hippocampus. *J. Biomed. Sci.* **2015**, *22*, 1–14. [CrossRef] [PubMed]
45. Fenn, A.M.; Gensel, J.C.; Huang, Y.; Popovich, P.G.; Lifshitz, J.; Godbout, J.P. Immune Activation Promotes Depression 1 Month After Diffuse Brain Injury: A Role for Primed Microglia. *Biol. Psychiatry* **2013**, *76*, 575–584. [CrossRef]
46. Muccigrosso, M.M.; Ford, J.; Benner, B.; Moussa, D.; Burnsides, C.; Fenn, A.M.; Popovich, P.G.; Lifshitz, J.; Walker, F.R.; Eiferman, D.S.; et al. Cognitive deficits develop 1 month after diffuse brain injury and are exaggerated by microglia-associated reactivity to peripheral immune challenge. *Brain Behav. Immun.* **2016**, *54*, 95–109. [CrossRef] [PubMed]
47. Manninen, E.; Chary, K.; Lapinlampi, M.N.; Andrade, P.; Paananen, T.; Sierra, A.; Tohka, J.; Gröhn, O.; Pitkänen, A. Early Increase in Cortical T2 Relaxation Is a Prognostic Biomarker for the Evolution of Severe Cortical Damage, but Not for Epileptogenesis, after Experimental Traumatic Brain Injury. *J. Neurotrauma* **2020**, *37*, 2580–2594. [CrossRef]
48. Vuokila, N.; Das Gupta, S.; Huusko, R.; Tohka, J.; Puhakka, N.; Pitkänen, A. Elevated Acute Plasma miR-124-3p Level Relates to Evolution of Larger Cortical Lesion Area after Traumatic Brain Injury. *Neuroscience* **2020**, *433*, 21–35. [CrossRef]
49. Barros, V.N.; Mundim, M.; Galindo, L.T.; Bittencourt, S.; Porcionatto, M.; Mello, L.E. The pattern of c-Fos expression and its refractory period in the brain of rats and monkeys. *Front. Cell. Neurosci.* **2015**, *9*, 72. [CrossRef]
50. Dragunow, M.; Robertson, H. Brain injury induces c-fos protein(s) in nerve and glial-like cells in adult mammalian brain. *Brain Res.* **1988**, *455*, 295–299. [CrossRef]
51. Yang, K.; Mu, X.; Xue, J.; Whitson, J.; Salminen, A.; Dixon, C.; Liu, P.; Hayes, R. Increased expression of c-fos mRNA and AP-1 transcription factors after cortical impact injury in rats. *Brain Res.* **1994**, *664*, 141–147. [CrossRef]
52. Raghupathi, R.; Welsh, F.A.; Lowenstein, D.H.; Gennarelli, T.A.; McIntosh, T.K. Regional Induction of c-Fos and Heat Shock Protein-72 mRNA following Fluid-Percussion Brain Injury in the Rat. *Br. J. Pharmacol.* **1995**, *15*, 467–473. [CrossRef] [PubMed]
53. Raghupathi, R.; McIntosh, T.K. Regionally and temporally distinct patterns of induction of c-fos, c-jun and junB mRNAs following experimental brain injury in the rat. *Mol. Brain Res.* **1996**, *37*, 134–144. [CrossRef]
54. Gass, P.; Herdegen, T. Neuronal expression of AP-1 proteins in excitotoxic-neurodegenerative disorders and following nerve fiber lesions. *Prog. Neurobiol.* **1995**, *47*, 257–290. [CrossRef]

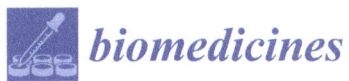

Article

MRI-Guided Electrode Implantation for Chronic Intracerebral Recordings in a Rat Model of Post−Traumatic Epilepsy—Challenges and Gains

Xavier Ekolle Ndode-Ekane *, Riikka Immonen, Elina Hämäläinen, Eppu Manninen, Pedro Andrade, Robert Ciszek, Tomi Paananen, Olli Gröhn and Asla Pitkänen

A.I. Virtanen Institute for Molecular Sciences, University of Eastern Finland, P.O. Box 1627, FI-70211 Kuopio, Finland
* Correspondence: xavier.ekollendode-ekane@uef.fi; Tel.: +358-442707689

Abstract: Brain atrophy induced by traumatic brain injury (TBI) progresses in parallel with epileptogenesis over time, and thus accurate placement of intracerebral electrodes to monitor seizure initiation and spread at the chronic postinjury phase is challenging. We evaluated in adult male Sprague Dawley rats whether adjusting atlas-based electrode coordinates on the basis of magnetic resonance imaging (MRI) increases electrode placement accuracy and the effect of chronic electrode implantations on TBI-induced brain atrophy. One group of rats (EEG cohort) was implanted with two intracortical (anterior and posterior) and a hippocampal electrode right after TBI to target coordinates calculated using a rat brain atlas. Another group (MRI cohort) was implanted with the same electrodes, but using T2-weighted MRI to adjust the planned atlas-based 3D coordinates of each electrode. Histological analysis revealed that the anterior cortical electrode was in the cortex in 83% (25% in targeted layer V) of the EEG cohort and 76% (31%) of the MRI cohort. The posterior cortical electrode was in the cortex in 40% of the EEG cohort and 60% of the MRI cohort. Without MRI-guided adjustment of electrode tip coordinates, 58% of the posterior cortical electrodes in the MRI cohort will be in the lesion cavity, as revealed by simulated electrode placement on histological images. The hippocampal electrode was accurately placed in 82% of the EEG cohort and 86% of the MRI cohort. Misplacement of intracortical electrodes related to their rostral shift due to TBI-induced cortical and hippocampal atrophy and caudal retraction of the brain, and was more severe ipsilaterally than contralaterally ($p < 0.001$). Total lesion area in cortical subfields targeted by the electrodes (primary somatosensory cortex, visual cortex) was similar between cohorts ($p > 0.05$). MRI-guided adjustment of coordinates for electrodes improved the success rate of intracortical electrode tip placement nearly to that at the acute postinjury phase (68% vs. 62%), particularly in the posterior brain, which exhibited the most severe postinjury atrophy. Overall, MRI-guided electrode implantation improved the quality and interpretation of the origin of EEG-recorded signals.

Keywords: cortical atrophy; hippocampal atrophy; intracerebral electrode; magnetic resonance imaging; posttraumatic epilepsy; traumatic brain injury

Citation: Ndode-Ekane, X.E.; Immonen, R.; Hämäläinen, E.; Manninen, E.; Andrade, P.; Ciszek, R.; Paananen, T.; Gröhn, O.; Pitkänen, A. MRI-Guided Electrode Implantation for Chronic Intracerebral Recordings in a Rat Model of Post−Traumatic Epilepsy—Challenges and Gains. *Biomedicines* **2022**, *10*, 2295. https://doi.org/10.3390/biomedicines10092295

Academic Editor: Jun Lu

Received: 8 August 2022
Accepted: 9 September 2022
Published: 15 September 2022

Publisher's Note: MDPI stays neutral with regard to jurisdictional claims in published maps and institutional affiliations.

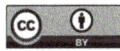

Copyright: © 2022 by the authors. Licensee MDPI, Basel, Switzerland. This article is an open access article distributed under the terms and conditions of the Creative Commons Attribution (CC BY) license (https://creativecommons.org/licenses/by/4.0/).

1. Introduction

Traumatic brain injury (TBI) is an alteration in brain function or brain pathology caused by an external force [1]. Postimpact secondary pathologies include axonal injury, neurodegeneration, blood–brain barrier dysfunction, and neuroinflammation, which can progress over days to weeks to years [2–7]. The progressive reorganization of neuronal networks can result in chronic comorbidities that compromise the quality of life, such as posttraumatic epilepsy (PTE) [8,9].

The risk of PTE increases with the severity of the TBI, and is approximately 16% after severe TBI [10]. The risk of epilepsy post-TBI increases with impact severity in both humans and animal models [11]. Clinical and experimental studies show that the seizure focus and epileptogenic network locate in cortical structures, including the cerebral cortex and hippocampus [12–14]. As epileptogenesis occurs over a period of weeks to months and the frequency of unprovoked seizures is low, mechanistic studies of the evolution of PTE require chronic electroencephalogram (EEG) recordings of the severely damaged brain with an ongoing progressive secondary pathology [11]. On the other hand, to detect unprovoked seizures (i.e., epilepsy diagnosis), electrodes are often implanted months to weeks after the injury. The usefulness of atlas coordinates for electrode placement into the atrophied cortical structures long after the occurrence of TBI and the effect of the presence of chronic intracerebral electrodes on brain pathology, however, are unknown.

In patients with epilepsy, advanced structural magnetic resonance imaging (MRI) techniques are used extensively in the clinic to facilitate intracerebral navigation during implantation of intracerebral EEG electrodes for identifying epileptic foci or for stimulation therapy [15,16]. To our knowledge, MRI guidance has not been applied in preclinical studies. One of the objectives of the National Institutes of Health (NIH)-funded Centers without Walls project EpiBioS4Rx (https://epibios.loni.usc.edu/; access on 14 March 2022) is to perform chronic intracerebral EEG recordings over the course of epileptogenesis after lateral fluid-percussion injury (FPI)-induced TBI. Lateral FPI is a widely used preclinical model of TBI, leading to epilepsy in approximately 25% of animals within 6 to 7 months postinjury [7,11,17,18]. Like in humans with PTE, progressive brain damage involves epileptogenic regions, including the cerebral cortex and hippocampus [7,19,20]. The progression of cortical and hippocampal atrophy and spatial distortion, however, varies significantly between animals over time [7,21–23].

Epileptogenesis studies often require large animal cohorts, and therefore optimizing the quality of EEG recordings and their interpretation in atrophied brain is critical for maintaining the feasibility and affordability of the studies [24]. As such, we aimed to develop methodologies to (a) maximize the accuracy of recording-electrode placement into the atrophied brain using preimplantation in vivo MRI, (b) reliably assess electrode locations to correctly interpret the origin of the EEG-recorded signal, and (c) respond to concerns related to the effect of chronic electrode implantations on TBI-induced brain atrophy. We hypothesized that (a) MRI-guided electrode implantation will improve the accuracy of perilesional intracortical and intrahippocampal electrode placements at a chronic postinjury time point, and (b) chronic electrode implantation does not worsen lateral FPI-induced cortical damage. The data presented include analysis of 297 electrode locations in 25 sham-operated experimental controls and 74 rats with severe TBI induced by lateral FPI in the University of Eastern Finland (UEF) subcohort of the EpiBioS4Rx Project 1. In 57 rats, electrode implantation was performed immediately after the injury (EEG cohort). In 42 rats, the electrodes were implanted after MRI was performed at 5 months postinjury (MRI cohort). At the end, all animals were perfused for ex vivo MRI and histology.

2. Materials and Methods

This study is part of the National Institutes of Health funded Centers without Walls international multicenter project EpiBioS4Rx, which aims to identify biomarkers for post-traumatic epileptogenesis (https://epibios.loni.usc.edu/, accessed 14 March 2022). We report data from the University of Eastern Finland (UEF) subcohort, including histological sections and MRI findings for assessing electrode locations.

2.1. Animals and Study Design

Animals. Adult male Sprague Dawley rats (300–350 g at the time of injury) were used. Animals were quarantined for 1 week (3–6 per cage) upon arrival at the animal facility. Thereafter, they were individually housed in a controlled environment (temperature 22 ± 1 °C; humidity 50–60%; lights on from 07:00 to 19:00 h) until the end of the experiments. Food and water were provided ad libitum for the duration of the study. All animal procedures were approved by the Animal Ethics Committee of the Provincial

Government of Southern Finland and carried out in accordance with the guidelines of European Community Council Directives 2010/63/EU.

Study design (Figure 1). The study design, randomization, and interventions performed in the 2 study cohorts are summarized in Figure 1. The rats were divided into EEG (14 sham, 43 TBI) and MRI (11 sham, 31 TBI) cohorts. In the EEG cohort, electrodes were implanted immediately after the induction of lateral FPI. Starting immediately after the TBI, video-EEG was performed first for 1 month and then during the 1st week of months 2 through 6. In the 7th post-TBI month, the rats underwent a 24 h/7 days video-EEG to record unprovoked spontaneous seizures (i.e., confirm epilepsy diagnosis). In the MRI cohort, the rats were imaged at 2, 9, and 30 days and at 5 months post-TBI; electrodes were implanted 14.02 ± 1.34 days (range: 4–40 days) after the last MRI, and video-EEG monitoring was performed during the 7th post-TBI month to detect unprovoked seizures (Figure 1A). Both groups were killed at the end of the 7-month follow-up, and the brains were processed for ex vivo MRI and histological analysis (Figure 1).

The EEG cohort was used to assess the sensitivity and specificity of ex vivo MRI to determine the electrode tip locations compared with histology. The MRI cohort was used to assess both (a) the accuracy of in vivo MRI-guided electrode implantation at the chronic phase and (b) the sensitivity and specificity of ex vivo MRI to detect electrode tip locations. Finally, we compared the accuracy of early (EEG cohort) and late (MRI cohort) electrode implantations.

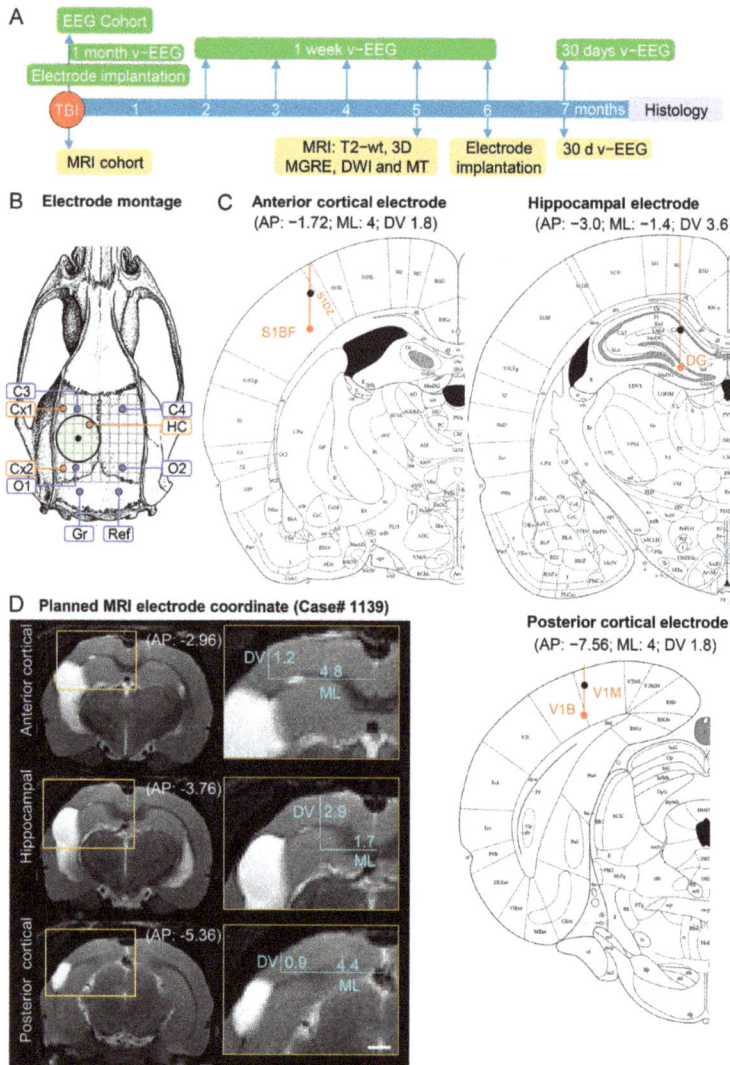

Figure 1. Study design, electrode montage, and atlas or MRI-planned electrode coordinates. (**A**) Study design. Following TBI, rats were divided into either the EEG or MRI cohort. The rats of the EEG cohort were implanted with electrodes after fully righting themselves following induction of TBI. The rats were followed up immediately afterward with 1 month video-EEG and then for 1 week monthly until the 6th post-TBI month. The rats of the MRI cohort were magnetic resonance-imaged at 5 months post-TBI and T2-wt images were used to calculate the coordinates of the intracerebral electrodes implanted at 6 months post-TBI. Both cohorts were continuously monitored with video-EEG for 30 days at 7 months post-TBI to diagnose epilepsy. At the end of the 7-month follow-up period, all rats were euthanized and the brains processed for histological identification of the location of the intracerebral electrodes. (**B**) Electrode montage used in the study. Four epidural screw electrodes (C3, C4, O1 and O2), 3 intracerebral bipolar wire electrodes (anterior cortical Cx1, posterior cortical Cx2, and hippocampal HC), a ground (Gr) and reference (Ref) electrode. (**C**) Atlas plates demonstrating the planned coordinates used in the EEG cohort to implant the anterior cortical, hippocampal, and

posterior cortical electrodes. The black dot refers to the upper tip and the red dot to the lower tip of the bipolar electrode (1 mm apart). Reprinted/adapted with permission from [25]. 2007, Elsevier Inc. (**D**) MRI T2-wt images of rat 1139 demonstrating the planned-MRI coordinates of the intracerebral anterior cortical, hippocampal, and posterior cortical electrodes. The anteroposterior (AP) coordinate was determined by aligning the MR images with the atlas [25]. The mediolateral (ML) and dorsoventral (DV) coordinates were determined using ImageJ software (version 1.47v, Wayne Rasband and contributors, National Institute of Health, USA).

2.2. Induction of Lateral FPI

Severe TBI was induced by lateral FPI as previously described [26,27]. The rat was placed into an anesthesia induction chamber and isoflurane anesthesia was induced at 5% (room air as carrier gas; Somnosuite, SS6069B, Kent Scientific, Torrington, CT, USA). The anesthetized rat was mounted in a stereotaxic frame, a probe was inserted into the rectum to continuously assess core temperature, and a heating pad was placed below the abdomen. The temperature of the heating pad was regulated based on the animal core temperature (max 38 °C). Isoflurane was delivered via a nose cone mounted on the stereotaxic frame and maintained at 1.9% throughout the surgery. The scalp incision site was shaved and cleaned using sterile 0.9% NaCl before subcutaneous injection with 0.5% lidocaine (7 mg/kg). Approximately 3 to 5 min later, a midline incision was made, and the surface of the skull was cleaned. A craniotomy 5 mm in diameter (center coordinate: anteroposterior [AP] −4.5 mm from the bregma; mediolateral [ML] 2.5 mm) was made over the left cortex using a handheld trephine with the dura left intact. A plastic female Luer lock connector was inserted into the craniotomy vertical to the skull surface, and its edges were sealed with tissue adhesive glue (3M Vetbond, 3M Deutschland GmbH, Neuss, Germany). Dental acrylate was spread around the Luer lock and the connector setup was secured to the skull with an ipsilateral frontal screw. To induce TBI, the Luer lock was filled with saline and the rat was connected to a straight-tipped fluid-percussion device (model FP 302, AmScien Instruments, Richmond, VA, USA). The pressure was adjusted to produce severe injury with an anticipated mortality rate of 20% to 30% within the first 48 h. The mean impact pressure was 2.9 ± 0.01 atm (range: 2.4–3.3 atm). The duration of the impact was <1 s. After injury, the rat was disconnected from the device, placed on a heating pad, and a rectal temperature probe was inserted. Occurrence of postimpact seizure-like behavior and its duration, duration of postimpact apnea, and time to return of the righting reflex were recorded. Sham-operated controls underwent all surgical procedures except exposure to FPI. To reduce impact of experimenter-induced variability in the experimental outcome, all surgical procedures, including TBI induction and electrode implantation, were performed by the same person.

2.3. Electrode Implantation

EEG cohort. Electrodes were implanted immediately after the lateral FPI using coordinates based on a rat brain atlas (Figure 1B,C) [25]. In brief, after return of the righting reflex, the rat was reanesthetized with isoflurane and placed in a stereotaxic frame. Four recording epidural stainless-steel screw electrodes (EM12/20/SPC; P1 Technologies, Roanoke, VA, USA) were implanted into the skull: 2 ipsilaterally (frontal cortex; C3, AP: −1.7, ML: left 2.5 and parieto-occipital cortex; O1, AP: −7.6, ML: left 2.5) and 2 contralaterally (frontal cortex; C4, AP: right 1.7; ML: −2.5 and parieto-occipital cortex; O2, AP: −7.6; ML: right 2.5; Figure 1B). Three intracerebral tungsten bipolar recording electrodes (EM12/3-2TW/SPC; P1 Technologies.; Ø 0.5 mm, tip separation 1.0 mm) were implanted ipsilaterally in the anterior perilesional cortex (AP: −1.72; ML: −4.0; DV: 1.8), septal hippocampus (AP: −3.0; ML: −1.4; DV: 3.6), and posterior perilesional cortex (AP: −7.56; ML: −4.0; DV: 1.8; Figure 1C). In addition, 1 epidural screw electrode serving as a ground was placed ipsilaterally posterior to lambda, and another serving as a reference electrode was placed contralaterally. Atlas-based placement of electrodes relies on calculating the target coordinates based on fixed skull surface landmarks, i.e., identification of bregma and midline sutural landmarks.

Thus, the coordinates are defined independently of the intracranial changes in brain volume and orientation, which progress over time after TBI.

MRI cohort. Electrodes were implanted approximately 6 months (164 ± 1.4 days, range: 156–195 days) post-TBI. The locations of the epidural recording screws, ground, and reference electrodes were the same as in the EEG cohort described above. Due to progressive brain atrophy and ventricle enlargement, we first assessed the severity of cortical and hippocampal atrophy in each rat on MRI T2-weighted (T2-wt) images to define the AP, ML, and DV coordinates to avoid electrode misplacements (see below) (Figure 1D). Based on the analysis, the distance between the tips of the bipolar electrodes was reduced from 1.0 mm to 0.5 mm to fit within the atrophied cortex (upper tip in layer I, lower tip in layer V) or hippocampus (upper tip in CA1, lower tip in hilus).

2.4. Postoperative Care and Body Weight Monitoring

After surgery, rats were placed on a body-temperature–regulated heating pad (+38 °C) controlled by the SomnoSuite system (SS6069B, Kent Scientific). A subcutaneous injection of buprenorphine (0.01 mg/kg, Temgesic®, Reckitt&Colman Products Ltd., Hull, UK) and 0.9% NaCl (saline) was administered. Analgesia treatment was repeated based on animal well-being. Upon return to the home cage, rats received either powder or soft pellet food (until they could eat on their own) and saline (twice daily for 3 days). Rats were weighed daily for the first 14 days post-TBI, weekly until 30 days post-TBI, and then once a month throughout the 6-month follow-up. Adverse complications following TBI were monitored using a strict physiologic monitoring paradigm to assess general appearance; hair, coat and skin condition; bowel and gastrointestinal function; body conditioning score; condition of injury scar; and external bleeding. Any identified complication was treated according to the laboratory animal center's guidelines.

2.5. Video-EEG Monitoring and Analysis

The video-EEG monitoring schedule is summarized in Figure 1. In the EEG cohort, monitoring was started immediately after surgery. In the MRI cohort, video-EEG monitoring was started at 6 months postinjury.

Monitoring. For video-EEG monitoring, the electrode headset attached to the rat skull was connected to a 12-pin swivel commutator (SL12C, PlasticsOne Inc., Roanoke, VA, USA) via a flexible shielded cable (363/2-363/2, PlasticsOne Inc.), allowing the rat to move freely during the EEG recordings. The commutator was connected to an amplifier with a flexible shielded cable 363/2-441/12 (PlasticsOne Inc). High-fidelity electrical brain activity was monitored using a 320-channel Digital Lynx 16SX amplifier (Neuralynx, Bozeman, MT, USA) with a 10 kHz sampling rate. The amplifier had an analogue bandwidth between DC to 80 kHz. It had 80 independent analogue references, allowing for a configuration of independent references for each animal. Data from each channel were converted individually into 24 bits. Each animal was video-monitored with a single high-resolution camera (Basler acA1300-75gm GigE, Basler, Germany) configured to record 30 frames per second (maximum 75) with a resolution of 1.3 megapixels and compressed using H.264. At night, cameras recorded under cage-specific infrared illumination (24 V, 150 mA). The EEG and video were synchronized using the precision time protocol IEEE-1588. The entire system generated approximately 1.5 TB of data every 24 h. For data storage, the video-EEG system was connected to network-attached storage (Synology RS4017xs+) comprising 200 TB of storage configured at RAID6 for redundancy and checksum for data integrity. The video-EEG recorded starting at 7 days after electrode implantation was analyzed for unprovoked seizures.

Analysis of EEG. Seizures were detected from video-EEG recordings by browsing the files visually and using the semiautomatic seizure detection algorithm [28]. A seizure was defined as a high-amplitude rhythmic discharge with frequency and amplitude modulation that clearly represented an abnormal EEG pattern (repetitive spikes, spike-and-wave discharges, polyspike-and-wave, or slow waves) and lasted at least 10 s. Behavioral severity of electrographic seizures was scored according to Racine [29]. Rats were defined as having epilepsy if at least 1 unprovoked electrographic seizure occurred during the 6-month EEG recording [30]. Seizure frequency was calculated as the number of unprovoked seizures/number of recording days.

2.6. MRI Acquisition

The animals were imaged in vivo using a 7-Tesla Bruker PharmaScan MRI scanner (Bruker BioSpin MRI GmbH, Ettlingen, Germany). The animals were anesthetized using 1% to 2% isoflurane mixed with carrier gas (70% N2, 30% O2), keeping their breathing rate at 50–70 breaths/min. The animal bed was heated to maintain the core temperature at 36–37 °C.

The MRI sequences used were described previously [31] [https://doi.org/10.1016/j.eplepsyres.2019.01.001, accessed 7 August 2022]. Briefly, T2-wt images were acquired using a 2D multislice fast-spin echo sequence with a repetition time of 3.4 s and an effective echo time of 45 ms. The image stack included 23 coronal slices with 800 μm thickness and an in-plane resolution of 117 μm × 117 μm. Additionally, 3D multigradient echo (MGRE) images with whole brain coverage at resolution 160 μm × 160 μm × 160 μm were acquired. Thirteen echoes with echo times between 2.7 ms and 40 ms were collected with a repetition time of 66 ms and a flip angle of 16°. The echo images were summed to create a high signal-to-noise ratio anatomic image.

2.7. MRI-Based Adjustment of Electrode Coordinates

As post-TBI cortical atrophy is common in the lateral FPI model, especially in the caudal aspects of the cortex [32], T2-wt MR images obtained at 5 months post-TBI were used to determine the anteroposterior (AP), mediolateral (ML), and dorsoventral (DV) coordinates of the depth electrodes in the MRI cohort. The aim was to position both tips of each bipolar depth electrode (0.5 mm vertical tip separation) in the rostral and caudal perilesional cortex or the septal hippocampus, instead of the lesion cavity or enlarged ventricles.

Intracortical electrodes. The 800 μm-thick in vivo T2-wt MRI coronal slices (11 slices from bregma to lambda) were converted to TIFF images. The images were uploaded into ImageJ software (version 1.47v, Wayne Rasband and contributors, National Institute of Health, USA), and scaled and aligned with the coronal plates of the rat brain atlas [25]. Then, the AP level (slice) near the planned anterior/posterior electrode location in which the cortex around the lesion cavity was thick enough to harbor both electrode tips (i.e., about 1 mm) was determined. The TIFF image (MR image) of that slice was used to define the ML and DV coordinates of the lower electrode tip using the ImageJ software line tool. First, a horizontal line was drawn from the pial surface of the brain midline laterally until its perpendicular vertical level reached layer V of the perilesional cortex approximately 500 μm from the lesion edge (Figure 1D). The horizontal length of the line was recorded as the ML coordinate. Then, the length of the vertical line to layer V was recorded as the DV coordinate (see details in [33]).

Intrahippocampal electrodes. An MRI T2-wt slice of the septal hippocampus approximately 3 to 4 mm from the bregma was selected. The MRI slice was opened in ImageJ as a TIFF file. To determine the ML coordinate, a horizontal line was drawn from the pial surface of the brain midline laterally until its perpendicular vertical level reached the hilus of the dentate gyrus. The horizontal length of the line was recorded as the ML coordinate (Figure 1D). The length of the vertical line to the hilus was recorded as the DV coordinate (see details in [33]).

The procedures were repeated for each rat because the lesion distribution as well as the cortical and hippocampal atrophy varied between rats.

2.8. MRI-Based Estimation of Cortical and Hippocampal Shrinkage

In the initial MRI-guided calculations of the AP and ML electrode coordinates, we did not consider tissue shrinkage or hippocampal transformation (rotation, tilting), which occurred over the follow-up and apparently contributed to some electrode misplacements. To improve the success rate, we next assessed the AP and ML shrinkage of both the ipsilateral and contralateral cortex and the hippocampi to further adjust the calculations for optimizing the electrode positions in the MRI cohort.

AP shrinkage. The coronal, sagittal, and horizontal in vivo MR 3D MGRE slices (160 μm thick) of each animal in the MRI cohort were opened in the medical images analysis application Aedes (version 1.0 rev 218, GitHub: aedes_getfilefilter.m, Juha-Pekka Niskanen, University of Eastern Finland, Finland), using MATLAB software (version R2019b, The MathWork, Inc, Natick, MA, USA). In the sagittal slices 4 mm from the midline (i.e., ML coordinate of the anterior intracortical electrode), the AP length of the ipsilateral and contralateral cortex was measured by calculating the geometric distance between the 2 points (160 × 160 × 160 μm resolution images) in Aedes (see detail in Section 3.4.1)

ML shrinkage. To set the ML level for the measurement, the targeted AP location of the rostral intracortical electrode was used as a reference (AP -1.72). Typically, it was located in a slice that was 1.56 mm (i.e., approximately ten 160 μm-thick MRI slices) caudal to the level where the ipsilateral and contralateral legs of the anterior commissure fuse, which occurs approximately at the level of the bregma (see detail in Section 3.4.1). Then, the ML distance from the midline to the lateral edge of the cortex was measured in a horizontal slice 1.7 mm below the surface of the brain (targeted DV location of the lower electrode tip; see detail in Section 3.4.1).

Hippocampal shrinkage. The AP hippocampal distortion was measured in the sagittal slice 1.4 mm from the midline as the distance from the rostral edge of the frontal cortex to the rostral edge of the hippocampus (see detail in Section 3.4.2) The ML shrinkage was measured as the distance from the brain midline to the lateral edge of the hippocampus in a horizontal slice at 2.8 mm below the brain surface (see details in Section 3.4.2).

2.9. Histology

At the end of the 7-month follow-up period, all rats were transcardially perfused with saline (5 min, 30 mL/min) followed by cold 4% paraformaldehyde (PFA; 30 min, 30 mL/min). The brain was removed from the skull, postfixed in 4% PFA (2 h at 4 °C), and cryoprotected by immersing in 20% glycerol for 36 h (4 °C). The brains were then frozen on dry ice and stored at -70 °C until further processing. The brains were sectioned at 30 μm in a 1-in-5 series using a sliding microtome.

The first series of sections was stained with thionine, mounted on glass slides, and cover-slipped from xylene. The mounted thionine-stained sections were scanned at 40× magnification with a digital slide scanner (Hamamatsu C12000-02 model) and analyzed using the Hamamatsu NDP viewer 2® software (Hamamatsu Photonics K.K., Hamamatsu City, Japan).

2.10. Generation of Unfolded Cortical Maps

The unfolded cortical maps were generated from coronal histological sections using software developed in-house, as described previously [32,34,35]. The unfolded maps were used to determine (a) the location of the cortical lesion in various cytoarchitectonic fields of the cortical mantle, (b) the total lesion area, (c) the lesion area within different cortical cytoarchitectonic subareas, (d) the planned vs. final AP and DV coordinates of the intracerebral electrodes, and (e) the distance of the electrode tips from the lesion edge. The unfolded map software is openly available at https://www.unfoldedmap.org/ (accessed 30 November 2020) [34] and the source code at https://github.com/UEFepilepsyAIVI/CortexMap (accessed 30 November 2020) [35].

Histological sections. To determine the final AP and DV locations of the electrode tip(s), the digitized image of the histological section(s) containing a trace of the electrode tip was matched with the best-fitting level of the rat brain atlas.

As the ML coordinate cannot be easily determined based on the atlas due to shrinkage related to histological processing, we first estimated the shrinkage factor for each animal by measuring the distance from the midline to the rhinal fissure in the histological section containing the electrode tip. The midline-hinal fissure distance was then measured at the matching atlas plate (EEG cohort) or T2-wt MRI slice (MRI cohort) and divided by the corresponding histological measure, resulting in a shrinkage factor specific for each brain (sham: 1.08 ± 0.01, range: 1.02–1.2, $n = 25$; TBI: 1.08 ± 0.01, range: 1.01–1.2, $n = 74$). Cortical and hippocampal electrode tip distances from the midline were then measured in histological sections and multiplied by the shrinkage factor to obtain the normalized ML distance.

To measure the distance of the electrode tip from the lesion cavity edge, a straight line was drawn from the tip to the lesion edge along layer V.

2.11. Statistical Analysis

Data were analyzed using GraphPad Prism (version 9.3.1, GraphPad Software, LLC, USA) and IBM SPSS Statistics (version 27, IBM Corp., USA). A Shapiro–Wilk test was performed to test for normality. The data were not normally distributed. Thus, the Mann–Whitney U test was used to analyze (1) the difference between the atlas, histological, and/or MRI-based coordinates (sham vs. TBI rats, EEG and MRI cohorts), (2) the difference in the distance of the electrode tip from the lesion edge (TBI rats, EEG vs. MRI cohorts), and (3) the difference in cortical and hippocampal shrinkage (sham vs. TBI rats, MRI cohort). The Wilcoxon signed-rank test was used to test the difference between the targeted and "true" histologically verified tip coordinates between the anterior and posterior cortical electrodes ipsilateral vs. contralateral cortical and hippocampal shrinkage. The Pearson chi-squared statistic was used to test the difference in the distribution of the DV location (layers) of the lower tip of the intracortical electrodes (sham vs. TBI rats, anterior vs. posterior cortical electrodes, separately in the EEG and MRI cohorts). All data are presented as means $\pm$ SEM.

3. Results

Altogether, the analysis included the location of 99 anterior intracortical, 99 posterior intracortical, and 99 intrahippocampal electrodes implanted in 99 rats (57 in the EEG cohort and 42 in the MRI cohort). In the EEG cohort, electrodes were implanted immediately after the lateral FPI using coordinates based on a rat brain atlas (Figure 1A–C). In the MRI cohort, electrodes were implanted approximately 6 months post-TBI using MRI T2-weighted (T2-wt) images from each rat to define the AP, ML, and DV coordinates to avoid electrode misplacements (see below) (Figure 1A,B,D).

3.1. Success in Positioning the Anterior Intracortical Electrode

3.1.1. Electrode Locations—An Overview

EEG cohort. Histological analysis indicated that the tip of the anterior intracortical electrode was within the cerebral cortex in 83% (47/57) of the cases. In the remaining 17% (10/57), the tip was located in either the external capsule or the corpus callosum. The histologically verified AP and ML electrode tip locations were within 0.5 mm of the targeted atlas-based coordinates in 11% (6/57) and 65% (37/57) of the rats, respectively (Figure 2A,B). The histological DV location of the cortical electrode tip was in the planned target (i.e., layer V) in 28% (16/57) of the animals. In the remaining 72% (41/57), the tip was located in either layer VI, the external capsule, or the corpus callosum (Figure 2C and summary Table 1).

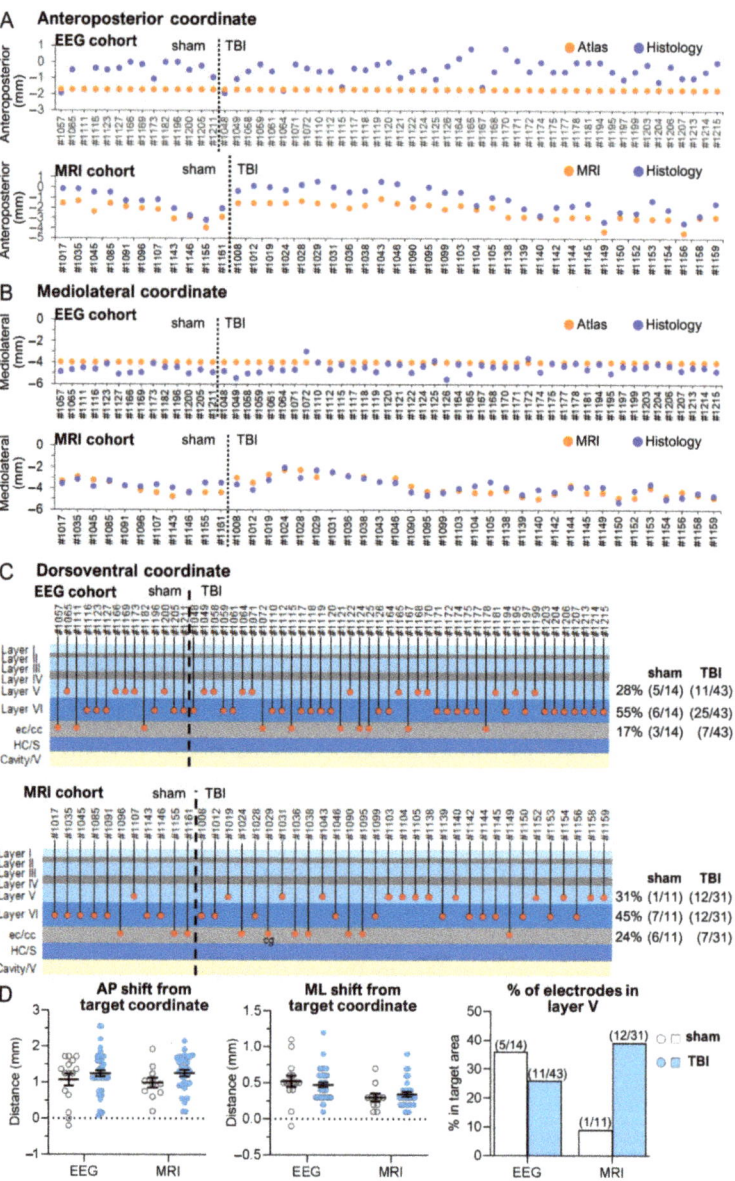

Figure 2. Anterior intracortical electrode—schematic representations of the atlas, histological, and MRI-guided coordinates in each rat of the EEG and MRI cohorts. (**A**) Anteroposterior (AP) coordinate. In the EEG cohort (electrode operation right after injury), the fixed atlas-based target AP coordinate of −1.72 mm from the bregma was applied to implant the electrodes (orange dots). In the MRI cohort (electrode operation 5 months after injury), the target AP coordinate was individually determined using the 5-month in vivo T2-weighted MR images. The target coordinate fluctuated depending on the extent of the TBI (traumatic brain injury)-induced lesion. Note the anterior shift (y-axis) in the histologically verified "true" AP coordinate (blue dots) relative to the target coordinate (orange dots) in both cohorts. The deviations were comparable between the sham and TBI animals ($p > 0.05$).

Animal numbers are shown on the x-axis. (**B**) Mediolateral (ML) coordinate. In the EEG cohort, the fixed atlas-based target ML coordinate at 4 mm lateral to midline was targeted. In the MRI cohort, the target ML coordinate was individually determined using the 5-month in vivo MRI. Note a small deviation of the histologically verified "true" ML coordinate from the target coordinate in both cohorts. (**C**) Dorsoventral (DV) coordinate. In both cohorts, the lower tip of the bipolar electrode was aimed to layer V in the selected AP and ML coordinates (see above). Electrode tips were located in the cortex in 83% (36/43) of the EEG cohort and 77% (24/31) of the MRI cohort. Importantly, even though the lower tip in the remaining cases went down into the external capsule or corpus callosum, the upper tip of the bipolar electrode, being 1 mm higher in the EEG and 0.5 mm in the MRI cohort, was still recording in the cortex. The percentages of electrode locations in the sham-operated and TBI animals are shown on the right side of the panel. (**D**) Dot plots of the AP and ML shift in the histological AP and ML coordinate, and % of electrode in the targeted layer V (number of cases in brackets). Note posterior and medial shift of some cases from the target (vertical dashed line). y-axis represents distance from target coordinate (Y = 0) or % of cases in targeted area. Abbreviations: cavity, cortical lesion cavity; cc, corpus callosum; cg, cingulum; S, subiculum; ec, external capsule; HC, hippocampus; and V, ventricle.

Table 1. Summary of the location of the dorsoventral tip of the intracerebral electrodes.

	EEG Cohort Atlas-Based % (n)			MRI Cohort Atlas-Based without MRI Guidance % (n)			MRI Cohort with MRI Guidance % (n)			EEG and MRI Cohorts % (n)		
	Sham	TBI	All	Sham	TBI	All	Sham	TBI	All	Sham	TBI	All
Anterior cortical electrode												
Within 1 mm of target coordinate [#]	29% (4/14)	26% (11/43)	26% (15/57)	100% (11/11)	100% (31/31)	100% (42/42)	55% (6/11)	32% (10/31)	38% (16/42)	42% (10/25)	28% (21/74)	31% (31/99)
In cortex	79% (11/14)	84% (36/43)	83% (47/57)	100% (11/11)	32% (10/31)	50% (21/42)	73% * (8/11)	77% *** (24/31)	76% (32/42)	76% (19/25)	81% (60/74)	78% (79/99)
In brain	100% (14/14)	100% (43/43)	100% (57/57)	100% (11/11)	52% (16/31)	64% (27/42)	100% (11/11)	100% *** (31/31)	100% (42/42)	100% (25/25)	100% (74/74)	100% (99/99)
Not recording in brain	0% (0/14)	0% (0/43)	0% (0/57)	0% (0/111)	48% (15/31)	36% (15/42)	0% (0/11)	0% *** (0/31)	0% (0/42)	0% (0/25)	0% (0/74)	0% (0/99)
Hippocampal electrode												
Within 1 mm of target coordinate [#]	93% (13/14)	77% (33/43)	81% (46/57)	100% (11/11)	100% (31/31)	100% (42/42)	82% (9/11)	52% (16/31)	60% (25/42)	88% (22/25)	66% (49/74)	72% (71/99)
In hippocampus proper/DG	86% (12/14)	81% (35/43)	82% (47/57)	100% (11/11)	100% (31/31)	100% (42/42)	100% (11/11)	81% * (25/31)	86% (36/42)	92% (23/25)	81% (60/74)	84% (83/99)
In brain	93% (13/14)	93% (41/43)	95% (54/57)	100% (11/11)	100% (31/31)	100% (42/42)	100% (11/11)	84% * (26/31)	88% (37/42)	96% (24/25)	91% (67/74)	92% (91/99)
Not recording in brain	7% (1/14)	5% (2/43)	5% (3/57)	0% (0/111)	0% (0/31)	0% (42/42)	0% (0/11)	16% * (5/39)	12% (5/42)	28% (7/25)	10% (7/74)	8% (8/99)
Posterior cortical electrode												
Within 1 mm of target coordinate [#]	43% (6/14)	51% (20/39)	49% (26/53)	100% (11/11)	100% (31/31)	100% (42/42)	36% (4/11)	21% (6/29)	25% (10/40)	40% (10/25)	38% (26/68)	41% (38/93)
In cortex	21% (3/14)	46% (18/39)	40% (21/53)	91% (10/11)	42% (13/31)	55% (23/42)	46% * (5/11)	66% * (19/29)	60% (24/40)	32% (8/25)	54% (37/68)	48% (45/93)
In brain	100% (14/14)	97% (34/35)	90% (48/53)	100% (11/11)	42% (13/31)	57% (24/42)	100% (11/11)	93% *** (27/29)	95% (38/40)	100% (25/25)	90% (61/68)	92% (86/93)
Not recording in brain	0% (0/14)	13% (5/39)	10% (5/53)	0% (0/11)	58% (18/31)	43% (18/42)	0% (0//11)	7% *** (2/29)	5% (2/40)	0% (0/25)	10% (7/68)	8% (7/93)

[#] Within <1 mm radius from the atlas-planned anteroposterior and mediolateral coordinate. The success rate was evaluated based on the location of the lower tip of bipolar electrode. Abbreviations: DG, dentate gyrus. Statistical significance: * $p < 0.05$; *** $p < 0.001$ compared to MRI cohort atlas-based without MRI guidance (X^2 test).

MRI cohort. Histological analysis indicated that the tip of the anterior intracortical electrode was within the cerebral cortex in 76% (32/42) of the cases. In the remaining 24% (10/42), the tip was located in either the external capsule or the corpus callosum. The histological AP and ML electrode tip locations were within 0.5 mm of the targeted atlas-based coordinates in 10% (4/42) and 86% (36/42) of the rats, respectively (Figure 2A,B). The histological DV location of the cortical electrode tip was in the planned target (i.e., layer V) in 31% (13/42) of the animals. In the remaining 69% (29/42), the tip was located in either layer VI, the external capsule, or the corpus callosum (Figure 2C and summary Table 1).

3.1.2. Anteroposterior Location of the Anterior Intracortical Electrode Tips

Based on estimation of the progression of the cortical lesion [7,27,32], the anterior intracortical electrode was aimed to the atlas-based AP level 1.72 mm from the bregma (primary somatosensory cortex, S1) to ensure proper EEG recording in the lesion vicinity during the 7th post-TBI month (Figure 1C).

EEG cohort. Histological examination showed neurodegeneration along the electrode path and around the electrode tip, often accompanied by iron deposits (Figure 3A,D,F). Occasionally, the electrode-associated lesion merged with the TBI-induced lesion cavity. The unfolded cortical map indicated that 100% of the electrode tracks were in S1. Further, 83% (47/57) of the electrode tips (at least one of the tips) were found in S1 (Figure 4A,B). The remaining 17% (10/57) of the lower electrode tips were located in either the external capsule or the corpus callosum (Figures 2C and 4A,B). The upper tip of the bipolar electrode (1.0 mm from the ventral tip), however, recorded in the targeted S1 cortex. In most of the rats, the histological AP electrode location was anterior to the targeted atlas-defined coordinate (-1.7 mm) (Figure 2A,D), the average deviation being 1.21 ± 0.07 mm (range: 0–2.56 mm, median: 1.24 mm). The rostral shift was comparable between the sham-operated experimental controls and TBI rats (sham 1.16 ± 0.15 mm vs. TBI 1.22 ± 0.09 mm; $p > 0.05$) (Figure 2A,D).

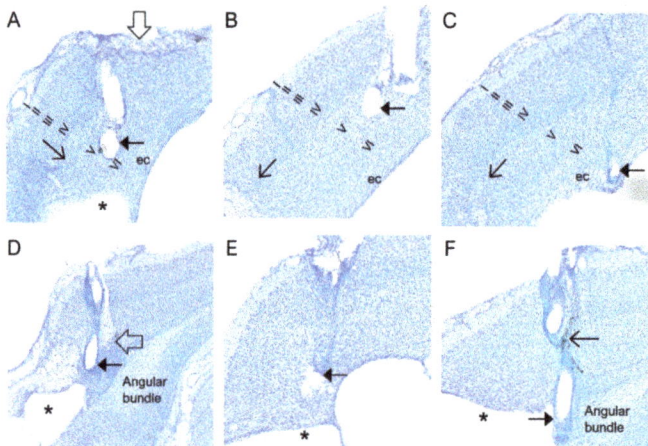

Figure 3. (**A–F**) Electrode tracts. Histological images from the coronal thionine-stained sections of 6 rats, showing the tracts of the bipolar intracortical electrodes and location of the lower electrode tip (filled arrowhead). Roman numerals indicate the cortical layers. In panels (**A,B**) the electrode tip is located in layer V of the perilesional cortex. Note the electrode track-related lesion on the surface of the brain in panel (**A**) (open filled arrow). In panel (**A**), the electrode tip is within 500 μm from the edge of the TBI-induced lesion cavity (asterisk). In panel (**C**), the electrode tip is in the external capsule (ec). In panel (**D**) the electrode tip is within the cortical lesion, close to the angular bundle. Open arrow points to the electrode path associated neurodegeneration. In panel (**E**), the electrode tip is close to the edge of the lesion cavity (asterisk). In panel (**F**), the electrode tip is within the angular bundle (closed arrowhead). The open arrowhead points to the location of the upper electrode in layer IV (open arrow). The dark staining indicates iron deposits (arrowheads) adjacent to the electrode path. Scale bar = 500 μm.

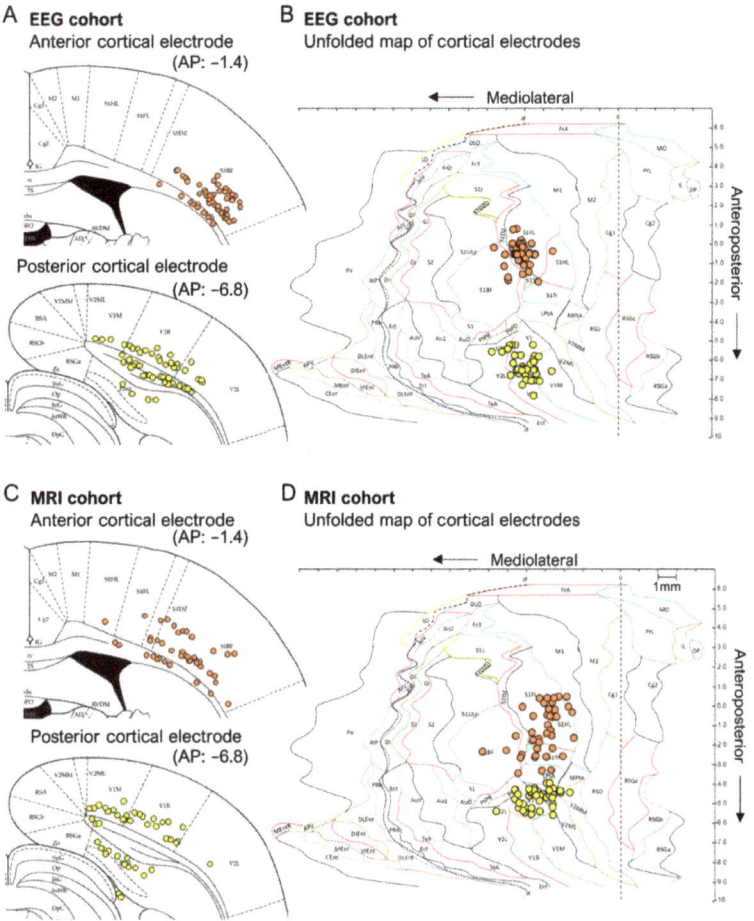

Figure 4. Location of the lower tip of the anterior and posterior intracortical electrodes on atlas plates and unfolded cortical maps. (**A**) In the EEG cohort (upper panel), the dorsoventral (DV) location of at least 1 of the tips of all anterior bipolar electrodes (atlas plate: bregma −1.4 mm) was within the primary somatosensory cortex (S1) and that of the posterior electrode (lower panel; atlas plate: bregma −6.8 mm) was within the visual cortex. Each dot represents 1 bipolar electrode. (**B**) An unfolded map (UFM) showing the location of electrode tracks in the EEG cohort as seen from the surface of the brain. The intersection of the electrode path with cortical layer V was used as reference. The UFMs confirmed the location of the anterior electrode paths in the S1 and posterior electrode paths in the visual cortex. (**C**) Atlas plate showing the DV locations of the anterior (upper panel) and posterior (lower panel) intracortical electrodes in the MRI cohort. As in the EEG cohort, the anterior electrode was in S1 and the posterior electrode was in the visual cortex. (**D**) A UFM showing the location of electrode tracks in the MRI cohort as seen from the surface of the brain. All electrode tracks were within S1 or the visual cortex. Note that in the MRI cohort, we used the 5-month in vivo MRI to adjust the electrode coordinates to target the perilesional cortex and to avoid lesion cavities, underlying brain areas, or ventricles. As expected, this resulted in a more heterogeneous distribution of electrode paths than in the EEG cohort with atlas-based fixed coordinates. Atlas plates and UFMs were generated using the Paxinos rat brain atlas (6th edition).

MRI cohort. Electrode-associated cortical lesions were rare in the MRI cohort (Figure 3A,D). As summarized in the cortical unfolded map, 100% of the electrode tracks (100%) and 76% (32/42) of the electrode tips were within S1 (Figure 4C,D). In the remaining cases, the lower tip was located within the external capsule or the corpus callosum (Figure 4C,D). Still, the upper tip of the bipolar electrode (0.5 mm from ventral tip) should have recorded in the targeted S1 cortex. As in the EEG cohort, the histological electrode location was anterior to the targeted MRI-guided AP coordinate, the average being 1.18 ± 0.08 mm (range: 0.2–2.16 mm, median: 1.19 mm) (Figure 2A,D). The rostral shift was comparable between the sham-operated controls and TBI groups (sham 0.99 ± 0.14 mm vs. TBI 1.25 ± 0.09 mm; $p > 0.05$) (Figure 2A,D).

3.1.3. Mediolateral Location of the Anterior Intracortical Electrode Tips

EEG cohort. Histological assessment revealed that the tip was lateral in 93% (53/57) of the cases and medial to the atlas-based coordinates (4 mm from midline) in 7% (4/57) of the cases (Figure 2B). The mean distance between the histological and MRI-guided ML coordinate was 0.58 ± 0.05 mm (range: 0–1.50 mm, median: 0.5 mm) (Figure 2D). The distance was comparable between sham-operated controls (0.68 ± 0.09 mm) and TBI (0.55 ± 0.06 mm) rats ($p > 0.05$) (Figure 2D).

MRI cohort. Histological assessment revealed that the tip was lateral to the MRI-based coordinates in 41% (17/42) of the cases and medial in 59% (25/42) of the cases (Figure 2B). The mean distance between the histological and MRI-guided ML coordinate was 0.44 ± 0.04 mm (range: 0–1.0 mm, median: 0.4 mm) (Figure 2D). The distance was comparable between the sham-operated controls (0.48 ± 0.09 mm) and TBI rats (0.42 ± 0.05 mm; $p > 0.05$) (Figure 2D).

3.1.4. Dorsoventral Location of the Anterior Intracortical Electrode Tips

Cortical layer V was set as the DV target for the lower tip of the bipolar intracerebral electrode in both cohorts.

EEG cohort. Histological analysis revealed that 83% (47/57) of the electrodes had at least one tip within the cerebral cortex. Of the 47 electrodes, 28% (16/57) were in layer V and 55% (31/57) were in layer VI. In the remaining 17% (10/57), the tip was identified in either the external capsule or the corpus callosum (Figure 2C). The DV distribution of the electrode tips was comparable between sham and TBI rats (χ^2 test; $p > 0.05$) (Supplementary Table S1).

MRI cohort. The DV location of the electrode tip was within the cortex in 76% (32/42) of rats, being in layer V in 31% (13/42) and layer VI in 45% (19/42) of the cases. In the remaining 24%, the tip was located in either the corpus callosum (7%, 3/42) or the external capsule (17%, 7/42) (Figure 2C). The DV distribution of the electrode tips was comparable between sham and TBI rats (χ^2 test; $p > 0.05$).

3.2. Success in Positioning the Posterior Intracortical Electrode

3.2.1. Electrode Locations—An Overview

EEG cohort. The electrode tip was within the cortex in 40% (21/53) of the rats. In the remaining 60% (31/53), it was either in the angular bundle, dorsal subiculum, or cortical lesion cavity (Figure 5 and Table 1). In four rats, the quality of the histological sections was not sufficient to determine the electrode location. The histological AP tip and ML electrode tip locations were within a 0.5-mm radius of the planned atlas coordinates in 19% (10/53) and 89% (47/53) of the rats, respectively (Figure 5A,B). The DV tip location was in the planned depth (layer V) in only 6% (3/53) of the rats. In the remaining 94% (50/53), it was either in layer VI, the angular bundle, dorsal subiculum, or cortical lesion cavity (Figure 5C).

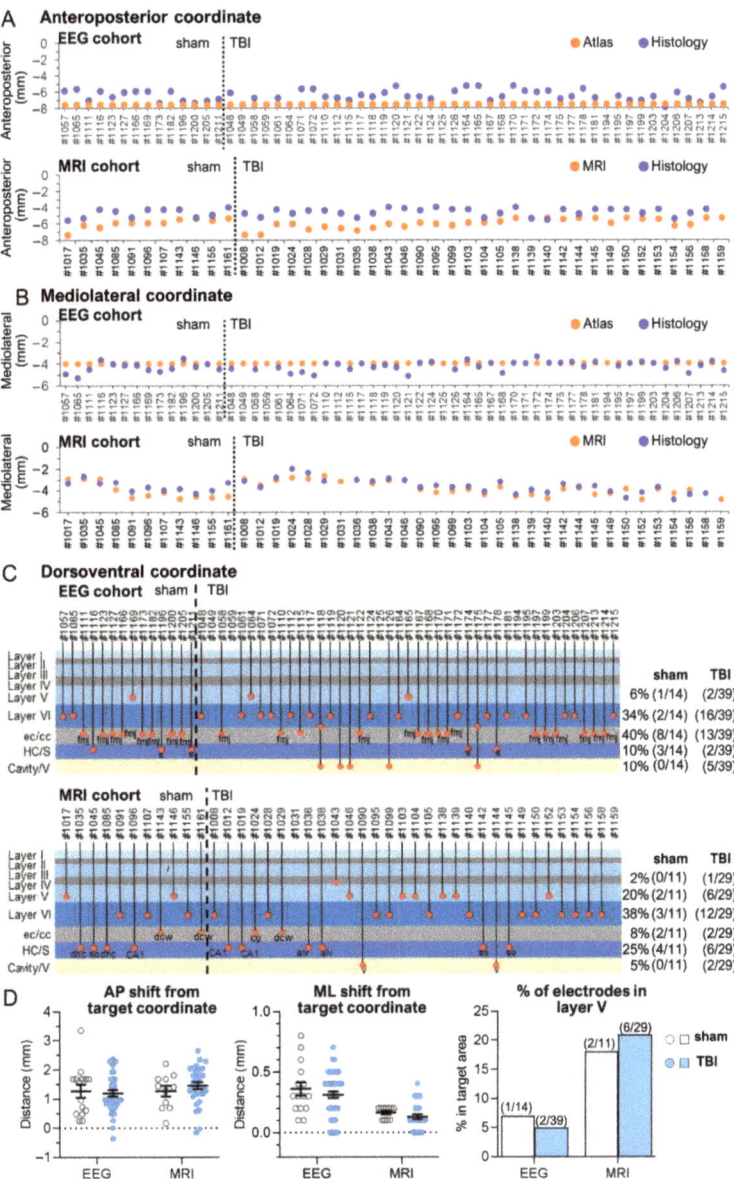

Figure 5. Posterior intracortical electrode—schematic representations of the atlas-based, histological, and MRI-guided coordinates in each rat of the EEG and MRI cohorts. (**A**) Anteroposterior (AP) coordinate. In the EEG cohort (*n* = 47, electrode operation right after injury), the fixed atlas-based target AP coordinate of −7.56 mm from the bregma was applied to implant the electrodes (orange dots). In the MRI cohort (*n* = 40, electrode operation at 5 months postinjury), the target AP coordinate was individually determined using the in vivo 5-month T2-weighted MR images. The target coordinate fluctuated depending on the TBI (traumatic brain injury)-induced lesion extent. Note a mild anterior shift (*y*-axis) in the histologically verified "true" AP coordinate (blue dots) relative to the target

coordinate (orange dots) in both cohorts. In general, the anterior shift was less than that in a case of the anterior intra-cortical electrode (compare to Figure 1). Animal numbers are shown on the x-axis. (**B**) Mediolateral (ML) coordinate. In the EEG cohort (n = 47), the fixed atlas-based ML coordinate at 4 mm lateral to midline was targeted. In the MRI cohort (n = 40), the target ML coordinate was individually determined using the 5-month MRI. Note almost a negligible deviation of the histologically verified "true" ML coordinate from the atlas-based (EEG cohort) or MRI-guided (MRI cohort) coordinates. (**C**) Dorsoventral (DV) coordinate. In both cohorts, the lower tip of the bipolar electrode was targeted to layer V in the selected AP and ML coordinates (see above). In the EEG cohort, 46% (18/39), and in the MRI cohort, 66% (19/29) of the electrode tips in injured animals were in the cortex. Importantly, even though the lower tip in the remaining cases went down into the external capsule or corpus callosum, the upper tip of the bipolar electrode, being 1 mm higher in the EEG and 0.5 mm in the MRI cohort, was still recording in the cortex in 79% (31/39) of the rats in the EEG cohort and in 72% (21/29) in the MRI cohort. In 5 rats (3 sham, 2 TBI) in the EEG cohort and 10 rats (4 sham, 6 TBI) in the MRI cohort, the electrode was recording hippocampal rather than cortical activity, which affected the interpretation of the EEG data. The percentages of electrode locations in the sham-operated and TBI animals are shown on the right side of the panel. (**D**) Dot plots of the AP and ML shift in the histological AP and ML coordinate, and % of electrode in the targeted layer V (number of cases in brackets). Note posterior shift of some TBI cases from the target (Y = 0). The y-axis represents distance from target coordinate (Y = 0) or % of cases in targeted area. Note that in 4 animals in the EEG cohort and 2 in the MRI cohort, the DV location of the electrode tip could not be reliably determined in histological sections. Abbreviations: cavity, cortical lesion cavity; cc, corpus callosum; cg, cingulum; dcw, deep cerebral white matter; ec, external capsule; fmj, forceps major corpus callosum; HC, hippocampus; S, subiculum; V, ventricle.

MRI cohort. The electrode tip was within the cortex in 60% (24/40) of the rats. In the remaining 40% (16/40), it was either in the external capsule, corpus callosum, dorsal subiculum, hippocampus, or ventricle. In two rats, the quality of the histological sections was not sufficient to determine the electrode location. The histological AP and ML electrode tip locations were within a 0.5 mm radius of the planned MRI coordinates in 8% (3/40) and 100% (40/40) of the rats, respectively (Figure 5A,B and Table 1). The DV tip location was in the planned depth (layer V) in only 20% (8/40) rats. In the remaining 80% (32/40), the tip was located in either layer IV or VI, the external capsule, corpus callosum, dorsal subiculum, hippocampus, or ventricle (Figure 5C).

3.2.2. Anteroposterior Location of the Posterior Intracortical Electrode Tips

Based on estimation of the progression of the cortical lesion, which tends to be more extensive caudally than rostrally [7,27,32], the posterior intracortical electrode was targeted to the atlas-based AP level −7.56 from the bregma (primary visual cortex, V1) to ensure proper EEG recording in the lesion vicinity during the 7th post-TBI month (Figure 1A).

EEG cohort. The unfolded cortical map indicated that all electrode tracks passed through the visual cortex. The electrode tips were in the visual cortex in only 40% (21/53) of the rats. In the remaining 60% (31/53), they were in the angular bundle, dorsal subiculum, or cortical lesion cavity (Figure 4A,B and Figure 5C). Typically, the tip location was anterior to the targeted atlas-based AP coordinate, the average deviation being 1.16 ± 0.09 mm (range: 0–2.28 mm, median: 0.96 mm) (Figure 5A,D). The rostral shift was comparable between the sham-operated controls and TBI rats (1.11 ± 0.17 mm vs. 1.18 ± 0.10 mm; $p > 0.05$) (V). The rostral shift of the posterior intracortical electrode was comparable to that of the anterior intracortical electrode ($p > 0.05$).

MRI cohort. As in the EEG cohort, histological analysis revealed that most of the posterior intracortical electrodes (60%, 24/40) were in the visual cortex. In the remaining 40% (16/40) of rats, the electrode track was in the visual cortex, but the tip penetrated either the deep cerebral white matter, cingulum, dorsal hippocampal commissure, hippocampus proper, or ventricle (Figure 4C,D and Figure 5C). In 95% (38/40) of the rats, the electrode tip was anterior to the targeted MRI-guided AP coordinate (Figure 5A,D and Figure 6A,B,D,E), the average deviation being 1.39 ± 0.09 mm (range: 1.28–2.64 mm, median: 1.42 mm). The rostral shift was comparable between the sham-operated controls and TBI rats (sham 1.26 ± 0.18 vs. TBI 1.45 ± 0.12; $p > 0.05$) (Figure 5D). The rostral shift of the posterior intracortical electrode was comparable to that of the anterior intracortical electrode ($p > 0.05$).

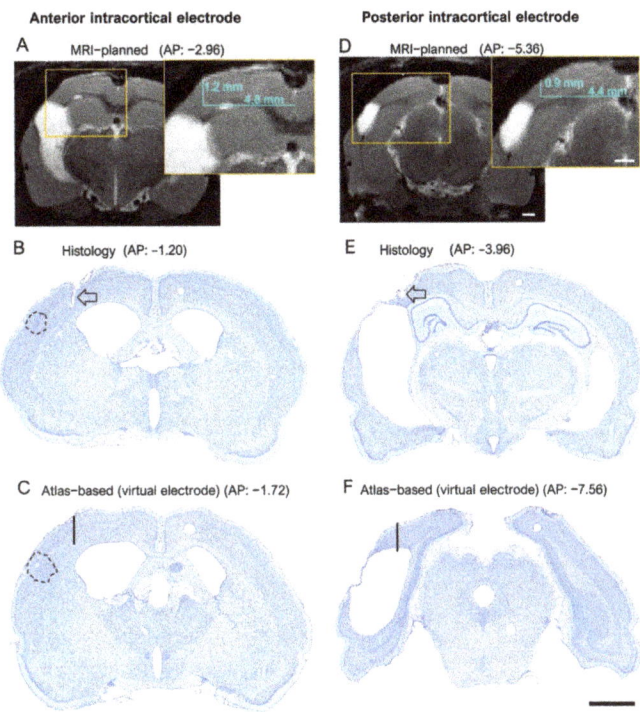

Figure 6. Histological confirmation of the success of MRI-guided electrode placement. Left panel (**A–C**): Anterior intracortical electrode MRI-planned coordinate, histological confirmation, and "virtual" electrode. Right panel: Posterior intracortical electrode MRI-panned coordinate histological confirmation, and "virtual" electrode. (**A**) T2-weighted MRI and (**B**) histological images showing the MRI-guided (insert) and histology-confirmed "true" location of the anterior intracortical electrode in rat 1139. The anteroposterior (AP) coordinate was estimated by aligning the magnetic resonance images with the rat brain atlas [25]. The mediolateral (ML) and dorsoventral (DV) coordinates (inserts in (**A,D**)) were determined using ImageJ software (version 1.47v, Wayne Rasband and contributors, National Institute of Health, USA). Note that in this case, the confirmed AP location was about 1.8 mm more rostral than the planned location (−1.20 mm vs. −2.96). Lesion area is denoted in black-dashed-line circle. (**C**) A "virtual" location of the electrode tip (black line) if the electrode had been implanted to the targeted atlas-based coordinate (−1.75 mm from bregma, 4 mm from midline, 1.8 mm from the surface of the brain). (**D**) MRI-guided (insert) AP, ML and DV coordinates and (**E**) histology-confirmed "true" location of the posterior intracortical electrode tip in rat 1139. The black-dashed-line circle denotes the lesion area. Note that the confirmed AP location was approximately 1.4 mm more rostral than the planned location (−3.96 vs. −5.36). Thus, even though both the anterior and posterior intracortical electrodes were more rostral than planned, their tips were recording EEG signals in the perilesional cortex. (**F**) A "virtual" electrode (black line) at the atlas-based coordinates would have ended up in the lesion cavity. Scale bar in (**A,D**) = 1 mm, and in (**B,C,E,F**) = 2 mm.

3.2.3. Mediolateral Location of the Posterior Intracortical Electrode Tips

EEG cohort. The histological ML tip coordinate was lateral to the targeted atlas-based coordinate in 62% (33/53), on target in 2% (1/83), and medial in 36% (19/53) of the rats (Figure 4B). The mean deviation from the atlas-based ML coordinate (0.38 ± 0.05 mm, range: 0–1.26 mm, median: 0.3 mm) was less than that of the anterior intracortical electrode (0.58 ± 0.05 mm, range: 0–1.50 mm; $p < 0.05$) (Figure 5D). The average deviation was comparable between sham-operated controls (0.45 ± 0.09 mm) and TBI rats (0.35 ± 0.05 mm; $p > 0.05$) (Figure 5D).

MRI cohort. The histological ML tip coordinate was lateral to the MRI-guided coordinate in 25% (10/40) and medial in 75% (30/40) of the rats (Figure 4B). The mean distance between the histological ML and MRI-guided coordinate was 0.45 ± 0.04 mm (range: 0.03–1.29 mm, median: 0.4 mm). The deviation was comparable between sham-operated controls (0.62 ± 0.09 mm) and TBI rats (0.39 ± 0.04 mm; $p > 0.05$) (Figure 5D). Also, the deviation from the MRI-based ML did not differ from that of the anterior intracortical electrode (0.44 ± 0.04 mm; $p > 0.05$) (Figure 5D).

3.2.4. Dorsoventral Location of the Posterior Intracortical Electrode Tips

EEG cohort. The histologically verified DV location of the lower tip of the posterior intracortical electrode was more diverse compared with the anterior electrode, with only 40% (21/52) within the cortical layers (6% in layer V, 34% in layer VI) (Figure 5C and Table 1). Moreover, 40% (21/52) of the tips had traveled down to the angular bundle, 10% (5/53) to the dorsal subiculum, and 10% (5/52) to the underlying cortical lesion cavity (Figure 5C).

Further analysis indicated that the laminar location of the electrode tips differed between the posterior and anterior electrodes (χ^2 test; $p < 0.001$). The overall percentage of posterior electrode tips in the cortex was less than that of the anterior electrode (40% vs. 83%; $p < 0.001$) (Table 1). Also, fewer posterior electrode tips were located in the targeted layer V compared with anterior cortical electrode tips (9% vs. 28%; $p < 0.01$) (Figure 5C, Supplementary Table S1). Surprisingly, the overall percentage of posterior cortical electrodes in the cortex was comparable between sham (46%; 5/11) and TBI rats (67%, 19/29; $p > 0.05$). Also, there was no difference in the overall DV distribution of the locations of the posterior intracortical electrode tips between sham and TBI rats (χ^2 test; $p > 0.05$) (Supplementary Table S1).

MRI cohort. Altogether, 60% (24/40) of the posterior intracortical electrodes had the lower tip within the cortex, of which 2% (1/40) were in layer IV, 20% (8/40) in layer V, and 38% (15/40) in layer VI (Figure 5C and Table 1). The tip had reached the external capsule or cingulum in 8% (4/40), the angular bundle or hippocampus proper in 27% (11/40), and the ventricle in 5% (2/40). Unlike in the EEG cohort, none of the electrode tips appeared to enter the lesion cavity (Figure 5C). The overall DV tip distributions did not differ between sham-operated controls and TBI rats (χ^2 test; $p > 0.05$) (Supplementary Table S1).

The overall percentage of tips in the cortex was comparable between the anterior and posterior cortical electrodes (76% vs. 60%, χ^2 test; $p > 0.05$), and between sham and TBI rats (46% vs. 66%, χ^2 test; $p > 0.05$) (Table 1). Like in the EEG cohort, however, the overall DV distribution of the electrode tips differed between the anterior and posterior intracortical electrodes (χ^2 test; $p < 0.01$). Particularly, the percentage of electrodes entering into the septal hippocampus was greater in the TBI rats than in the sham group (27% vs. 0%, χ^2 test; $p < 0.001$).

3.3. Success in Positioning the Intrahippocampal Electrode

3.3.1. Electrode Locations—An Overview

The lower tip of the hippocampal electrode was targeted to the hilus of the septal end of the dentate gyrus (AP: −3.0; ML: −1.4; DV: 3.6) in both the EEG and MRI cohorts.

EEG cohort. The electrode tip was in the hippocampus or dentate gyrus in 82% (47/57) of the rats (Table 1). In the remaining 18% (10/57), the tip was located in either the fimbria, ventricle, dorsal thalamus, or out of the hippocampus (unidentified tip location) (Figure 7). The histologically verified AP and ML electrode tip locations were within 0.5 mm of the planned atlas coordinates in 65% (37/57) and 100% (56/56) of rats, respectively (Figure 7A,B). In one rat, the quality of the histological sections was not sufficient to determine the electrode location. The DV tip location was in the dentate gyrus in 54% (31/57) of rats. In the remaining 46% (26/57), the tip was located in either the CA1 or CA3 subfield of the hippocampus proper, fimbria, ventricle, or dorsal thalamus (Figure 7C).

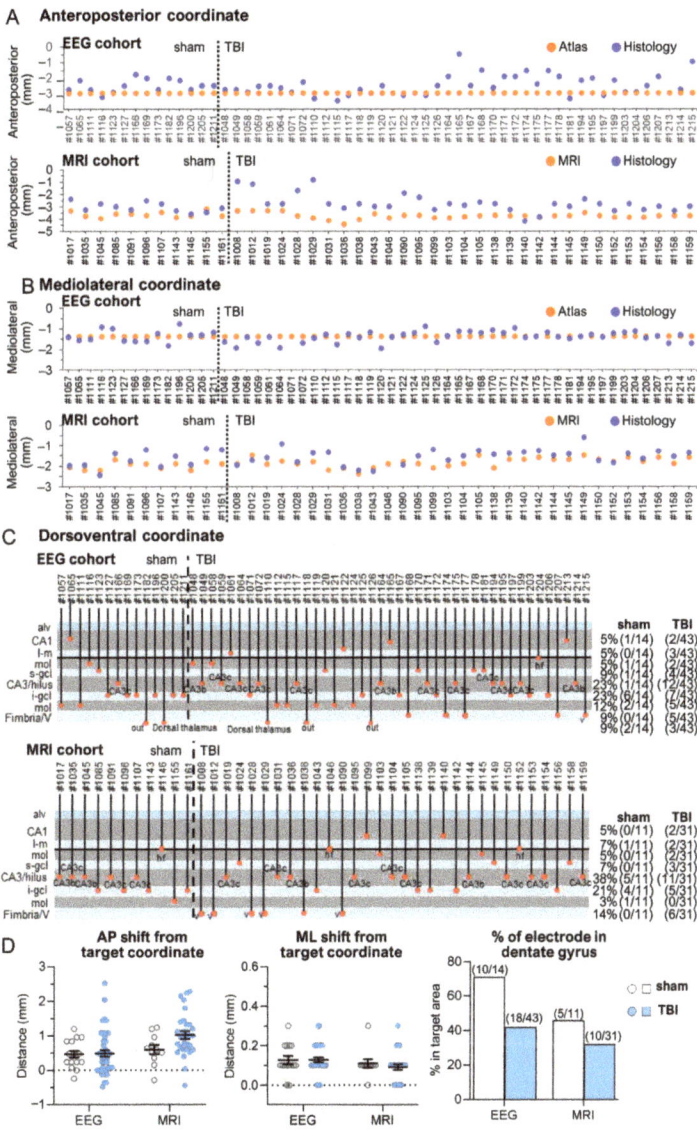

Figure 7. Hippocampal electrode—schematic representations of the atlas-based, histological, and

MRI-guided coordinates in each rat of the EEG and MRI cohorts. (**A**) Anteroposterior (AP) coordinate. In the EEG cohort (electrode operation right after injury), the fixed atlas-based target AP coordinate of −3 mm from the bregma was applied to implant the electrodes (orange dots). In the MRI cohort (electrode operation 5 months after injury), the target AP coordinate was individually determined using the 5-month in vivo T2-weighted MR images. The target coordinate fluctuated, depending on the TBI-induced hippocampal structural abnormality. Note the anterior shift (y-axis) in the histologically verified "true" AP coordinate (blue dots) relative to the aimed target coordinate (orange dots) in both cohorts. Note the great variability in the anterior shift from animal to animal, particularly in the MRI cohort. Animal numbers are shown on the x-axis. (**B**) Mediolateral (ML) coordinate. In the EEG cohort, the fixed atlas-based target ML coordinate at 1.4 mm lateral to midline was targeted. In the MRI cohort, the target ML coordinate was individually determined using the 5-month MRI. Note only a very small deviation of the histologically defined "true" ML coordinate from the atlas-based (EEG cohort) or MRI-guided (MRI cohort) coordinates. (**C**) Dorsoventral (DV) coordinate. In both cohorts, the lower tip of the bipolar electrode was aimed at the hilus in the selected AP and ML coordinates (see above). In the EEG cohort, most of the tips were recording in the hippocampus proper or the dentate gyrus. In the EEG cohort, in only 19% (8/43) of TBI cases, the tip was either in fimbria, ventricle, or went through the septal hippocampus to the dorsal thalamus or to an unidentified location. In the MRI cohort, in only 14% (6/31) of TBI cases, the tip was outside the hippocampus or the dentate gyrus. The percentages of electrode locations in the sham-operated and TBI animals are shown on the right side of the panel. (**D**) Dot plots of the AP and ML shift in the histological AP and ML coordinate, and % of electrodes in the targeted dentate gyrus (number of cases in brackets). Note posterior shift of some cases from the target (vertical dashed line). The y-axis represents distance from target coordinate (Y = 0) or % of cases in targeted area. Abbreviations: alv, alveus; CA1, CA1 subfield of the hippocampus; CA3, CA3 (CA3b, CA3c) subfield of the hippocampus; gcl, granule cell layer (s-gcl, suprapyramidal blade, i-gcl, infrapyramidal blade); hf, hippocampal fissure; l-m, stratum lacunosum moleculare of CA1; mol, molecular layer of the dentate gyrus; V, ventricle.

MRI cohort. The electrode tip was in the hippocampus proper or dentate gyrus in 86% (36/42) of rats (Table 1). In the remaining 14% (6/42), the tip was located in either the ventricle or fimbria (Figure 7). The histologically verified AP and ML electrode tip locations were within 0.5 mm of the planned atlas coordinates of the MRI-guided location in 14% (6/43) and 100% (42/42) of rats, respectively (Figure 7A,B). The electrode tip was in the planned DV coordinate in 38% (16/42) of the rats. In the remaining 62% (26/42), the tip was located in either the hippocampal CA1 or CA3 subfields, hippocampal fissure, fimbria, or ventricle (Figure 7C).

3.3.2. Anteroposterior Location of Hippocampal Electrode Tips

EEG cohort. Only 9% (5/57) of the electrode tips were in the planned atlas-based coordinate (AP: 3.0 mm). The remaining 77% (44/57) were positioned rostrally and 14% (8/57) were positioned caudally (Figure 7A). The mean deviation of the histologically verified coordinate from the atlas-based coordinate was 0.57 ± 0.07 mm (range: 0–2.52 mm, median: 0.48 mm). The deviation was comparable between sham-operated controls and TBI rats (0.54 ± 0.09 mm vs. 0.58 ± 0.09 mm; $p > 0.05$) (Figure 7D).

MRI cohort. The AP distribution of MRI-guided hippocampal electrode tip placements was anterior in 93% (39/42) and posterior in 7% (2/42) of the cases (Figure 7A). The average deviation of the histologically verified coordinate from the MRI-guided coordinate was 0.95 ± 0.08 mm (range: 0.04–2.28, median: 0.84) (Figure 7D). The deviation was comparable between sham-operated controls and TBI rats (0.66 ± 0.11 mm vs. 1.06 ± 0.10 mm; $p > 0.05$) (Figure 7D).

3.3.3. Mediolateral Location of Hippocampal Electrode Tips

EEG cohort. The hippocampal electrode was located anterior to the atlas-defined target in 48% (27/56), medial in 50% (28/56), and on target in 2% (1/56) of the rats (Figure 5B). The mean deviation of the histologically defined coordinate from the atlas-defined coordinate was 0.21 ± 0.02 mm (range: 0–0.63 mm, median: 0.2 mm) (Figure 7D). The deviation was comparable between sham-operated controls and TBI rats (0.24 ± 0.04 mm vs. 0.19 ± 0.03 mm; $p > 0.05$) (Figure 7D).

MRI cohort. The histologically defined tip coordinate was lateral to the MRI-guided coordinate in 17% (7/42) and medial in 83% (34/42) of the rats. The average deviation of the histologically defined coordinate from the MRI-guided coordinate was 0.34 ± 0.04 mm (range: 0–0.9 mm, median: 0.3 mm) (Figure 7D). The deviation was comparable between sham-operated controls and TBI rats (0.35 ± 0.07 mm vs. 0.34 ± 0.05 mm; $p > 0.05$) (Figure 7D).

3.3.4. Dorsoventral Location of Hippocampal Electrode Tips

EEG cohort. Histology revealed electrode path-associated lesions (see details in Section 3.4.2). In some TBI rats, the electrode path appeared slanted rather than vertical, probably due to hippocampal distortion related to enlarged ventricles.

The electrode tip was in the dentate gyrus in 49% (28/57) of the rats, locating in the molecular layer of the dentate gyrus in 17% (10/57) and in the granule cell layer in 32% (18/57) of the cases. No tips were observed in the hilus (Figure 7C). In the remaining rats, the tip was located in the hippocampus proper in 33% (5% [3/57] in the stratum lacunosum moleculare or hippocampal fissure, 5% [3/57] in CA1, 23% [13/57] in CA3), most of the tips in the CA3 subfield being in the CA3c subfield (Figure 5C). In 9% (5/57) of the cases, the tip was in the fimbria or ventricle. In 9% (5/57), the electrode went through the septal hippocampus and ended in the dorsal thalamus ($n = 2$) or in an unidentified location ($n = 3$) (see details in Section 3.4.2). The DV distribution of the electrode tips was comparable between sham-operated controls and TBI rats (χ^2 test; $p > 0.05$).

MRI cohort. Unlike in the EEG cohort, electrode path-associated lesions were small. Also, the electrode paths were vertical rather than slanted.

The electrode tip was in the targeted dentate gyrus in 36% (15/42) of animals, being 8% (3/42) in the molecular layer and 28% (12/42) in the granule cell layer (Figure 7C). No electrode tips were observed in the hilus. In 50% of the rats, the tip was in the hippocampus proper (7% [3/42] in the stratum lacunosum moleculare or hippocampal fissure, 5% [2/42] in CA1, and 38% [16/42] in CA3). Like in the EEG cohort, most of the tips in the CA3 were in the CA3c subfield (Figure 7C). In the remaining 14% (6/42), the tip was located in either the fimbria ($n = 1$) or the ventricle ($n = 5$) (Figure 7C). The DV distribution of tip locations was comparable between sham-operated controls and TBI rats (χ^2 test; $p = 0.741$).

3.4. Cortical and Hippocampal Atrophy after TBI

3.4.1. Cortical Atrophy

Anteroposterior. In sham-operated controls, there was no difference in the cortical AP length at 4 mm lateral to the midline between the ipsilateral (13.89 ± 0.19 mm, range: 12.48–0.56 mm, median: 14.1 mm) and contralateral hemispheres (13.70 ± 0.09 mm, range: 13.12–14.24 mm, median: 13.6 mm; $p > 0.05$) (Figure 8A1,B,C).

In TBI rats, the cortical AP length was shorter ipsilaterally (12.37 ± 0.16 mm, range: 10.08–13.76 mm, median: 12.23 mm) than contralaterally (13.13 ± 0.17, range: 11.04–14.72 mm, median: 13.12 mm; $p < 0.001$) (Figure 8A2–A4,B). Both the ipsilateral ($p < 0.001$) and contralateral ($p > 0.05$) AP lengths were shorter in the TBI rats than in the sham group (Figure 8B,C).

Mediolateral. In sham-operated controls, the ML length was similar ipsilaterally (5.62 ± 0.06 mm, range: 5.28–6.08 mm, median: 5.6 mm) and contralaterally (5.51 ± 0.06 mm, range: 5.12–5.76 mm, median: 5.6 mm; $p > 0.05$).

In the TBI group, the ML length was shorter ipsilaterally (5.03 ± 0.03 mm, range: 4.64–5.44, median: 4.96 mm) than contralaterally (5.27 ± 0.04 mm, range: 4.80–5.92 mm, median: 5.28 mm; $p < 0.001$). Both the ipsilateral ($p < 0.001$) and contralateral ($p < 0.05$) ML lengths were shorter in the TBI rats than in the sham group (Figure 8D).

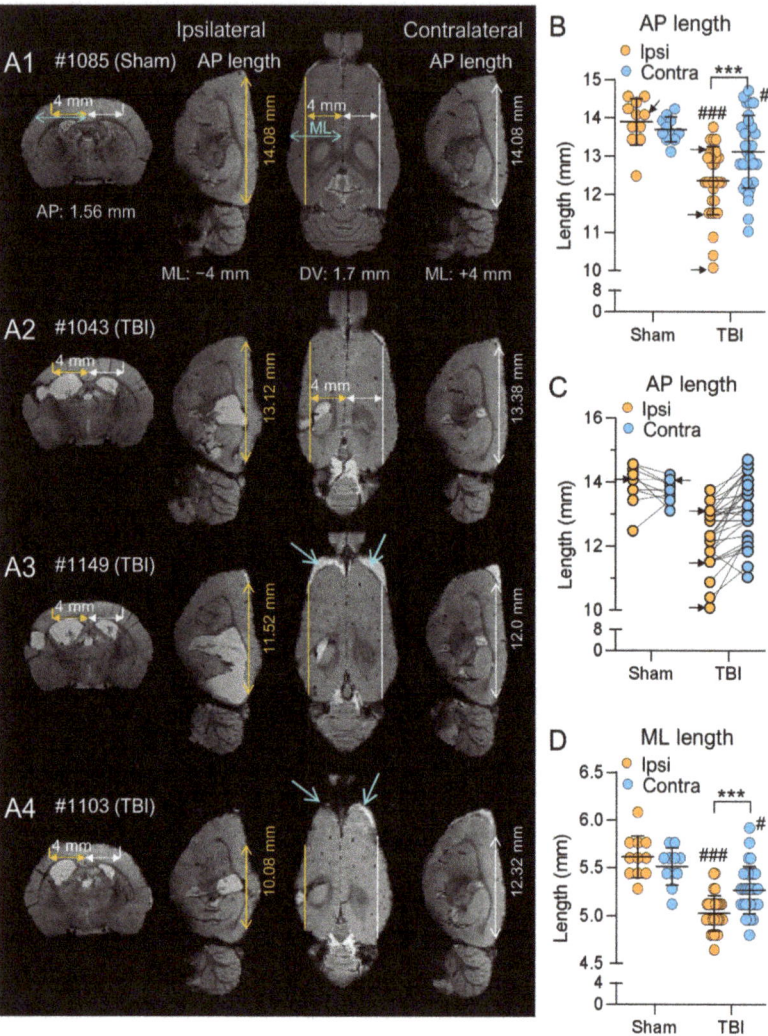

Figure 8. Anteroposterior and mediolateral shrinkage of the brain. In vivo magnetic resonance 3D multigradient echo (MGRE) images acquired at 5 months after TBI were used to estimate cortical shrinkage in the MRI cohort. (**A1–A4**) coronal, sagittal (ipsilateral and contralateral) and horizontal MGRE images of a sham rat (**A1**) and TBI rats (**A2–A4**). Anteroposterior (AP) cortical shrinkage was estimated by measuring the distance between the rostral and caudal cortical surface (double-headed arrows) in the sagittal slice at 4 mm from the midline both ipsilaterally (orange) and contralaterally (white). Note the change in the shape of the ipsilateral cortex (sagittal images) in TBI rats, indicating the TBI-induced cortical atrophy (see also turquoise arrows in (**A3,A4**)). Mediolateral (ML) shrinkage was assessed by measuring the distance between the midline and the lateral edge of the cortex (turquoise double headed arrow) in a horizontal slice at 1.7 mm below the pial surface at AP level −1.56 (corresponding to the targeted location of the anterior intracortical electrode tip). (**B**) A dot plot showing the ipsilateral (orange) and contralateral (blue) cortical AP lengths (*y*-axis) in the sham and TBI groups (*x*-axis). Note that both the ipsilateral and contralateral cortical AP lengths were reduced

in TBI rats compared with sham-operated animals. Also, in the TBI group, the cortical AP length was shorter ipsilaterally than contralaterally. (**C**) A paired dot plot showing that the ipsilateral vs. contralateral shrinkage in each rat. The greater the ipsilateral shrinkage, the greater the contralateral shrinkage in the TBI compared with sham group. Arrows point to the 3 cases illustrated in panels (**A1–A4**). (**D**) A dot plot showing the ipsilateral and contralateral cortical ML lengths in sham-operated and TBI rats. Note that both the ipsilateral and contralateral cortical ML lengths were reduced in TBI rats compared with sham-operated animals. Also, in the TBI group, the cortical ML length was shorter ipsilaterally than contralaterally. Statistical significance: *** $p < 0.001$ compared with the contralateral hemisphere (Wilcoxon signed-rank test); ### $p < 0.001$, # $p < 0.05$ compared with the sham group (Mann–Whitney U test).

3.4.2. Hippocampal Atrophy

Anteroposterior. In the sham group, the average AP length was similar ipsilaterally (7.40 ± 0.12 mm, range: 6.88–8.0 mm, median: 7.36 mm) and contralaterally (7.36 ± 0.09 mm, range: 7.04–8.0 mm, median: 7.36 mm; $p > 0.05$) (Figure 9D1,E,F).

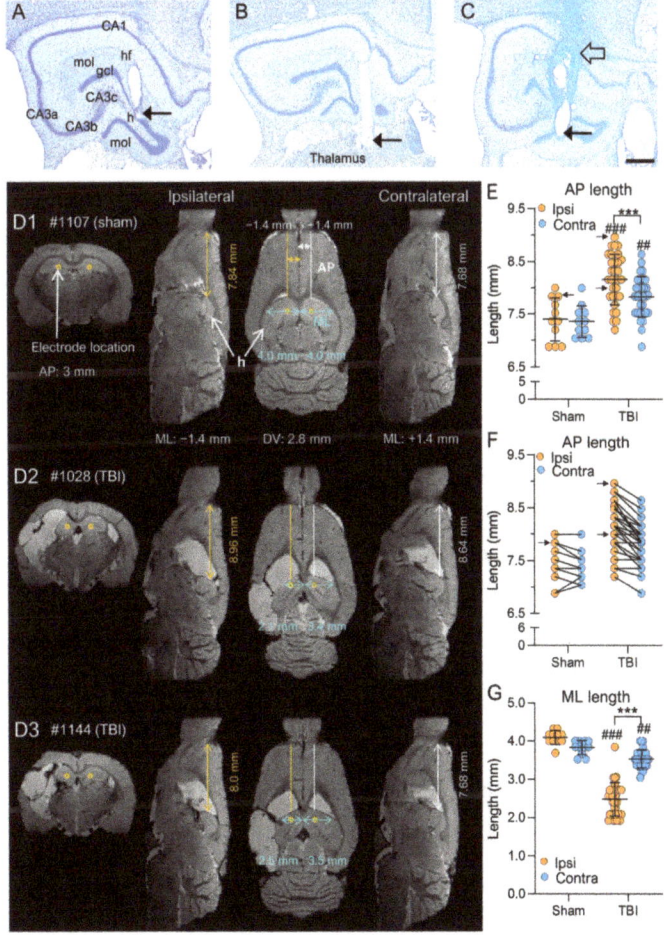

Figure 9. (**A–C**) Electrode tracts. Histological images from the coronal thionine-stained sections of 3 rats,

showing the tracts of the bipolar intracortical electrodes and locations of the lower electrode tip (filled arrowhead). The target of the lower tip was the hilus. In panel (**A**), the electrode tip is in the suprapyramidal blade of the granule cell layer. In panel (**B**), the tip went through the dentate gyrus down to the dorsal thalamus. In panel (**C**), the tip is in the infrapyramidal blade of the granule cell layer. Note the electrode-path associated lesion in CA1 (open arrow). (**D1–D3**) Coronal, sagittal and horizontal in vivo magnetic resonance 3D multigradient echo (MGRE) images of the ipsilateral and contralateral hippocampus were used to assess hippocampal shrinkage after traumatic brain injury (TBI). (**D1–D3**) Hippocampal distortion and shrinkage. Panel (**D1**): A sham-operated experimental control (1107). Panels (**D2,D3**): Two rats with TBI (1028, 1144). The anteroposterior (AP) shift of the hippocampus was assessed by measuring the distance from the rostral edge of the frontal cortex to the rostral edge of the hippocampus at 1.4 mm from the midline in the horizontal slice 2.8 mm below the surface of the brain (left hemisphere: orange double-headed arrow; right hemisphere: white double-headed arrow). Mediolateral (ML) shrinkage was assessed by measuring the distance from the brain midline to the lateral edge of the hippocampus in the same horizontal plane (2.8 mm below the surface of the brain, turquoise double-headed arrow) in a slice sampled at AP level −2.8 mm, corresponding to the AP level of the atlas-based target coordinate. In both TBI rats (**D2,D3**), the distance from the frontal pole to the rostral edge of the hippocampus was longer than that in the sham-operated animal, indicating retraction of the septal hippocampus caudally. The ML length in TBI rats (**D2,D3**) was shorter than that in the sham-operated animal (**D1**), indicating a shift toward midline. (**E**) A dot plot showing the ipsilateral (orange) and contralateral (blue) anteroposterior lengths (y-axis) in the sham and TBI groups (x-axis). Note that both the ipsilateral and contralateral cortical AP lengths were increased in TBI rats compared with sham-operated animals. Also, in the TBI group, the cortical AP length was greater ipsilaterally than contralaterally. (**F**) A paired dot plot showing the ipsilateral vs. contralateral backward "movement" in each rat. The greater the ipsilateral "movement", the greater the contralateral "movement". Arrows point to the 3 cases illustrated in panels (**D1–D3**). (**G**) A dot plot showing the ipsilateral and contralateral hippocampal ML lengths in sham-operated and TBI rats. Note that both the ipsilateral and contralateral cortical ML lengths were reduced in TBI rats compared with sham-operated animals. Also, in the TBI group, the ML length was shorter ipsilaterally than contralaterally. Statistical significance: ##, $p < 0.05$; ###, $p < 0.001$ as compared to the sham group (Mann–Whitney U test); *** $p < 0.001$ compared with the contralateral hemisphere (Wilcoxon signed-rank test). Scale bar in (**A–C**) = 500 µm.

In the TBI group, the AP length was greater ipsilaterally (8.16 ± 0.09 mm, range: 7.2–8.96 mm, median: 8.16 mm) than contralaterally (7.83 ± 0.07 mm, range: 6.88–8.64 mm, median: 7.84 mm; $p < 0.001$) (Figure 9D2,D3,E,F). Both the ipsilateral ($p < 0.001$) and contralateral ($p < 0.01$) AP lengths were greater in the TBI rats than in the sham group.

Mediolateral. In the sham group, the ML length was comparable ipsilaterally (4.09 ± 0.05 mm, range: 3.68–4.32 mm, median: 4.16 mm) and contralaterally (3.83 ± 0.06 mm, range: 3.52–4.0 mm, median: 3.84 mm; $p > 0.05$) (Figure 9D1,G).

In the TBI group, the ML length was shorter ipsilaterally (2.48 ± 0.08 mm, range: 1.92–3.84 mm, median: 2.4 mm) than contralaterally (3.53 ± 0.04 mm, range: 3.04–4.0 mm, median: 3.52 mm; $p < 0.001$) (Figures 7G and 9D2,D3). Both ipsilateral ($p < 0.001$) and contralateral ($p < 0.01$) ML lengths were shorter in the TBI rats than in the sham group (Figure 9).

3.5. "Virtual Electrode"—Comparison of Success Rate in Atlas-Based vs. MRI-Guided Electrode Placements

Finally, to assess whether the MRI images indeed improved the targeting of the electrode tip to the perilesional cortex, and not, for example, to the lesion cavity, we reexamined the histological sections of TBI rats in the MRI cohort. We focused on the caudal aspect of the brain, as targeting this area without the use of MRI was challenging due to remarkable TBI-related cortical atrophy.

A hypothetical "virtual" electrode was placed at the atlas-defined coordinate of the posterior intracortical electrode (Figure 10). We then reconstructed the destination of the electrode tip in the available histological sections by assessing (a) whether it was located in the cortex or lesion cavity and (b) the distance of the tip from the lesion edge. We found that by using the atlas-based coordinate (AP −7.56), 58% (18/31) of the electrodes had been in the lesion cavity compared with 0% for the MRI-guided implantations (Figures 5C and 10 and Table 2). The remaining 42% (13/31) of the "virtual" electrodes were located medial to the lesion cavity, except in one case (rat 1103), in which the tip location was caudal to the lesion. The average distance of the electrode tip to the lesion edge was 0.64 ± 0.1 mm (range: 0–1.3 mm) (see also Supplementary Table S2 for further details).

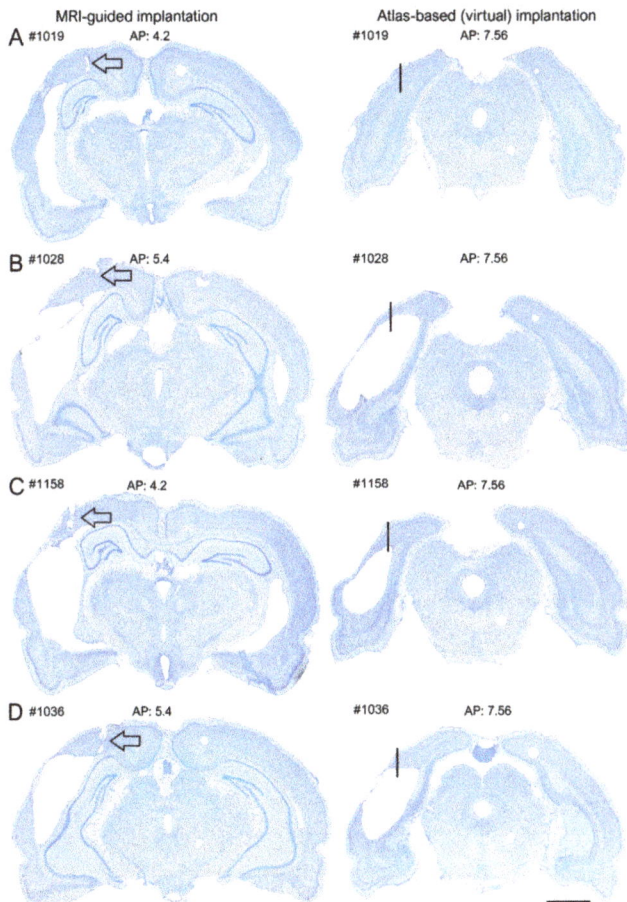

Figure 10. Location of electrode tip at 5 months postinjury without prior MRI analysis. Photomicrographs of thionine-stained coronal brain sections of 4 animals; (**A**) #1019, (**B**) #1139, (**C**) #1158 and (**D**) #1036 in the MRI cohort with electrode implantations at 5 months after TBI. Left panels: MRI-guided placement of the posterior cortical electrode. Note that all electrodes are within the perilesional cortex. Right panels: The location of the electrode tip (arrow), if the electrode was implanted according to the targeted atlas-based coordinates (−7.56 mm from bregma, 4 mm from midline, 1.8 mm from the surface of the brain). Note that in all rats except 1019, the electrode tip ended in the lesion cavity. Table 2 summarizes the locations for all cases. Scale bar = 2 mm.

Table 2. Location of the "virtual electrode". Summary of the locations of the posterior intracortical electrodes in the MRI cohort, if implanted according to the atlas-based coordinates. Note that 58% (18/31) of the lower electrode tips were in the cortex while 42% (13/31) of the lower tips were in the lesion cavity. After MRI-guidance, 71% (22/31) of the lower tips were recording in the cortex. In 5 additional cases, the upper tip (0.5 dorsal to the lower tip) was expected to record in the cortex, resulting in a total of 87% (27/31) of the electrodes recording in the cortex. Only 1 electrode was not recording in the brain.

	Atlas-Based		MRI-Guided	
Animal	AP Level	DV Location (Distance from Lesion Edge)	AP Level	DV Location
1008	7.56	Lesion cavity	−4.68	Layer VI
1012	7.56	Lesion cavity	−5.20	CA1
1019	7.56	Perilesional cortex (medial, 0 mm)	−4.20	Layer V
1024	7.56	Lesion cavity	−4.68	angular bundle
1028	7.56	Lesion cavity	−4.36	Layer VI
1029	7.56	Lesion cavity	−4.36	corpus callosum
1031	7.56	Lesion cavity		not found
1036	7.56	Lesion cavity	−5.28	Layer VI
1038	7.56	Perilesional cortex (medial, 0.7 mm)	−4.68	alveus of the hippocampus
1043	7.56	Lesion cavity	−3.96	Layer IV
1046	7.56	Lesion cavity	−4.08	Layer V
1090	7.56	Perilesional cortex (medial, 0.53 mm)	−4.36	Layer VI
1095	7.56	Perilesional cortex (medial, 0.32 mm)	−3.96	Layer VI
1099	7.56	Perilesional cortex (medial, 0.93 mm)	−4.20	Layer VI
1103	7.56	Perilesional cortex (caudal, 0.2 mm)	−4.20	Layer V
1104	7.56	Perilesional cortex (medial, 0.73 mm)	−5.28	Layer V
1105	7.56	Lesion cavity	−4.68	Layer VI
1138	7.56	Perilesional cortex (medial, 0.71 mm)	−3.96	Layer V
1139	7.56	Lesion cavity	−5.40	Layer V
1140	7.56	Perilesional cortex (medial, 1.1 mm)	−5.52	Layer VI
1142	7.56	Lesion cavity	−4.20	corpus callosum
1144	7.56	Lesion cavity	−4.80	ventricle
1145	7.56	Perilesional cortex (medial, 0.63 mm)	−4.20	CA1
1149	7.56	Lesion cavity	−4.20	Layer VI
1150	7.56	Lesion cavity	−4.20	Layer VI
1152	7.56	Perilesional cortex (medial, 0.91 mm)	−4.68	Layer V
1153	7.56	Lesion cavity	−4.20	Layer VI
1154	7.56	Lesion cavity	−5.40	Layer VI
1156	7.56	Perilesional cortex (medial, 0.28 mm)	−4.68	Layer VI
1158	7.56	Lesion cavity	−4.20	Layer VI
1159	7.56	Perilesional cortex (medial, 1.3 mm)		not found

4. Effect of Electrode Implantation on Progression of the Cortical Lesion

Next, we assessed whether a 6-month-long presence of intracortical electrodes enhanced cortical atrophy. We hypothesized that (1) the lesion area would be greater in the EEG cohort than in the MRI cohort and (2) the cortical electrode tips would be closer to the lesion cavity (expected distance $\geq$ 500 µm) in the EEG cohort than in the MRI cohort.

Lesion area and location. The cortical lesion spread laterally and caudally, typically involving the sensory, auditory, and visual cortices, as previously described [32] (Figure 11A). The average total lesion area was comparable between the EEG (27.31 $\pm$ 2.29 mm^2, range: 1.72–93.8 mm^2, median: 25.8 mm^2) and MRI (25.69 $\pm$ 2.32 mm^2, range: 5.7–47.6 mm^2, median: 26.1 mm^2) cohorts ($p > 0.05$) (Figure 11B). Also, the mean lesion area in the primary somatosensory (4.89 $\pm$ 0.41 mm^2 vs. 5.16 $\pm$ 0.55 mm^2; $p > 0.05$) and visual cortex (7.73 $\pm$ 0.72 mm^2 vs. 7.37 $\pm$ 0.51 mm^2; $p > 0.05$) was similar in the EEG and MRI cohorts (Table 3). In the secondary somatosensory cortex (S2) (0.56 $\pm$ 0.07 mm^2 vs. 1.07 $\pm$0.17 mm^2; $p < 0.01$)

and the primary auditory cortex (Au1) (3.77 ± 0.20 mm^2 vs. 4.32 ± 0.30 mm^2; $p < 0.05$) the lesion area was smaller in the EEG cohort than in the MRI cohort (Table 3).

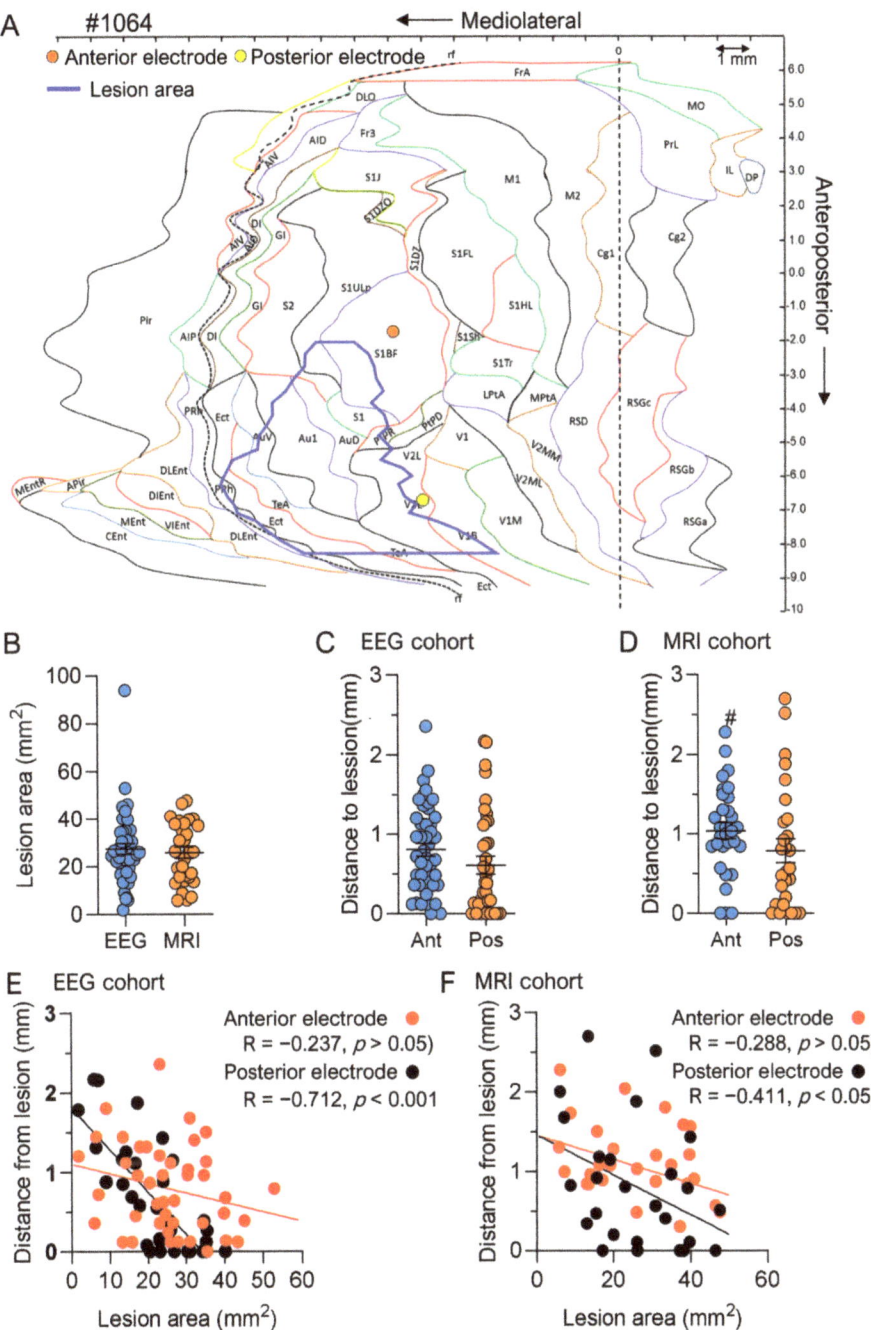

Figure 11. Distance of the intracortical electrodes from the edge of the cortical lesion cavity. (**A**) An

unfolded cortical map of a rat 1064, showing the cytoarchitectonic distribution of the cortical lesion (blue outline) and the location of the anterior (brown filled circle in the S1BF) and posterior (yellow filled circle in the V2L) intracortical electrodes. Note that the lesion had progressed laterally and caudally. Consequently, the posterior electrode was closer to the lesion cavity edge than the anterior electrode. (**B**) A scatter plot showing the cortical lesion area in the EEG and MRI cohorts (each dot represents 1 rat). The lesion area was comparable between cohorts ($p > 0.05$). (**C**) In the EEG cohort, the distance from the electrode tip to the lesion cavity edge (layer V intersection was used as reference) was similar between the anterior and posterior intracortical electrodes ($p > 0.05$). (**D**) In the MRI cohort, the distance from the anterior intracortical electrode tip to the cavity edge was slightly greater than that from the EEG cohort ($p < 0.05$). (**E**) In the EEG cohort, the larger the lesion, the closer the posterior electrode tip to the lesion cavity edge ($p < 0.001$). (**F**) In the MRI cohort, the larger the lesion, the closer the posterior electrode tip to the cavity edge ($p < 0.001$). Abbreviations: S1BF, primary somatosensory barrel field; V2L, secondary visual cortex lateral area. Statistical significance: #, $p < 0.05$ compared with the EEG cohort (Mann–Whitney U test).

Electrode distance from the lesion cavity. In the EEG cohort, 54% of the anterior intracortical electrodes were located anterior to the rostral edge of the lesion and 46% were located medial to the lesion. The average distance to the lesion edge was 0.79 ± 0.08 mm (range: 0–2.36 mm, median: 0.71 mm) (Figure 11C). All posterior intracortical electrodes were located medial to the lesion; 33%, however, were observed on the edge of the lesion or in the lesion cavity. The mean distance to the lesion edge was 0.63 ± 0.11 mm (range: 0–2.17 mm, median: 0.38 mm), comparable to that of the anterior intracortical electrode ($p > 0.05$).

In the MRI cohort, 41% of the anterior intracortical electrodes were located anterior to the rostral edge of the lesion and 59% were located medial to the lesion. The distance to the lesion edge was greater in the MRI (1.038 ± 0.10 mm, range: 0–2.3 mm, median: 1.03 mm) than in the EEG cohort ($p < 0.05$). All posterior intracortical electrodes (100%) were located medial to the lesion. Unlike in the EEG cohort, none of the tips was at the lesion edge or in the cavity. The distance of the posterior electrode tip to the lesion edge (0.79 ± 0.15 mm, range: 0–2.7 mm, median: 0.54 mm) was comparable to that of the anterior intracortical electrode ($p > 0.05$) (Figure 11D) or the posterior intracortical electrode in the EEG cohort ($p > 0.05$).

In both cohorts, we were unable to verify the hypothesis that the greater the lesion, the closer the tip of the anterior intracortical electrode to the lesion edge as there was no correlation between lesion size and the distance of the anterior intracortical electrode from the lesion edge (EEG cohort: $R = -0.237$; $p > 0.05$; MRI cohort: $R = -0.288$; $p > 0.05$) (Figure 9E,F). In the case of posterior cortical electrodes, however, the larger the lesion, the closer the tip to the lesion edge (EEG cohort: $R = -0.712$; $p < 0.0001$, MRI cohort: $R = -0.411$; $p < 0.05$) (Figure 9E,F).

Table 3. Cytoarchitectonic distribution of the TBI-induced cortical lesion in the EEG and MRI cohorts.

Cortical Area	EEG Cohort Area (mm²) (Mean ± SEM)	Min–Max	% of Rats	MRI Cohort Area (Mean ± SEM)	Min–Max	% of Rats
DLEnt	0.27 ± 0.01	0.27–0.27	5 (2/43)			0 (0/30)
PRh	0.44 ± 0.11	0.01–1.35	44 (19/43)	0.79 ± 0.16	0.10–1.61	37 (11/30)
Ect	1.47 ± 0.20	0.01–3.82	77 (33/43)	1.77 ± 0.33	0.08–5.11	70 (21/30)
DI			0 (0/43)	0.18	0.18–0.18	3 (1/30)
GI			0 (0/43)	0.12 ± 0.05	0.03–0.24	13 (4/30) [#]
TeA	2.35 ± 0.17	0.01–3.92	91 (39/43)	2.33 ± 0.26	0.01–3.92	87 (26/30)
AuV	0.91 ± 0.09	0.01–2.45	93 (40/43)	1.22 ± 0.15	0.02–2.62	90 (27/30)
Au1	3.77 ± 0.20	0.86–5.78	100 (43/43)	4.32 ± 0.30 *	0.66–5.86	100 (30/30)
AuD	2.31 ± 0.06	0.58–2.61	100 (43/43)	2.32 ± 0.09	1.04–2.61	100 (30/30)
S1ULp	0.75 ± 0.09	0.03–1.98	93 (40/43)	1.14 ± 0.12 *	0.13–2.52	80 (24/30)
S1	1.16 ± 0.03	0.49–1.23	98 (42/43)	1.09 ± 0.05	0.02–1.23	97 (29/30)
S1BF	3.79 ± 0.36	0.56–10.44	98 (42/43)	3.42 ± 0.41	0.16–8.68	93 (28/30)
S1DZ	0.19 ± 0.06	0.02–0.3	9 (4/43)	0.01	0.01–0.01	3 (1/30)
PtPR	0.61 ± 0.03	0.06–0.75	95 (41/43)	0.61 ± 0.04	0.01–0.75	97 (29/30)
PtPD	0.47 ± 0.05	0.01–0.97	86 (37/43)	0.47 ± 0.05	0.01–0.96	83 (25/30)
V2L	4.62 ± 0.27	0.02–6.28	100 (43/43)	4.60 ± 0.32	0.87–6.48	100 (30/30)
V1B	2.12 ± 0.23	0.02–4.59	81 (35/43)	2.19 ± 0.30	0.15–4.81	80 (24/30)
V1	0.73 ± 0.16	0–2.13	56 (24/43)	0.37 ± 0.09	0.05–1.21	60 (18/30)
V1M	1.42 ± 0.26	0.01–3.98	47 (20/43)	1.32 ± 0.28	0.12–3.54	53 (16/30)
V2ML	0.68 ± 0.29	0.03–2.7	21 (9/43)	0.24 ± 0.14	0.01–0.76	17 (5/30)
V2MM	0.76 ± 0.50	0.04–2.26	9 (4/43)	0.28 ± 0.15	0.02–1.01	20 (6/30)
MPtA	0.04 ± 0.02	0.02–0.06	5 (2/43)			0 (0/30)
LPtA	0.83 ± 0.22	0.06–1.62	16 (7/43)	0.04 ± 0.03	0.01–0.09	10 (3/30)
S1Tr	0.54 ± 0.27	0.2–1.09	7 (3/43)			0 (0/30)
S1Sh	0.01	0.01–0.01	2 (1/43)			0 (0/30)
S1FL	0.12	0.12–0.12	2 (1/43)			0 (0/30)
S2	0.56 ± 0.07	0.04–2.10	95 (41/43)	1.07 ± 0.17 *	0.38–3.09	80 (24/30) [#]
RSD	1.09 ± 0.91	0.17–2.0	5 (2/43)	0.20 ± 0.08	0.02–0.42	13 (4/30)
RSGc	0.37	0.37–0.37	2 (1/43)			0 (0/30)
Sum of S1	4.89 ± 0.41	0.00–12.09	(43/43)	5.16 ± 0.55	0.00–11.55	(30/30)
Total S	5.43 ± 0.44	0.00–13.22	(43/43)	6.01 ± 0.65	0.00–12.59	(30/30)
Sum of V1	2.80 ± 0.46	0.00–10.20	(43/43)	2.68 ± 0.49	0.00–9.12	(30/30)
Sum of V2	4.84 ± 0.31	0.02–10.76	(43/43)	4.69 ± 0.34	0.87–7.71	(30/30)
Total V	7.63 ± 0.72	0.02–20.95	(43/43)	7.37 ± 0.78	0.87–15.82	(30/30)
Total Au	6.93 ± 0.34	1.44–10.84	(43/43)	7.73 ± 0.51	1.86–11.08	(30/30)
Total Area	25.33 ± 1.74	1.72–52.88	(43/43)	25.69 ± 2.32	5.66–47.61	(30/30)

Abbreviations: Au1, primary auditory cortex; AuD, secondary auditory cortex, dorsal area; AuV, secondary auditory cortex, ventral area; DLEnt, dorsolateral entorhinal cortex; DI, dysgranular insular cortex; Ect, ectorhinal cortex; GI, granular insular cortex; LPtA, lateral parietal association cortex; MPtA, medial parietal association cortex; PRh, perirhinal cortex; PtPD, parietal cortex, posterior area, dorsal part; PtPR, parietal cortex; RSD, retrosplenial dysgranular cortex; RSGc, retrosplenial granular cortex, c region; S1, primary somatosensory cortex; S2, secondary somatosensory cortex; S1BF, primary somatosensory cortex, barrel field; S1DZ, primary somatosensory cortex, dysgranular zone; S1FL, primary somatosensory cortex, forelimb region; S1Sh, primary somatosensory cortex, shoulder region; S1Tr, primary somatosensory cortex, trunk region; S1ULp, primary somatosensory cortex, upper lip region; TeA, temporal association cortex; V1, primary visual cortex; V1M, primary visual cortex, monocular area; V1B, primary visual cortex, binocular area; V2L, secondary visual cortex, lateral area; V2ML secondary visual cortex, mediolateral area; V2MM, secondary visual cortex, mediomedial area. Area is shown as a mean ± standard error of the mean (SEM). Animal numbers are in parenthesis. Statistical significances: *, $p < 0.05$ as compared to the area in the EEG cohort (Mann-Whitney U); [#], $p < 0.05$ as compared to the percentage of rats in the EEG cohort (X^2 test).

5. Discussion

To address the challenges related to chronic implantation of electrodes in brain-damaged rats, our objective was to develop methodologies to maximize the accuracy of chronic recording-electrode placements using preimplantation structural MRI. In the material available, we also assessed the effect of chronic electrode implantations on TBI-induced brain atrophy. Our data revealed that (1) animal-dependent progression of the cortical lesion after TBI compromises the placement accuracy of depth electrodes implanted at later time-points when only atlas-based coordinates are used; (2) MRI-guided adjustment of atlas-based coordinates increases the placement accuracy of intracerebral electrodes at the chronic post-TBI phase, particularly in the perilesional cortex; and (3) chronically implanted electrodes do not increase cortical and/or hippocampal atrophy.

5.1. Electrode Implantation Immediately after TBI Resulted in Good Location Accuracy of Intracerebral Electrode Tips Rostrally, but Was Less Accurate Caudally

In the EEG cohort, we implanted two bipolar intracortical and one bipolar hippocampal electrode ipsilateral to the lesion immediately after TBI to monitor the acute post-TBI electrophysiologic events and followed up the evolution of epileptiform activities over the following 7 months [36,37]. We assumed that the deformation and atrophy of the brain were not compromising the electrode placement accuracy at this early postinjury time-point, and thus we could rely on the rat brain atlas designed for the normal brain in defining the AP and DV coordinates for electrode placements. The fixed atlas-based cortical and hippocampal AP coordinates were chosen based on our previous observations that the cortical lesion progresses laterally and caudally [32]. In particular, it is critical to position the electrode tip in the anticipated epileptogenic area in the perilesional cortex, but avoid the lesion cavity [13].

Despite the unpredictable caudal progression of the cortical lesion, 83% of the anterior and 40% of the posterior cortical electrodes were within the cortex, and there was no difference in the overall DV distribution of the electrode tips between sham-operated controls and TBI rats. In 10% of the animals, however, the electrode tip of the posterior cortical electrodes had entered the lesion cavity when assessed at 7 months after implantation. This was particularly evident in cases with a large lesion size, which associated with robust cortical thinning. Also, 10% of the posterior cortical electrodes had entered the hippocampus, and consequently, recorded hippocampal EEG instead of cortical EEG. Progression of cortical lesions in the lateral FPI model is known to be variable and unpredictable [7,21,32,38]. It is possible that the progressive cortical atrophy "melting" of the brain around the electrode tips may have caused many of the electrode tips to end in the lesion cavity or subcortical areas, including the angular bundle and hippocampus. Even in the presence of an acute preimplantation MRI of the rats included in the EEG cohort, it was difficult to estimate the correct location for the intracerebral cortical electrodes 7 months later.

Although we were quite successful in implanting the electrode tips in the cortical tissue, both the anterior and posterior electrodes tended to locate slightly more anterior than planned. The anterior deviation from the target was typically less than 1 mm, however, and the mediolateral deviation was even smaller. We assume that the use of the Sprague Dawley strain in the present experiments instead of Wistar rats, which were used in the atlas preparation, and also mild human errors in reading bregma, could have affected the accuracy of the electrode placements. It is also important to note that depending on the skull size, the location of the 5 mm-diameter craniotomy slightly varied, which could also affect electrode insertion.

The target of the lower hippocampal electrode tip was at the hilus of the dentate gyrus. Consequently, the upper tip was expected to be in the CA1 subfield. As such, we aimed to have at least one electrode tip recording hippocampal epileptiform activity. Although in previous studies we noticed the development of hippocampal atrophy and deformations over months postinjury, we had no quantitative data to estimate the adjustments needed to fix the atlas-guided electrode tip coordinates. Somewhat disappointingly, at 7 months after the electrode implantation in the EEG cohort, the electrode tip was outside the dentate gyrus in half of the cases. In the remaining cases, the electrode tips were mainly in the CA3c subfield of the hippocampus proper. Only 7% of the electrodes were outside the hippocampus and not recording. In two cases, the electrodes were recording in the thalamus. We assume that postimpact subdural hematoma and/or edema affected the reading of the pial surface, which is used to calculate the DV coordinate, leading to mild misplacement of the hippocampal electrode in the TBI rats, particularly as the CA3c misplacement was observed in 1 sham rat only. Moreover, the implantation was technically challenging, as the AP coordinate of the hippocampal electrode was very close to the rostromedial edge of the craniotomy, leading in some cases to more rostral electrode repositioning of the AP coordinate planned during the surgery.

Taken together, our data show that the location of intracortical electrodes implanted immediately after TBI in the lateral FPI model, particularly to the posterior parts of the brain, can be compromised by unpredictable caudolateral progression of the cortical lesion and cortical thinning, leading to electrode misplacement affecting the EEG recordings. The hippocampal electrode placements immediately after TBI for chronic EEG follow-up are generally more stable and less affected by post-TBI hippocampal morphologic transformations; even the acute cortical swelling and subdural hematoma can affect DV electrode placement. As 30% of the 297 intracortical or hippocampal electrodes were recording outside the target tissue (cortex or hippocampus/dentate gyrus), verification of the electrode tip locations is needed for accurate interpretation of chronic EEG recordings even when the electrode implantations are performed in the early postinjury time period.

5.2. Preimplantation Structural MRI Improved the Accuracy of Electrode Implantations at 5 Months Postinjury

The interim review of MRIs imaged during the 5-month follow-up of animals in the MRI cohort confirmed our previous observations of the progression of cortical lesion in injured rats and raised concerns about the accuracy of electrode placements for the 1-month 24 h/7-day high-density video-EEG recordings, which was critical for the epilepsy phenotyping in our animal cohorts. It is generally recognized that proper electrode placement is a basis for accurate EEG data interpretation. To maximize the success rate of electrode implantations, we used images of coronal in vivo MR T2-wt slices obtained at 5 months post-TBI to generate rat-specific AP, ML, and DV coordinates for the anterior and posterior cortical electrodes, as well as the hippocampal electrodes. The aim was to place the cortical electrodes in the perilesional cortex within 500 μm of the lesion cavity, similar to that in the EEG cohort. Moreover, we wanted to get the DV coordinate of the ventral electrode tip to layer V of the sometimes very atrophied cortex. As in the EEG cohort, the hippocampal electrode tip was targeted to the dentate gyrus.

Analysis of histological sections prepared from the same rats approximately 1 month after the MRI, i.e., right after finishing the 1-month video-EEG monitoring, revealed a rostral shift of both the cortical and hippocampal electrodes relative to the MRI-guided coordinate. These data suggest that cortical atrophy, retracting the brain backwards may have contributed to the anterior shift and low accuracy of the cortical electrodes, particularly the posterior cortical electrode, in injured animals [7,17,39]. In case of hippocampal electrodes, the anterior shift was clearer in TBI rats than in sham animals, similar to the EEG cohort. Even though deviation of the hippocampal electrodes from the planned position can also relate to hippocampal atrophy, changes in its septotemporal orientation, rotation, and medial shift toward midline can contribute to electrode misplacements [23].

Generally, despite the unexpected divergence between the MRI-defined and histologically verified "true" coordinates, our data demonstrate that the MR images were useful when targeting the perilesional cortex for EEG recordings during the chronic phase post-TBI. Our "simulation" revealed that most (60%) of the MRI-guided posterior cortical electrode placements were in the cortex compared with 42% of the posterior cortical electrode placements when only the atlas-based coordinate was used. Moreover, with MRI-guided implantation, we were able to avoid the cortical lesion cavity. Additionally, the effect of cortical thinning on the DV location of the posterior electrode was mitigated, as the percentage of electrodes in the cortex was comparable between sham and TBI rats. Moreover, there was a 40% increase in cases with a cortical electrode location and a 14% increase in reaching the target layer V compared with the EEG cohort. We also demonstrated that despite the inaccuracy in adjusting the hippocampal AP coordinate when using MRI guidance, 36% of the hippocampal electrodes were recording in the dentate gyrus in the MRI cohort compared with 49% in the EEG cohort. This finding suggests that a 3D change in hippocampal orientation, which was less evident in the 2D MR images used in this study, compromised the estimation of the hippocampal AP coordinate. The 2D images were effective for determining the DV hippocampal target as the overall DV distribution of the electrode tip in the dentate gyrus was the same between sham and TBI rats.

One question is: Would presurgery MRIs help to improve the interpretation of postsurgery MRIs and the accuracy of electrode placements? In addition to the cost, it is important to note that unlike MRI, the histology-based rat brain atlas offers a benefit of using skull landmarks for calculation of coordinates for electrode positioning, that is, using the bregma as a reference point. Histological sections also give a higher spatial resolution and possibility to also assess the laminar placement of electrode tips.

Taken together, MR images were useful in targeting the AP and DV locations of perilesional intracortical electrodes in the chronic post-TBI phase. For hippocampal electrode implantations, the MR images were not as useful in targeting the AP location, but improved the precision of targeting the DV electrode tip into the dentate gyrus. To increase the accuracy of estimating the AP coordinate for intracerebral electrode implantation at the chronic post-TBI phase, we suggest using a 3D reconstruction of the brain to fully understand the effect of the ipsilateral cortical and hippocampal atrophy and orientation affecting the electrode placements. We propose the following MRI protocol for estimating the adjustments needed for atlas-based coordinates to successfully and accurately implant electrodes in the chronic post-TBI phase (see also Supplementary Figure S1):

1. Acquire T2-weighted MRI and 3D MGRE datasets.
2. Select the coronal T2-weighted and/or MGRE images containing the target region of the intracerebral electrode (e.g., perilesional cortex or hippocampus).
3. In each MGRE image selected in step 2, calculate the ML distance of the intended electrode tip location (e.g., perilesional cortex). Select the sagittal MGRE image at that ML coordinate. In MGRE sagittal images, calculate the DV distance (from the brain surface) to which the tip of the electrode will be targeted, and select the MGRE horizontal images at that depth.
4. In the sagittal and horizontal images selected in step 3, estimate the cortical AP (in the sagittal plane) and ML (in the horizontal plane) distances (shrinkage) for a given rat as described in this study, using available 3D slice viewer and analysis software
5. Determine the ratio of the AP distance based on the atlas coordinates/AP distance measured in the sagittal slice in a given rat (estimated in step 4).
6. To determine the final MRI AP coordinate, align the selected coronal images (step 2) with the atlas. Multiply the atlas AP coordinate at this location with the ratio determined in step 5.
7. To determine the final MRI ML location, repeat steps 5 and 6 in the horizontal plane.

5.3. Chronic Intracerebral Electrode Implantation Did Not Affect the Cortical Lesion Area or Cortical and Hippocampal Atrophy over the 7-Month Follow-Up

Chronic electrode implantation has been proposed to add tissue damage due to blood–brain barrier damage and chronic inflammation in the electrode path [40]. Therefore, we expected to see more cortical atrophy in the EEG than the MRI cohort. The cortical lesion areas were comparable in the EEG and MRI cohorts. Also, the percentage of the lesion area in cytoarchitectonic areas targeted by the electrode tips did not differ between the EEG cohort and MRI cohort. Taken together, the progression of the cortical lesion in the EEG cohort was not augmented by the chronically implanted electrodes.

We recently demonstrated that the hippocampus undergoes a series of post-TBI morphologic transformations, including atrophy and orientation changes due to neurodegeneration, white-matter atrophy, and expanding ventricles [23]. The present analysis revealed a caudal shift of the hippocampus. Apparently, the expanding ventricles pushed the hippocampus backward and toward the midline.

6. Conclusions

Our study demonstrates the benefit of using MR images for adjusting atlas-based coordinates to improve the accuracy in chronic intracerebral electrode placements into atrophied and distorted brain areas, which is critical, e.g., for a high-quality recording of various epileptiform activities in candidate epileptogenic regions after TBI. Future studies should consider using T2-wt MRI slices much thinner than 800 µm or 3D spatial encoding with close to isotropic resolution to allow for accurate visualization in coronal, sagittal, and horizontal planes to enhance the accuracy of MRI-guided electrode implantations. Importantly, comparison of the cortical lesion area and cytoarchitectonic distribution between cohorts with 7-month- or 1-month-long electrode implantations did not reveal any worsening of brain atrophy by the chronic electrode implantation.

Supplementary Materials: The following supporting information can be downloaded at: https://www.mdpi.com/article/10.3390/biomedicines10092295/s1. Supplementary Table S1. The distribution of the dorsoventral location of the lower tip of the anterior and posterior intracortical electrodes in sham-operated and TBI rats. Supplementary Table S2. Location of the "virtual electrode". Summary of the locations of the anterior and posterior intracortical, and hippocampal electrodes in the MRI cohort, if implanted according to the atlas-based coordinates. Supplementary Figure S1. A schematic presentation of the MRI protocol for estimating the adjustments needed for atlas-based coordinates (See discussion for further details).

Author Contributions: Conceptualization, X.E.N.-E., O.G. A.P.; formal analysis, X.E.N.-E. and E.H.; funding acquisition, A.P. and O.G.; investigation, X.E.N.-E., R.I., E.H., E.M., P.A., R.C. and T.P.; methodology, X.E.N.-E., R.I. and O.G.; project administration, X.E.N.-E.; resources, O.G. and A.P.; software, P.A., R.C. and T.P.; supervision, O.G. and A.P.; visualization, X.E.N.-E. writing—original draft, X.E.N.-E. and A.P.; writing—review and editing, X.E.N.-E. and A.P. All authors have read and agreed to the published version of the manuscript.

Funding: This study was supported by the European Union's Seventh Framework Programme (FP7/2007-2013) under grant agreement 602102 (EPITARGET)(AP), the Medical Research Council of the Academy of Finland (grants 272249, 273909, and 2285733-9) (AP), the National Institute of Neurological Disorders and Stroke (NINDS) Center without Walls of the National Institutes of Health (NIH) under award U54NS100064 (EpiBioS4Rx) (AP), and the Sigrid Jusélius Foundation (AP).

Institutional Review Board Statement: The study was conducted according to the guidelines of the Declaration of Helsinki. All animal procedures were approved by the Animal Ethics Committee of the Provincial Government of Southern Finland and carried out in accordance with the guidelines of European Community Council Directives 2010/63/EU.

Informed Consent Statement: Not applicable.

Data Availability Statement: The data presented in this study are available on request from the corresponding author.

Acknowledgments: We thank Jarmo Hartikainen and Merja Lukkari for their excellent technical help.

Conflicts of Interest: The authors declare no conflict of interest.

References

1. Menon, D.K.; Schwab, K.; Wright, D.W.; Maas, A.I. Demographics and Clinical Assessment Working Group of the International and Interagency Initiative toward Common Data Elements for Research on Traumatic Brain Injury and Psychological Health. Position Statement: Definition of Traumatic Brain Injury. *Arch. Phys. Med. Rehabil.* **2010**, *91*, 1637–1640. [CrossRef] [PubMed]
2. Mckee, A.C.; Daneshvar, D.H. The Neuropathology of Traumatic Brain Injury. *Handb. Clin. Neurol.* **2015**, *127*, 45–66. [PubMed]
3. Thapa, K.; Khan, H.; Singh, T.G.; Kaur, A. Traumatic Brain Injury: Mechanistic Insight on Pathophysiology and Potential Therapeutic Targets. *J. Mol. Neurosci.* **2021**, *71*, 1725–1742. [CrossRef] [PubMed]
4. Graham, N.S.; Sharp, D.J. Understanding Neurodegeneration After Traumatic Brain Injury: From Mechanisms to Clinical Trials in Dementia. *J. Neurol. Neurosurg. Psychiatry* **2019**, *90*, 1221–1233. [CrossRef] [PubMed]

5. MacKenzie, J.D.; Siddiqi, F.; Babb, J.S.; Bagley, L.J.; Mannon, L.J.; Sinson, G.P.; Grossman, R.I. Brain Atrophy in Mild Or Moderate Traumatic Brain Injury: A Longitudinal Quantitative Analysis. *AJNR Am. J. Neuroradiol.* **2002**, *23*, 1509–1515. [PubMed]
6. Sidaros, A.; Skimminge, A.; Liptrot, M.G.; Sidaros, K.; Engberg, A.W.; Herning, M.; Paulson, O.B.; Jernigan, T.L.; Rostrup, E. Long-Term Global and Regional Brain Volume Changes Following Severe Traumatic Brain Injury: A Longitudinal Study with Clinical Correlates. *Neuroimage* **2009**, *44*, 1–8. [CrossRef]
7. Immonen, R.J.; Kharatishvili, I.; Niskanen, J.P.; Grohn, H.; Pitkanen, A.; Grohn, O.H. Distinct MRI Pattern in Lesional and Perilesional Area After Traumatic Brain Injury in Rat–11 Months Follow-Up. *Exp. Neurol.* **2009**, *215*, 29–40. [CrossRef]
8. Haarbauer-Krupa, J.; Pugh, M.J.; Prager, E.M.; Harmon, N.; Wolfe, J.; Yaffe, K. Epidemiology of Chronic Effects of Traumatic Brain Injury. *J. Neurotrauma* **2021**, *38*, 3235–3247. [CrossRef]
9. Lowenstein, D.H. Epilepsy After Head Injury: An Overview. *Epilepsia* **2009**, *50* (Suppl. 2), 4–9. [CrossRef]
10. Annegers, J.F.; Hauser, W.A.; Coan, S.P.; Rocca, W.A. A Population-Based Study of Seizures After Traumatic Brain Injuries. *N. Engl. J. Med.* **1998**, *338*, 20–24. [CrossRef]
11. Dulla, C.G.; Pitkanen, A. Novel Approaches to Prevent Epileptogenesis after Traumatic Brain Injury. *Neurotherapeutics* **2021**, *18*, 1582–1601. [CrossRef] [PubMed]
12. Gupta, P.K.; Sayed, N.; Ding, K.; Agostini, M.A.; Van Ness, P.C.; Yablon, S.; Madden, C.; Mickey, B.; D'Ambrosio, R.; Diaz-Arrastia, R. Subtypes of Post-Traumatic Epilepsy: Clinical, Electrophysiological, and Imaging Features. *J. Neurotrauma* **2014**, *31*, 1439–1443. [CrossRef] [PubMed]
13. Bragin, A.; Li, L.; Almajano, J.; Alvarado-Rojas, C.; Reid, A.Y.; Staba, R.J.; Engel, J., Jr. Pathologic Electrographic Changes after Experimental Traumatic Brain Injury. *Epilepsia* **2016**, *57*, 735–745. [CrossRef] [PubMed]
14. Kelly, K.M.; Miller, E.R.; Lepsveridze, E.; Kharlamov, E.A.; Mchedlishvili, Z. Posttraumatic Seizures and Epilepsy in Adult Rats After Controlled Cortical Impact. *Epilepsy Res.* **2015**, *117*, 104–116. [CrossRef]
15. Duncan, J.S. Imaging in the Surgical Treatment of Epilepsy. *Nat. Rev. Neurol.* **2010**, *6*, 537–550. [CrossRef]
16. Duncan, J.S.; Winston, G.P.; Koepp, M.J.; Ourselin, S. Brain Imaging in the Assessment for Epilepsy Surgery. *Lancet Neurol.* **2016**, *15*, 420–433. [CrossRef]
17. Thompson, H.J.; Lifshitz, J.; Marklund, N.; Grady, M.S.; Graham, D.I.; Hovda, D.A.; McIntosh, T.K. Lateral Fluid Percussion Brain Injury: A 15-Year Review and Evaluation. *J. Neurotrauma* **2005**, *22*, 42–75. [CrossRef]
18. Xiong, Y.; Mahmood, A.; Chopp, M. Animal Models of Traumatic Brain Injury. *Nat. Rev. Neurosci.* **2013**, *14*, 128–142. [CrossRef]
19. Bramlett, H.M.; Dietrich, W.D. Quantitative Structural Changes in White and Gray Matter 1 Year Following Traumatic Brain Injury in Rats. *Acta Neuropathol.* **2002**, *103*, 607–614. [CrossRef]
20. Rodriguez-Paez, A.C.; Brunschwig, J.P.; Bramlett, H.M. Light and Electron Microscopic Assessment of Progressive Atrophy Following Moderate Traumatic Brain Injury in the Rat. *Acta Neuropathol.* **2005**, *109*, 603–616. [CrossRef]
21. Manninen, E.; Chary, K.; Lapinlampi, N.; Andrade, P.; Paananen, T.; Sierra, A.; Tohka, J.; Grohn, O.; Pitkanen, A. Early Increase in Cortical T2 Relaxation is a Prognostic Biomarker for the Evolution of Severe Cortical Damage, but not for Epileptogenesis, after Experimental Traumatic Brain Injury. *J. Neurotrauma* **2020**, *37*, 2580–2594. [CrossRef] [PubMed]
22. Manninen, E.; Chary, K.; Lapinlampi, N.; Andrade, P.; Paananen, T.; Sierra, A.; Tohka, J.; Grohn, O.; Pitkanen, A. Acute Thalamic Damage as a Prognostic Biomarker for Post-Traumatic Epileptogenesis. *Epilepsia* **2021**, *62*, 1852–1864. [CrossRef] [PubMed]
23. De Feo, R.; Hamalainen, E.; Manninen, E.; Immonen, R.; Valverde, J.M.; Ndode-Ekane, X.E.; Grohn, O.; Pitkanen, A.; Tohka, J. Convolutional Neural Networks Enable Robust Automatic Segmentation of the Rat Hippocampus in MRI After Traumatic Brain Injury. *Front. Neurol.* **2022**, *13*, 820267. [CrossRef] [PubMed]
24. Galanopoulou, A.S.; Mowrey, W.B. Not all that Glitters is Gold: A Guide to Critical Appraisal of Animal Drug Trials in Epilepsy. *Epilepsia Open* **2016**, *1*, 86–101. [CrossRef] [PubMed]
25. Paxinos, G.; Watson, C. *The Rat Brain in Stereotaxic Coordinates*, 7th ed.; Elsevier Inc.: Amsterdam, The Netherlands, 2007.
26. McIntosh, T.K.; Vink, R.; Noble, L.; Yamakami, I.; Fernyak, S.; Soares, H.; Faden, A.L. Traumatic Brain Injury in the Rat: Characterization of a Lateral Fluid-Percussion Model. *Neuroscience* **1989**, *28*, 233–244. [CrossRef]
27. Kharatishvili, I.; Nissinen, J.P.; McIntosh, T.K.; Pitkanen, A. A Model of Posttraumatic Epilepsy Induced by Lateral Fluid-Percussion Brain Injury in Rats. *Neuroscience* **2006**, *140*, 685–697. [CrossRef]
28. Andrade, P.; Paananen, T.; Ciszek, R.; Lapinlampi, N.; Pitkanen, A. Algorithm for Automatic Detection of Spontaneous Seizures in Rats with Post-Traumatic Epilepsy. *J. Neurosci. Methods* **2018**, *307*, 37–45. [CrossRef]
29. Racine, R.J. Modification of Seizure Activity by Electrical Stimulation. II. Motor Seizure. *Electroencephalogr. Clin. Neurophysiol.* **1972**, *32*, 281–294. [CrossRef]
30. Fisher, R.S.; Acevedo, C.; Arzimanoglou, A.; Bogacz, A.; Cross, J.H.; Elger, C.E.; Engel, J., Jr.; Forsgren, L.; French, J.A.; Glynn, M.; et al. ILAE Official Report: A Practical Clinical Definition of Epilepsy. *Epilepsia* **2014**, *55*, 475–482. [CrossRef]
31. Immonen, R.; Smith, G.; Brady, R.D.; Wright, D.; Johnston, L.; Harris, N.G.; Manninen, E.; Salo, R.; Branch, C.; Duncan, D.; et al. Harmonization of Pipeline for Preclinical Multicenter MRI Biomarker Discovery in a Rat Model of Post-Traumatic Epileptogenesis. *Epilepsy Res.* **2019**, *150*, 46–57. [CrossRef]
32. Ekolle Ndode-Ekane, X.; Kharatishvili, I.; Pitkanen, A. Unfolded Maps for Quantitative Analysis of Cortical Lesion Location and Extent After Traumatic Brain Injury. *J. Neurotrauma* **2017**, *34*, 459–474. [CrossRef] [PubMed]

33. Santana-Gomez, C.; Andrade, P.; Hudson, M.R.; Paananen, T.; Ciszek, R.; Smith, G.; Ali, I.; Rundle, B.K.; Ndode-Ekane, X.E.; Casillas-Espinosa, P.M.; et al. Harmonization of Pipeline for Detection of HFOs in a Rat Model of Post-Traumatic Epilepsy in Preclinical Multicenter Study on Post-Traumatic Epileptogenesis. *Epilepsy Res.* **2019**, *156*, 106110. [CrossRef] [PubMed]
34. Andrade, P.; Ciszek, R.; Pitkanen, A.; Ndode-Ekane, X.E. A Web-Based Application for Generating 2D-Unfolded Cortical Maps to Analyze the Location and Extent of Cortical Lesions Following Traumatic Brain Injury in Adult Rats. *J. Neurosci. Methods* **2018**, *308*, 330–336. [CrossRef] [PubMed]
35. Ciszek, R.; Andrade, P.; Tapiala, J.; Pitkanen, A.; Ndode-Ekane, X.E. Web Application for Quantification of Traumatic Brain Injury-Induced Cortical Lesions in Adult Mice. *Neuroinformatics* **2020**, *18*, 307–317. [CrossRef] [PubMed]
36. Tubi, M.A.; Lutkenhoff, E.; Blanco, M.B.; McArthur, D.; Villablanca, P.; Ellingson, B.; Diaz-Arrastia, R.; Van Ness, P.; Real, C.; Shrestha, V.; et al. Early Seizures and Temporal Lobe Trauma Predict Post-Traumatic Epilepsy: A Longitudinal Study. *Neurobiol. Dis.* **2019**, *123*, 115–121. [CrossRef]
37. Andrade, P.; Banuelos-Cabrera, I.; Lapinlampi, N.; Paananen, T.; Ciszek, R.; Ndode-Ekane, X.E.; Pitkanen, A. Acute Non-Convulsive Status Epilepticus After Experimental Traumatic Brain Injury in Rats. *J. Neurotrauma* **2019**, *36*, 1890–1907. [CrossRef]
38. Kharatishvili, I.; Pitkanen, A. Association of the Severity of Cortical Damage with the Occurrence of Spontaneous Seizures and Hyperexcitability in an Animal Model of Posttraumatic Epilepsy. *Epilepsy Res.* **2010**, *90*, 47–59. [CrossRef] [PubMed]
39. Golarai, G.; Greenwood, A.C.; Feeney, D.M.; Connor, J.A. Physiological and Structural Evidence for Hippocampal Involvement in Persistent Seizure Susceptibility After Traumatic Brain Injury. *J. Neurosci.* **2001**, *21*, 8523–8537. [CrossRef] [PubMed]
40. Campbell, A.; Wu, C. Chronically Implanted Intracranial Electrodes: Tissue Reaction and Electrical Changes. *Micromachines* **2018**, *9*, 430. [CrossRef]

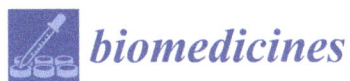

Review

The Neuroinflammatory Role of Pericytes in Epilepsy

Gaku Yamanaka [1,*], Fuyuko Takata [2], Yasufumi Kataoka [2], Kanako Kanou [1], Shinichiro Morichi [1], Shinya Dohgu [2] and Hisashi Kawashima [1]

1. Department of Pediatrics and Adolescent Medicine, Tokyo Medical University, Tokyo 160-8402, Japan; kanako.hayashi.0110@gmail.com (K.K.); s.morichi@gmail.com (S.M.); hisashi@tokyo-med.ac.jp (H.K.)
2. Department of Pharmaceutical Care and Health Sciences, Faculty of Pharmaceutical Sciences, Fukuoka University, Fukuoka 814-0180, Japan; ftakata@fukuoka-u.ac.jp (F.T.); ykataoka@fukuoka-u.ac.jp (Y.K.); dohgu@fukuoka-u.ac.jp (S.D.)
* Correspondence: gaku@tokyo-med.ac.jp; Tel.: +81-3-3342-6111; Fax: +81-3-3344-0643

Abstract: Pericytes are a component of the blood–brain barrier (BBB) neurovascular unit, in which they play a crucial role in BBB integrity and are also implicated in neuroinflammation. The association between pericytes, BBB dysfunction, and the pathophysiology of epilepsy has been investigated, and links between epilepsy and pericytes have been identified. Here, we review current knowledge about the role of pericytes in epilepsy. Clinical evidence has shown an accumulation of pericytes with altered morphology in the cerebral vascular territories of patients with intractable epilepsy. In vitro, proinflammatory cytokines, including IL-1β, TNFα, and IL-6, cause morphological changes in human-derived pericytes, where IL-6 leads to cell damage. Experimental studies using epileptic animal models have shown that cerebrovascular pericytes undergo redistribution and remodeling, potentially contributing to BBB permeability. These series of pericyte-related modifications are promoted by proinflammatory cytokines, of which the most pronounced alterations are caused by IL-1β, a cytokine involved in the pathogenesis of epilepsy. Furthermore, the pericyte-glial scarring process in leaky capillaries was detected in the hippocampus during seizure progression. In addition, pericytes respond more sensitively to proinflammatory cytokines than microglia and can also activate microglia. Thus, pericytes may function as sensors of the inflammatory response. Finally, both in vitro and in vivo studies have highlighted the potential of pericytes as a therapeutic target for seizure disorders.

Keywords: pericytes; mural cells; cytokine; blood-brain barrier; neuroinflammation

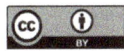

1. Introduction

Accumulating evidence has demonstrated that the pathogenesis of epilepsy is linked to neuroinflammation and cerebrovascular dysfunction [1–6]. Traditionally, microglia had been considered to be responsible for the cytokine-centered immune response in the central nervous system (CNS); however, brain pericytes can respond to inflammatory signals, such as circulating cytokines, and convey this information to surrounding cells through chemokine and cytokine secretions [7–10]. Recent studies have demonstrated that pericytes may act as sensors for the inflammatory response in the CNS, as pericytes react intensely to proinflammatory cytokines when compared to other cell types (e.g., microglia) that constitute the CNS and factor-induced reactive pericytes can also activate microglia in vitro [9,11–13].

Pericytes provide physical support to the blood–brain barrier (BBB) and play an integral role in CNS homeostasis and BBB function [14]. Pericyte degeneration and/or dysfunction contribute to the loss of BBB integrity, which is an early hallmark of several neurodegenerative and inflammatory conditions [8,15,16]. Another notable feature of pericytes is their ability to regulate the migration of leukocytes across the brain microvascular endothelial cell (BMVEC) barrier, which secretes key molecules that support the

BBB barrier [17,18]. Recent research on the pathogenesis of epilepsy has begun to elucidate the mechanisms mediating peripheral-to-CNS cell infiltration in human and mouse models [19,20]. Pericytes may contribute to the mechanisms, while emerging research is investigating the extent of peripheral immune cell involvement in the inflammatory pathology of epilepsy.

The various functions of pericytes and their involvement in CNS diseases, including ischemic stroke [21], spinal cord injury [22], brain injury [23], and multiple sclerosis [24], has been reported.

The association between pericytes and epilepsy has attracted attention, while several recent studies have illustrated the contributions of pericytes to the pathogenesis of epilepsy [2,25–32]. These studies suggested that pericytes might participate in the pathogenesis of epilepsy, consisting of neuroinflammation and BBB damage and the interaction between peripheral and central immunity. Thus, evidence on the relationship between pericytes and the pathogenesis of epilepsy is gradually accumulating. Therefore, this study aimed to investigate the pathogenesis of epilepsy and pericytes because none of the review articles focused on this, even though therapeutic targets for pericytes in neurological disorders were investigated [17,33,34].

This review (1) explores the current literature regarding the role of pericytes in the pathogenesis of epilepsy and (2) highlights novel directions for research on therapeutic interventions for epilepsy that target pericytes. Given the paucity of knowledge on pericyte function in seizures and epilepsy-related pathologies, further studies are warranted to investigate pericytes as a potential therapeutic target for epilepsy treatment.

2. What Are Pericytes?

Pericytes were first described by the French scientist Charles-Marie Benjamin Rouget and were originally called Rouget cells in 1873 [35]. Later, this population was rediscovered by Zimmermann as a cell that shows a specific morphology around microvessels, and became widely known as a "pericyte" [36]. Pericytes are mural cells that are implanted in the basal membrane surrounding endothelial cells in capillaries and small vessels, including precapillary arterioles and postcapillary venules. Although the origin of all pericytes has not been clarified, blood vessels in the CNS are predominantly covered by neural crest cell-derived pericytes, while mesoderm-derived pericytes mainly contribute to blood vessel coverage in the trunk [37]. In the brain, pericytes constitute a vital component of the BBB/neurovascular unit (NVU) and cover the BMVECs lining the capillaries on the parenchymal side, where there are astrocytic end feet that enclose cerebral vessels, perivascular microglia/macrophages, and neurons [17,38,39]. Pericytes form a crucial component of the brain microvasculature and play an integral role in CNS homeostasis and BBB function [14] in normal physiological (Figure 1) and pathological conditions (Figure 2). A potential mechanism of pericyte action is the regulation of signaling through platelet-derived growth factor receptor beta (PDGFRβ), which is commonly used as a marker of pericytes and regulates pericyte survival, proliferation, and migration signals [40]. In the CNS, platelet-derived growth factor-beta subunit (PDGF-BB) is released by endothelial cells and binds to PDGFRβ at the cell surface of pericytes to promote pericyte vascularization within the BBB [41]. The PDGFRβ signaling pathway is involved in pericyte survival and subsequent development as well as the function of the BBB during adulthood and senescence, as demonstrated by experiments in pericyte-deficient mice [17,38]. In addition to its role as a marker of CNS pericytes, PDGFRβ is expressed in oligodendrocyte precursor cell (OPC)/neuron-glial antigen 2 (NG2) parenchymal glial cells [2,25,42]. Other markers for pericytes exist (Table 1), but these remain inconclusive. Anatomical studies are required to investigate the characteristics of pericytes that possess longitudinal processes along vessels and contribute to BBB maintenance [15]. Pericytes in the brain are highly heterogeneous and have different morphologies as well as functions depending on their location in the vasculature [10]. Further, transgenic mice generated to study pericyte function may yield information on other cell types [43]. Therefore, "peripheral blood-specific" markers must be used with caution [44]. Although there is no scientific consensus on what constitutes true pericytes [45], the current review focuses on studies using definitive pericyte-related markers and anatomy.

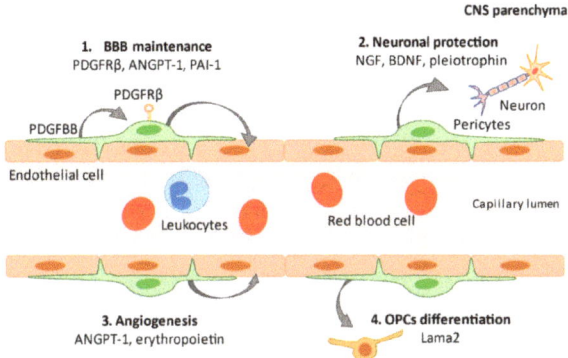

Figure 1. Regulatory functions of pericytes. In the central nervous system (CNS), platelet-derived growth factor-beta subunit (PDGF-BB) is released by endothelial cells and binds to PDGFRβ at the cell surface of pericytes to promote pericyte vascularization within the blood–brain barrier (BBB). Secretion of angiopoietin-1 (ANGPT-1) and plasminogen activator inhibitor type 1 (PAI-1) from pericytes promotes the development of vascular endothelial cells and contributes to the maintenance of the BBB (1). Pericytes maintain neuronal health by secreting factors such as nerve growth factor (NGF), brain-derived nerve growth factor (BDNF), and pleiotrophin (2). Pericytes are involved in angiogenesis by secreting ANGPT-1 and erythropoietin (3) and produce a factor (Lama2) that facilitates the differentiation of oligodendrocyte progenitor cells (OPCs) into mature oligodendrocytes (4).

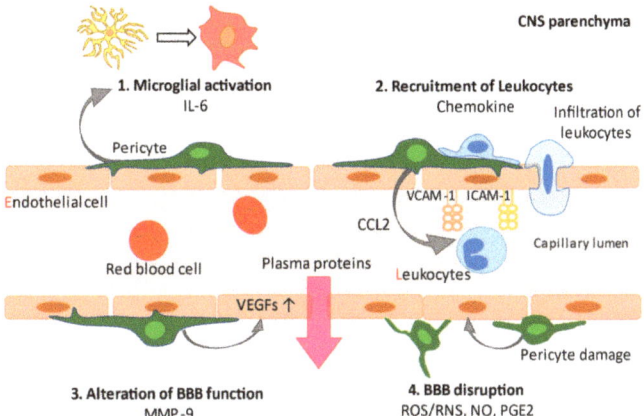

Figure 2. In pathological conditions, pericytes generate various inflammatory factors. Pericytes secrete IL-6 that can polarize parenchymal microglia to a proinflammatory phenotype to activate microglia (1). The secretion of chemokines (CCL2, CXCL1, CXCL8, and CXCL10) by pericytes recruits leukocytes to the CNS parenchyma via the upregulation of ICAM-1 and VCAM-1 adhesion molecules on the endothelium (2). MMP-9 secretion stimulates the production and secretion of vascular endothelial growth factor (VEGF), resulting in endothelial dysfunction (3). Secretion of reactive oxygen species/reactive nitrogen species (ROS/RNS), nitric oxide (NO), and prostaglandins (PGE2) by pericytes lead to vasodilation and breaching of the blood–brain barrier. Pericytes themselves are morphologically altered by inflammatory mediators (4).

Table 1. Common markers used to identify pericytes in the central nervous system of mice that also label other cell types.

Marker	Cells Labeled	Main Function	Reference(s)
PDGFRβ (platelet-derived growth factor receptor beta)	Fibroblasts, SMCs, pericytes	Tyrosine kinase receptor	[14,41]
NG2 (CSPG4; chondroitin sulfate proteoglycan 4)	OPCs, NSCs, SMCs, pericytes	Cell-membrane proteoglycan	[46]
CD13 (aminopeptidase N)	Fibroblasts, SMCs, pericytes	Cell-membrane aminopeptidase	[14]
αSMA (actin, aortic smooth muscle)	SMCs, myofibroblasts, pericytes	Cytoskeletal protein	[14]
Desmin	SMCs, pericytes	Intermediate filament	[14]
Rgs5 (regulator of G protein signaling 5)	SMCs, pericytes	Regulator of G protein	[47]
CD146 (cell surface glycoprotein MUC18)	SMCs, pericytes	Membrane proteins	[48]
SUR2 (sulfonylurea receptor 2)	SMCs, pericytes	Potassium-channel	[47,49]
Kir6.1 (K+ channel pore-forming subunit)	SMCs, fibroblasts, pericytes	Potassium-channel	[47,49]
NeuroTrace 500/525 (fluorescent Nissl dye/FluoroNissl Green)	Pericytes	-	[50]
Vitronectin	SMCs, Pericytes	Complement-binding protein	[49,51]

Note: NSCs, neural stem cells; OPCs, oligodendrocyte progenitor cells; SMCs, smooth muscle cells.

3. Pericytes and Neuroinflammation

Evidence accumulated from experimental models and human samples implicates immunological processes in the pathogenesis of epilepsy [1,4]. The involvement of pericytes in the CNS immune responses has attracted significant attention. Pericytes present heterogeneous signals to the surrounding cells and actively modulate inflammatory responses in a tissue- and context-dependent manner. The expression of various pattern-recognition receptors (PRRs), including toll-like receptors (TLRs) and nucleotide-binding and oligomerization domain (NOD)-like receptor families, has been detected in brain pericytes [52]. Given the abundance of surface receptors, pericytes can respond to inflammatory mediators, such as monocyte chemoattractant protein-1 (MCP-1/CCL2) and tumor necrosis factor (TNF)-α, which in turn induce the secretion of CCL2, nitric oxide (NO), and several cytokines [7–9,53]. Pericytes act as promoters of both the innate and adaptive immune system [43]. In the CNS, microglia are a hallmark of the immune response, which produce cytokines such as interleukin (IL)-1β, TNF-α, IL-6, and various other chemokines [54], and related effector pathways, including cyclooxygenase-2 (COX-2)/prostaglandin (PGE2) and complement factors [55]. The rapid activation of microglia impairs neuronal function by inducing inflammatory mediators, such as NO, reactive oxygen species (ROS), and proinflammatory cytokines [56,57].

Pericytes have been shown to be more sensitive to proinflammatory cytokines compared to other cells in the NVU [9,11–13]. Specifically, cytokine and chemokine release profiles from brain pericytes in response to TNF-α are distinct to those of other cell types comprising the NVU, and TNF-α-stimulated pericytes release macrophage inflammatory protein (MIP)-1α and IL-6. Among BBB cells, pericytes stimulated with TNF-α induced the highest levels of iNOS and IL-1β mRNA expression, which indicates the activation of BV-2 microglia [9]. The mechanism underlying TNF-α-induced IL-6 release involves the inhibitor kappa B (IκB)-nuclear factor kappa-light-chain-enhancer of activated B cells (NFκB) and the Janus family of tyrosine kinase (JAK)-signal transducer and activator of transcription (STAT) 3 pathways [13]. NFκB plays a key role in inflammation, immune, and stress-related responses, as well as in the regulation of cell survival and in the growth of neural processes in developing peripheral and central neurons [58]. These findings indicate that the activated brain pericytes trigger the development of uncoordinated NVU function, including glial activation, and may act as sensors at the BBB in TNF-α-mediated brain inflammation.

Pericytes also release anti-inflammatory factors, highlighting their involvement in regeneration and protection [7,59,60]. Pericytes respond to lipopolysaccharide (LPS), secrete anti-inflammatory cytokines such as IL-10 and IL-13 [61], and produce neurotrophins such as nerve growth factor (NGF) and brain-derived neurotrophic factor (BDNF), which regulate neuronal development [42,62]. Pericytes upregulate neurotrophin-3 production in response to hypoxia, resulting in increased NGF production in astrocytes, thereby protecting neurons from hypoxia-induced apoptosis [62]. These actions highlight the neuroprotective functions of pericytes under pathological conditions.

4. Pericytes and Epilepsy

Table 2 summarizes the research on pericytes and epilepsy.

Table 2. Research and key findings on pericytes and epilepsy.

No.	Patients/Model	Species	Key Findings	Reference
1	Intractable complex partial seizures	Humans	• Degeneration of pericytes (aggregates of cellular debris within the basement membrane) with the morphological changes in pericyte-basement membrane unit thickness and pericyte cytoplasmic density were observed in the spiking area of microvessels in an electron microscopy study of brain tissue	[63]
2	TLE with HS	Humans	• PDGFRβ+ cells are distributed around the cerebrovasculature and are present in the brain parenchyma of human TLE specimens	[2]
	NG2DsRed or C57BL/6J mice (intraperitoneal KA injections)	Mice	• Constitutive cerebrovascular NG2DsRed pericyte coverage is impaired in response to SE in vivo or seizure-like events in vitro • Redistribution of parenchymal and vascular PDGFRβ+ cells occurs in vitro and in vivo • Vascular and parenchymal PDGFRβ+ cells partially co-localize with NG2DsRed and NG2, but not with IBA-1 (indicators of microglia)	
3	FCD, TLE without HS, cryptogenic epilepsy	Humans	• FCD and TLE-HS display the highest PDGFRβ immunoreactivity at the microvasculature identifying pericytes • Cryptogenic epilepsy patients also showed a similar immune response pattern, although to a lesser extent than that in FCD • The amount of perivascular PDGFRβ immunoreactivity was found to be associated with increased hippocampal angiogenesis in tissues from patients with TLE-HS	[25]
	Neurovascular dysplasia rat model (Sprague-Dawley rats with pre-natal exposure to methyl-axozy methanoic acid), pilocarpine	Mice	• Pericyte-vascular dysplasia was detected in hippocampi corresponding to neuronal heterotopias • Severe SE was associated with a region-specific increase in PDGFRβ immunoreactivity	
4	TLE	Humans	• Chronic IFN-γ treatment blocks signaling through PDGFRβ by enhancing agonist PDGF-BB	[26]
5	Drug-resistant TLE (microarray analysis)	human	• TGFβ1 decreased pericyte proliferation and decreased phagocytosis • TGFβ1 also upregulates the expression of IL-6, MMP-2, and NOX4, which disrupt the function of the BBB, and these responses to TGFβ1 may not be therapeutic for the neurovascular system	[27]

Table 2. Cont.

No.	Patients/Model	Species	Key Findings	Reference
6	Dynamics of NG2 mural cells under SE with systemic KA injection in mice	Mice	• NG2 mural cells are added and removed from veins, arterioles, and capillaries after status epilepticus • Loss of NG2 mural cells is proportional to seizure severity and vascular pathology (e.g., rigidity, perfusion, and permeability) • Treatment with PDGF-BB reduced NG2 mural cell loss, vascular pathology, and epileptiform electroencephalogram activity	[28]
7	TLE with or without HS, FCD	Humans	• Pericyte-microglia assemblies with IBA1/HLA microglial cells outlining the capillary wall were observed in TLE-HS and FCD-IIb specimens • Proinflammatory cytokines such as IL-1β cause morphological changes and IL-6 causes cell damage in human-derived pericytes	[29]
	NG2DsRed/C57BL6 (unilateral intra-hippocampal KA injections)	Mice	• IL-1β elicited pericyte morphological changes and pericyte-microglia clustering in NG2DsRed hippocampal slices	
8	NG2DsRed/C57BL6 (unilateral intra-hippocampal KA injections)	Mice	• Multicellular scarring occurs at the outer capillary wall in the hippocampus during seizure progression • PDGFRβ stromal cells and collagens III and IV participate in the localized pericyte-glial scarring and capillary pathology in hippocampal subregions • PDGFRβ is a proposed anti-inflammatory entry point for chronic disease stages in vivo	[30]
9	Transgenic mice (4-aminopyridine or low-Mg^{2+} conditions)	Mice	• Pericytes regulate changes in vascular diameter in response to neuronal activity • Recurrent seizures are associated with impaired neurovascular coupling and increased BBB permeability in capillaries • Recurrent seizures lead to depolarization of pericytic mitochondria and subsequent vasoconstriction	[31]
10	Traumatic brain injury model (C57BL/6J mice with CCI and pilocarpine injections)	Mice	• PDGFRβ levels were increased from 1 h to 4 days after CCI in the injured ipsilateral hippocampus prior to increased expression of markers of microglia and astrocytes; this supports the postulated role of pericytes as initiators of the CNS immune response • Treatment with imatinib on postoperative days 0–4 reduced seizure susceptibility, demonstrating the usefulness of imatinib in vitro	[32]

CCI, controlled cortical impact; FCD, focal cortical dysplasia, HS, hippocampal sclerosis; IP, intraperitoneal; KA, kainic acid; PDGF-BB, platelet-derived growth factor-beta subunit; SE, status epilepticus; TBI, traumatic brain injury; TLE, temporal lobe epilepsy.

5. Blood-Brain Barrier Disruption in the Pathogenesis of Epilepsy

Experimental evidence of BBB impairment in the pathogenesis of epilepsy has been demonstrated in patients and animal models [64–67], which is a hallmark of epilepsy. BBB disruption can also directly induce seizure activity and exacerbate epileptogenesis; the relationship between epilepsy and BBB breakdown is bidirectional [64,65].

BBB dysfunction and subsequent infiltration of serum albumin into the brain leads to changes in epileptogenesis, including astrocyte changes, neuroinflammation, excitatory synapse formation, and pathological plasticity [68,69]. These BBB alterations are not only due to leakage, as demonstrated by Evans Blue staining [65]. There is involvement of various inflammatory mediators as nondisruptive changes at the molecular level of pericytes are also involved in the changes of the BBB; specifically, they secrete various mediators as follows: IL-1β, TNF-α, IFN-γ, matrix metalloproteinases (MMPs), ROS/reactive nitrogen species (RNS), (NO), and prostaglandin E2 (PGE2). Pericyte-derived MMP-9 upregulation in the cerebral microvasculature can cause endothelial dysfunction through degradation of tight junctions and extracellular matrices, resulting in subsequent pericyte loss from the microvasculature and BBB disruption [11,43]. Moreover, the secretion of ROS/RNS, NO, and PGE2 lead to vasodilation and breaching of the BBB [9]. Epileptic seizures can cause pericytes surrounding the blood vessels to rearrange [2] and morphologically alter, which is facilitated by the inflammatory mediators [29,30]. These series of alterations are thought to be linked to the pathogenesis of epilepsy, although further details are warranted.

6. Leukocyte Recruitment and Peripheral-to-Central Infiltration

Pericytes regulate the migration of leukocytes across the BMVEC barrier and secrete key molecules that support the BBB [17,18]. Chemokines (CCL2, CXCL1, CXCL8, and CXCL10) secreted by pericytes in both basal and inflammatory states recruit peripheral immune cells, including monocytes, B and T cells, and neutrophils, to the CNS parenchyma via upregulation of intercellular adhesion molecule-1 (ICAM-1) and vascular cell adhesion molecule-1 (VCAM-1) on the endothelium [7–9,70]. Although the human brain is considered an immune-privileged area [68,71], this is not preserved during inflammatory conditions. Analysis of brain parenchyma in patients with epilepsy showed that there have been both positive [72,73] and negative [74] reports on the occurrence of infiltration of peripheral leukocytes into the brain tissue. Recent experimental research demonstrated that peripheral-to-CNS cell infiltration, particularly monocytes, occurs in the status epilepticus (SE) model, without evidence of infections or immune disorders [20,75,76]. The possibility of classifying peripheral monocytes and indigenous microglia, which have been considered difficult to differentiate, has been increased using genetic engineering [75,77,78].

In chemokine receptor 2 (CCR2)-knockout mice, the CCL2 receptor, which blocks peripheral monocyte invasion into the brain tissue, attenuated neuronal damage in SE models [75]. Analysis of the brain tissue from pediatric patients with drug-resistant epilepsy (DRE) revealed that seizure frequency was correlated with the number of infiltrating peripherally activated CD3+ T cells and monocytes, but not microglia [19]. Current analysis of pediatric patients with DRE also demonstrated a correlation between the number of seizures and intracellular IL-1β levels in monocytes [79], while experimental data and human research attributed seizure-induced neuronal death to the activation of resident microglia [78,80]. Whether the peripheral monocytes or the resident microglia are the primary triggers of epilepsy, as well as the extent to which the infiltrated cells are significant, remains to be determined; nevertheless, the combination of the roles of the pericytes in maintaining the BBB integrity, producing inflammatory mediators, and recruiting leukocytes indicate that the pericytes could be intimately involved in the pathogenesis of epilepsy.

7. Clinical Evidence Links Pericytes to Epilepsy

The disarray of the pericyte-basal lamina interface in patients with epilepsy was first described in 1990 [63]. Evidence of pericyte degeneration with basement membrane unit thickness and cytoplasmic density has also been reported in most of the spiking area microvessels in human brain tissues of intractable complex partial seizures using an electron microscope [63].

With the advent of PDGFRβ, though a nonspecific CNS pericyte marker, the immunostaining reports of the presence of PDGFRβ+ cells have emerged in the brain specimens of patients with intractable epilepsy in focal cortical dysplasia (FCD) and temporal lobe seizures (TLE) [2,25,29]. In tissues from patients with refractory TLE and hippocampal sclerosis (HS), the presence of PDGFRβ+ cells associated with blood vessels and parenchyma was observed, although findings were heterogenous [2]. Indeed, the highest perivascular PDGFRβ immunoreactivity was detected in patients with TLE-HS, specifically in the microvasculature [2]. Tissue from patients with cryptogenic epilepsy has exhibited a similar immune response pattern, although to a lesser extent than that of FCD. Increased perivascular PDGFRβ immunoreactivity was associated with increased hippocampal vascularization in the cells of patients with TLE-HS [25].

Another study of TLE and FCD specimens revealed robust PDGFRβ-positive cell pericyte immunoreactivity surrounding the blood vessels, particularly in TLE with HS specimens, with aggregation of IBA1/HLA microglial cells and pericyte-microglia outlining the capillary wall [29]. The morphological changes in pericytes were induced by proinflammatory cytokines, including IL-1β, TNFα, and IL-6; in particular, IL-6 exposure was drastically associated with apoptosis, suggesting pericyte damage [29].

Collectively, the accumulation of pericytes (PDGFRβ-positive cells) in the cerebral vascular regions was consistently observed in patients with refractory epilepsy [2,25,29]. The degree of accumulation correlates to some extent with the clinical picture [25,29], and morphological changes of the pericytes might be due to proinflammatory cytokines [29]. In addition, the amount of angiogenesis, which is associated with epileptogenesis, was related to the number of PDGFRβ-positive cells [25], suggesting a relationship between PDGFRβ-positive cells and the pathogenesis of epilepsy.

8. Experimental Evidence Links Pericytes to Epilepsy

An in vivo study of NG2DsRed mice, which enabled the visualization of cerebrovascular pericytes, revealed heterogeneous perivascular prominence of NG2DsRed cells with PDGFRβ expression in an SE model induced by intraperitoneal kainic acid (KA) [2]. These heterogeneous perivascular patterns of PDGFRβ+ cells are inconsistent with the aforementioned human tissue findings [2,25,29], which have also been observed in a rat model of neurovascular dysplasia SE, particularly in the hippocampus with a neurovascular dysplasia SE rat model [25].

An in vitro and in vivo study by Milesi et al. demonstrated that the parenchymal and vascular PDGFRβ+ cells were redistributed, alongside partial colocalization of vascular and parenchymal PDGFRβ+ cells with NG2DsRed and NG2, but not with IBA-1 [2]. These findings, suggesting that the accumulation of pericytes and microglia is associated with epileptic seizure events, have been documented in recent studies [29,30].

Klement et al. employed a model of TLE (associated with HS) in NG2DsRed mice to assess the impact of seizure progression on capillary pericytes and surrounding glial cells [29]. In vivo, SE mice presenting with spontaneous recurrent seizures (SRS) exhibited disorganized NG2DsRed-positive pericyte somata in the hippocampus at 72 h and 1 week after SE (epileptogenesis) in the hippocampus. Pericyte modifications clustered with IBA1-positive microglia, surrounding capillaries, and overlapped topographically with pericytes lodged within microglial cells [29]. Residual microglial clustering was also observed surrounding NG2DsRed pericytes in SRS, proinflammatory mediators, such as IL-1β, IL-6, TNF-α, and particularly IL-1β; however, the in vitro study in humans revealed that IL-6 induced these morphological changes of pericyte-microglia clustering in NG2DsRed hippocampal slices [29]. In addition, Klement et al. also reported a pericyte-glia perivascular scar with capillary leaks in the hippocampus during seizure activity. These scars in the cornu ammonis region developed an abnormal distribution or accumulation of extracellular matrix collagen III/IV as the seizure progressed [30]. In vitro experiments induced by 4-aminopyridine and low-Mg^{2+} conditions repeated seizures that cause vasoconstriction associated with the depolarization of mitochondria in pericytes and gradual neurovascular disconnection, suggesting that the pericyte damage causes vascular dysfunction in epilepsy [31]. The gradual progression of neurovascular decoupling during recurrent seizures suggests that pericyte damage induces vascular dysfunction in epilepsy (Figure 3) [31].

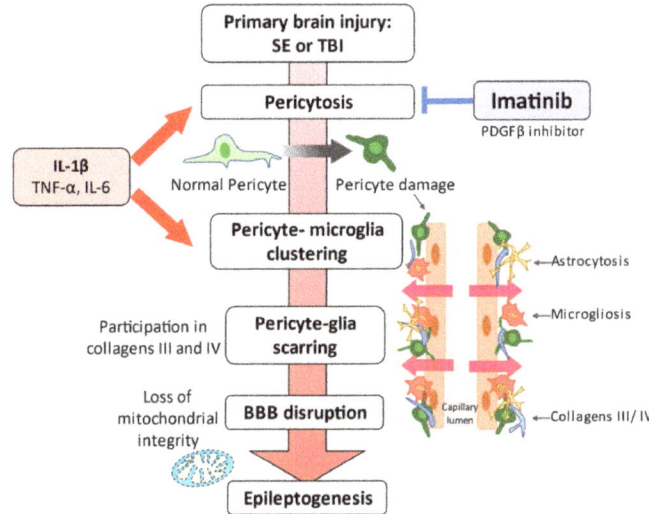

Figure 3. Schematic representation of the events linking pericytes to epilepsy. Status epilepticus leads to redistribution and remodeling of cerebrovascular pericytes, potentially contributing to blood–brain barrier permeability [2,28,29]. A significant clustering of microglia/macrophages around pericytes occurs one week after the attack, although pericyte proliferation is significantly increased as early as 72 h [29]. These series of pericyte-related modifications are promoted by proinflammatory cytokines, including IL-1β, TNFα, and IL-6. Alterations caused by IL-1β, which is one of the cytokines most deeply involved in the pathogenesis of epilepsy, were most pronounced. These pericyte-associated modifications and pericyte-microglia clustering may be facilitated by IL-1β [29], and pericyte-glial scarring with collagens III and IV process leaky capillaries during seizure progression [30]. Recurrent seizures can lead to pericytic injury with neurovascular decoupling and BBB dysfunction at the arterial and capillary levels. Moreover, capillary vasoconstriction is accompanied by a loss of mitochondrial integrity in pericytes [81]. In vitro and in vivo studies have highlighted the potential of pericytes as a therapeutic target for seizure disorders [28,30,32].

9. Prospects for Pericyte-Mediated Epilepsy Therapy

PDGFRβ can regulate pericyte survival, proliferation, and migration signals and is commonly used as a marker for pericytes [40]; PDGFRβ suppression has been proposed as a possible treatment for epilepsy [28,30,32].

As described above, a pericyte-glia perivascular scar with capillary leaks induced by seizures and a high expression of PDGFRβ transcript and protein levels were detected [30]. In the organotypic hippocampal cultures, PDGFRβ reactivity surrounding capillaries is also enhanced by electrographic activity and was reduced by PDGF-BB (a PDGFRβ agonist) and PDGFβ inhibitor imatinib [30]. Furthermore, PDGF-BB can reduce mural cell loss, vascular pathology, and epileptiform electroencephalography activity in a KA-induced SE model [28]. Recently, traumatic brain injury (TBI) has been highlighted as a major factor in epilepsy owing to certain intractable cases. The evaluation of the involvement of pericytes in the pathogenesis of epilepsy was performed using a controlled cortical impact (CCI) device. PDGFRβ levels were significantly increased following CCI in the injured ipsilateral hippocampus; pilocarpine-induced seizures can be regulated by imatinib treatment in this CCI model [32]. The efficacy of imatinib was also observed in vitro.

The findings from both in vitro and in vivo studies highlight the potential of pericytes as a therapeutic target for seizure disorders, as indicated by the efficacy of PDGF-BB and imatinib in blocking PDGFRβ. However, both PDGFRβ and PDGF-BB are required for the pericyte coating of the BBB in the developing CNS [38,41]. Under pathological conditions, mural cells in the immediate postacute phase (SE, ischemic stroke, and head trauma) require support from the PDGFRβ activation [28]; hence, the inflammatory involvement of PDGFRβ may be relevant in long-term progression as well as in chronic stages.

When considering the pharmacological modulation of pericyte signaling pathways as a means of attenuating disease progression and capillary pathology, the impact of pericyte modulation in the epileptic brain must consider the activation state of the glial cells and the disease stage (e.g., acute vs. chronic) [29]. Further, considering the distinct functions of PDGFRβ at different developmental stages, the timing of PDGFRβ inhibition needs to be carefully studied; moreover, avoiding imatinib in the acute phase of the disease may be considered. It remains debatable whether the changes in pericytes and accumulation of microglia associated with PDGFR expression in this series of studies should be suppressed.

Transforming growth factor-beta 1 (TGFβ1) is a multifaceted cytokine in the brain that plays a role in regulating cell proliferation, differentiation, survival, and scar formation [82,83]. Since 1989, the possibility of PDGF-induced TGF-β signaling has been suggested [84]; PDGFR-β and TGF-β with PDGFR-β might mediate the endothelial cell/pericyte interaction to protect the BBB integrity [33]. The potential involvement of TGF-β in epileptogenesis has been recognized from an experimental model showing TGF-β upregulation as part of the inflammatory response [85]. Microarray analysis of TGFβ1-stimulated human brain pericytes isolated from intractable TLE demonstrated inhibition of pericyte proliferation and phagocytosis by TGFβ1 [27]. However, TGFβ1 also enhanced the expression of IL-6, MMP-2, and NOX4, which can disrupt BBB functioning; thus, these reactions caused by TGFβ1 might not lead to the treatment of the neurovascular system [27].

Although the brain pericyte-derived TGF-β contributes to the upregulation of BBB functions [86], suppression of TGFβ1 indicates improvement in epilepsy [87]. Losartan, an angiotensin-type 1 receptor (AT1) antagonist, prevents phosphorylation of Smad proteins of TGF-β signaling [88,89], which has demonstrated both neuroprotective and antineuroinflammatory effects [90–92].

These in vitro studies also suggest that human-derived pericytes are morphologically altered by proinflammatory cytokines that induce apoptosis [29], indicating the potential of targeting IFN-γ for pericyte-mediated epilepsy treatment [26]. IFN-γ is a central component of the CNS inflammatory response and is secreted by microglia, astrocytes, endothelial cells, and circulating immune cells [93–95]. This classical inflammatory mediator has been implicated in CNS diseases, including epilepsy [96,97]. Altering the proportion of microglial phenotypes via IFN-γ treatment improved the prognosis in a mouse model of epilepsy [98].

Notably, in epileptiform conditions, IL-1β, a neurotoxic cytokine and one of the cytokines chiefly involved in the pathogenesis of epilepsy, prominently contributes to the morphological changes in the pericytes [29]. There is evidence that the IL-1/IL-1R1 axis plays an important role in the inflammatory response in epilepsy, as presented by Vezzani et al. in an excellent review [4,99]. IL-1β agonist, the IL-1 receptor antagonist (IL-1RA), has already been tested for clinical application for epileptic syndromes using anakinra, and has shown favorable clinical outcomes [100–103]. The use of anakinra on pericytes in status epilepticus has not yet been investigated. To ensure the involvement of pericytes in epilepsy, it is worthwhile to confirm that anakinra suppresses the morphological changes in pericytes and reduces seizures.

Previous reports have demonstrated that inhibition of pericytes could have positive effects of neuroprotection [26,28,30,32]; however, there is also a concern that the suppression of pericytes by TGFβ1 may not necessarily have a positive effect on the CNS [27]. Since TGFβ1 suppresses pericyte phagocytosis and reduces the expression of central leukocyte trafficking chemokines and adhesion molecules while increasing the expression of proinflammatory cytokines and enzymes that promote BBB disruption, a paradoxical reaction has been reported [27]. The TGFβ1 response of pericytes may differ from the anti-inflammatory response of microglia [104–107]; therefore, further studies are required to obtain any effect on this nonuniform response.

In the pathogenesis of epilepsy, pericytes adopt a phenotype that is neither solely pro- nor anti-inflammatory [27]. Merely suppressing pericytes may not be sufficient to improve the treatment of epilepsy, and it may be necessary to seek a treatment tailored to the affected child in combination with various therapies that have been introduced in recent reviews [108].

10. Conclusions

In this review, we present evidence for the substantive role of pericytes in the pathogenesis of epilepsy. The roles of pericytes in maintaining BBB integrity, producing inflammatory secretions, and recruiting leukocytes highlights the potential role of pericytes in the pathogenesis of epilepsy. Pericytes may also act as sensors of inflammatory processes in the CNS and regulating them may lead to the development of novel therapies for epilepsy. However, as there remains a lack of absolute molecular markers for pericytes, and since pericytes originate from multiple cellular sources and vary in morphology, localization as well as function in different tissues leaves several issues to be addressed. In addition, we are unable to determine whether brain inflammation is an initiator or a consequence of a systemic inflammatory process.

Several reports have suggested entry points that may also act as a basis for various neurovascular therapies, including anakinra [100,101] and losartan [87], though the level of evidence for both drugs is limited for the establishment of treatment for epilepsy. These drugs provide an avenue for novel therapeutic, anti-inflammatory, or cerebrovascular repair to mitigate epileptic pathophysiology. Unfortunately, definitive treatments for epilepsy are currently lacking. BBB integrity and systemic peripheral inflammation may contribute to epilepsy and hold potential for molecular biomarkers and targets in the treatment of epilepsy. Moreover, human pluripotent stem cell-derived brain pericyte-like cells induced BBB properties in BMECs, resulting in strengthening of the barrier and a reduction in transcytosis [109]. These stem cell techniques could be applied to examine the possibility of new strategies to selectively target pericytes and the role of pericytes in epilepsy more specifically. Novel tools to control pericytes should be developed to target inflammatory vascular-related processes during seizure progression or activity.

Author Contributions: Conceptualization, G.Y.; investigation, K.K. and S.M.; writing—original draft preparation, G.Y.; writing—review and editing, F.T.; visualization, S.D.; supervision, Y.K. and H.K. All authors have read and agreed to the published version of the manuscript.

Funding: This study was funded by the Kawano Masanori Memorial Foundation for Promotion of Pediatrics in Japan under grant number 30-7 and the Japan Epilepsy Research Foundation under grant number 20012. APC funded by the Japan Epilepsy Research Foundation.

Institutional Review Board Statement: We confirm that we have read the journal's position on the issues associated with ethical publication and affirm that this report is consistent with these guidelines.

Informed Consent Statement: Not applicable.

Data Availability Statement: The datasets generated and/or analyzed during the current study are available at the PubMed database repository (https://pubmed.ncbi.nlm.nih.gov/, accessed on 31 May 2021).

Conflicts of Interest: The authors declare no conflict of interest.

References

1. Vezzani, A.; Balosso, S.; Ravizza, T. The role of cytokines in the pathophysiology of epilepsy. *Brain. Behav. Immun.* **2008**, *22*, 797–803. [CrossRef] [PubMed]
2. Milesi, S.; Boussadia, B.; Plaud, C.; Catteau, M.; Rousset, M.C.; De Bock, F.; Schaeffer, M.; Lerner-Natoli, M.; Rigau, V.; Marchi, N. Redistribution of PDGFRβ cells and NG2DsRed pericytes at the cerebrovasculature after status epilepticus. *Neurobiol. Dis.* **2014**, *71*, 151–158. [CrossRef]

3. Marchi, N.; Banjara, M.; Janigro, D. Blood-brain barrier, bulk flow, and interstitial clearance in epilepsy. *J. Neurosci. Methods* **2016**, *260*, 118–124. [CrossRef]
4. Vezzani, A.; Balosso, S.; Ravizza, T. Neuroinflammatory pathways as treatment targets and biomarkers in epilepsy. *Nat. Rev. Neurol.* **2019**, *15*, 459–472. [CrossRef] [PubMed]
5. Löscher, W.; Friedman, A. Structural, Molecular, and Functional Alterations of the Blood-Brain Barrier during Epileptogenesis and Epilepsy: A Cause, Consequence, or Both? *Int. J. Mol. Sci.* **2020**, *21*, 591. [CrossRef]
6. Nishibori, M.; Wang, D.; Ousaka, D.; Wake, H. High Mobility Group Box-1 and Blood-Brain Barrier Disruption. *Cells* **2020**, *9*, 2650. [CrossRef] [PubMed]
7. Kovac, A.; Erickson, M.A.; Banks, W.A. Brain microvascular pericytes are immunoactive in culture: Cytokine, chemokine, nitric oxide, and LRP-1 expression in response to lipopolysaccharide. *J. Neuroinflamm.* **2011**, *8*, 139. [CrossRef] [PubMed]
8. Jansson, D.; Rustenhoven, J.; Feng, S.; Hurley, D.; Oldfield, R.L.; Bergin, P.S.; Mee, E.W.; Faull, R.L.; Dragunow, M. A role for human brain pericytes in neuroinflammation. *J. Neuroinflamm.* **2014**, *11*, 104. [CrossRef] [PubMed]
9. Matsumoto, J.; Takata, F.; Machida, T.; Takahashi, H.; Soejima, Y.; Funakoshi, M.; Futagami, K.; Yamauchi, A.; Dohgu, S.; Kataoka, Y. Tumor necrosis factor-α-stimulated brain pericytes possess a unique cytokine and chemokine release profile and enhance microglial activation. *Neurosci. Lett.* **2014**, *578*, 133–138. [CrossRef] [PubMed]
10. Rustenhoven, J.; Jansson, D.; Smyth, L.C.; Dragunow, M. Brain Pericytes as Mediators of Neuroinflammation. *Trends Pharmacol. Sci.* **2017**, *38*, 291–304. [CrossRef]
11. Takata, F.; Dohgu, S.; Matsumoto, J.; Takahashi, H.; Machida, T.; Wakigawa, T.; Harada, E.; Miyaji, H.; Koga, M.; Nishioka, T.; et al. Brain pericytes among cells constituting the blood-brain barrier are highly sensitive to tumor necrosis factor-α, releasing matrix metalloproteinase-9 and migrating in vitro. *J. Neuroinflamm.* **2011**, *8*, 106. [CrossRef]
12. Machida, T.; Takata, F.; Matsumoto, J.; Takenoshita, H.; Kimura, I.; Yamauchi, A.; Dohgu, S.; Kataoka, Y. Brain pericytes are the most thrombin-sensitive matrix metalloproteinase-9-releasing cell type constituting the blood-brain barrier in vitro. *Neurosci. Lett.* **2015**, *599*, 109–114. [CrossRef]
13. Matsumoto, J.; Dohgu, S.; Takata, F.; Machida, T.; Bölükbaşi Hatip, F.F.; Hatip-Al-Khatib, I.; Yamauchi, A.; Kataoka, Y. TNF-α-sensitive brain pericytes activate microglia by releasing IL-6 through cooperation between IκB-NFκB and JAK-STAT3 pathways. *Brain Res.* **2018**, *1692*, 34–44. [CrossRef] [PubMed]
14. Armulik, A.; Genové, G.; Mäe, M.; Nisancioglu, M.H.; Wallgard, E.; Niaudet, C.; He, L.; Norlin, J.; Lindblom, P.; Strittmatter, K.; et al. Pericytes regulate the blood-brain barrier. *Nature* **2010**, *468*, 557–561. [CrossRef] [PubMed]
15. Armulik, A.; Genové, G.; Betsholtz, C. Pericytes: Developmental, physiological, and pathological perspectives, problems, and promises. *Dev. Cell* **2011**, *21*, 193–215. [CrossRef] [PubMed]
16. Sweeney, M.D.; Zhao, Z.; Montagne, A.; Nelson, A.R.; Zlokovic, B.V. Blood-Brain Barrier: From Physiology to Disease and Back. *Physiol. Rev.* **2019**, *99*, 21–78. [CrossRef]
17. Winkler, E.A.; Bell, R.D.; Zlokovic, B.V. Central nervous system pericytes in health and disease. *Nat. Neurosci.* **2011**, *14*, 1398–1405. [CrossRef]
18. Stark, K.; Eckart, A.; Haidari, S.; Tirniceriu, A.; Lorenz, M.; von Brühl, M.L.; Gärtner, F.; Khandoga, A.G.; Legate, K.R.; Pless, R.; et al. Capillary and arteriolar pericytes attract innate leukocytes exiting through venules and 'instruct' them with pattern-recognition and motility programs. *Nat. Immunol.* **2013**, *14*, 41–51. [CrossRef]
19. Xu, D.; Robinson, A.P.; Ishii, T.; Duncan, D.S.; Alden, T.D.; Goings, G.E.; Ifergan, I.; Podojil, J.R.; Penaloza-MacMaster, P.; Kearney, J.A.; et al. Peripherally derived T regulatory and gammadelta T cells have opposing roles in the pathogenesis of intractable pediatric epilepsy. *J. Exp. Med.* **2018**, *215*, 1169–1186. [CrossRef] [PubMed]
20. Yamanaka, G.; Morichi, S.; Takamatsu, T.; Watanabe, Y.; Suzuki, S.; Ishida, Y.; Oana, S.; Yamazaki, T.; Takata, F.; Kawashima, H. Links between Immune Cells from the Periphery and the Brain in the Pathogenesis of Epilepsy: A Narrative Review. *Int. J. Mol. Sci.* **2021**, *22*, 4395. [CrossRef]
21. Fernández-Klett, F.; Potas, J.R.; Hilpert, D.; Blazej, K.; Radke, J.; Huck, J.; Engel, O.; Stenzel, W.; Genové, G.; Priller, J. Early loss of pericytes and perivascular stromal cell-induced scar formation after stroke. *J. Cereb. Blood Flow Metab.* **2013**, *33*, 428–439. [CrossRef]
22. Göritz, C.; Dias, D.O.; Tomilin, N.; Barbacid, M.; Shupliakov, O.; Frisén, J. A pericyte origin of spinal cord scar tissue. *Science* **2011**, *333*, 238–242. [CrossRef]
23. Reeves, C.; Pradim-Jardim, A.; Sisodiya, S.M.; Thom, M.; Liu, J.Y.W. Spatiotemporal dynamics of PDGFRβ expression in pericytes and glial scar formation in penetrating brain injuries in adults. *Neuropathol. Appl. Neurobiol.* **2019**, *45*, 609–627. [CrossRef]
24. Rivera, F.J.; Hinrichsen, B.; Silva, M.E. Pericytes in Multiple Sclerosis. *Adv. Exp. Med. Biol.* **2019**, *1147*, 167–187. [CrossRef] [PubMed]
25. Garbelli, R.; de Bock, F.; Medici, V.; Rousset, M.C.; Villani, F.; Boussadia, B.; Arango-Lievano, M.; Jeanneteau, F.; Daneman, R.; Bartolomei, F.; et al. PDGFRβ(+) cells in human and experimental neuro-vascular dysplasia and seizures. *Neuroscience* **2015**, *306*, 18–27. [CrossRef]
26. Jansson, D.; Scotter, E.L.; Rustenhoven, J.; Coppieters, N.; Smyth, L.C.; Oldfield, R.L.; Bergin, P.S.; Mee, E.W.; Graham, E.S.; Faull, R.L.; et al. Interferon-γ blocks signalling through PDGFRβ in human brain pericytes. *J. Neuroinflamm.* **2016**, *13*, 249. [CrossRef] [PubMed]

27. Rustenhoven, J.; Aalderink, M.; Scotter, E.L.; Oldfield, R.L.; Bergin, P.S.; Mee, E.W.; Graham, E.S.; Faull, R.L.; Curtis, M.A.; Park, T.I.; et al. TGF-beta1 regulates human brain pericyte inflammatory processes involved in neurovasculature function. *J. Neuroinflamm.* **2016**, *13*, 37. [CrossRef]
28. Arango-Lievano, M.; Boussadia, B.; De Terdonck, L.D.T.; Gault, C.; Fontanaud, P.; Lafont, C.; Mollard, P.; Marchi, N.; Jeanneteau, F. Topographic Reorganization of Cerebrovascular Mural Cells under Seizure Conditions. *Cell Rep.* **2018**, *23*, 1045–1059. [CrossRef]
29. Klement, W.; Garbelli, R.; Zub, E.; Rossini, L.; Tassi, L.; Girard, B.; Blaquiere, M.; Bertaso, F.; Perroy, J.; de Bock, F.; et al. Seizure progression and inflammatory mediators promote pericytosis and pericyte-microglia clustering at the cerebrovasculature. *Neurobiol. Dis.* **2018**, *113*, 70–81. [CrossRef]
30. Klement, W.; Blaquiere, M.; Zub, E.; deBock, F.; Boux, F.; Barbier, E.; Audinat, E.; Lerner-Natoli, M.; Marchi, N. A pericyte-glia scarring develops at the leaky capillaries in the hippocampus during seizure activity. *Epilepsia* **2019**, *60*, 1399–1411. [CrossRef] [PubMed]
31. Prager, O.; Kamintsky, L.; Hasam-Henderson, L.A.; Schoknecht, K.; Wuntke, V.; Papageorgiou, I.; Swolinsky, J.; Muoio, V.; Bar-Klein, G.; Vazana, U.; et al. Seizure-induced microvascular injury is associated with impaired neurovascular coupling and blood-brain barrier dysfunction. *Epilepsia* **2019**, *60*, 322–336. [CrossRef] [PubMed]
32. Sakai, K.; Takata, F.; Yamanaka, G.; Yasunaga, M.; Hashiguchi, K.; Tominaga, K.; Itoh, K.; Kataoka, Y.; Yamauchi, A.; Dohgu, S. Reactive pericytes in early phase are involved in glial activation and late-onset hypersusceptibility to pilocarpine-induced seizures in traumatic brain injury model mice. *J. Pharmacol. Sci.* **2021**, *145*, 155–165. [CrossRef]
33. Sweeney, M.D.; Ayyadurai, S.; Zlokovic, B.V. Pericytes of the neurovascular unit: Key functions and signaling pathways. *Nat. Neurosci.* **2016**, *19*, 771–783. [CrossRef]
34. Cheng, J.; Korte, N.; Nortley, R.; Sethi, H.; Tang, Y.; Attwell, D. Targeting pericytes for therapeutic approaches to neurological disorders. *Acta Neuropathol.* **2018**, *136*, 507–523. [CrossRef]
35. Rouget, C. Note sur le developpement de la tunique contractile des vaisseaux. *C. R. L'académie Sci.* **1874**, *59*, 559–562.
36. Zimmermann, K.W. Der feinere bau der blutcapillares. *Z. Anat. Entwicklungsgesch.* **1923**, *68*, 3–109. [CrossRef]
37. Ando, K.; Fukuhara, S.; Izumi, N.; Nakajima, H.; Fukui, H.; Kelsh, R.N.; Mochizuki, N. Clarification of mural cell coverage of vascular endothelial cells by live imaging of zebrafish. *Development* **2016**, *143*, 1328–1339. [CrossRef] [PubMed]
38. Winkler, E.A.; Bell, R.D.; Zlokovic, B.V. Pericyte-specific expression of PDGF beta receptor in mouse models with normal and deficient PDGF beta receptor signaling. *Mol. Neurodegen.* **2010**, *5*, 32. [CrossRef] [PubMed]
39. Thomsen, M.S.; Routhe, L.J.; Moos, T. The vascular basement membrane in the healthy and pathological brain. *J. Cereb. Blood Flow Metab.* **2017**, *37*, 3300–3317. [CrossRef] [PubMed]
40. Hellström, M.; Kalén, M.; Lindahl, P.; Abramsson, A.; Betsholtz, C. Role of PDGF-B and PDGFR-beta in recruitment of vascular smooth muscle cells and pericytes during embryonic blood vessel formation in the mouse. *Development* **1999**, *126*, 3047–3055. [CrossRef]
41. Lindahl, P.; Johansson, B.R.; Levéen, P.; Betsholtz, C. Pericyte loss and microaneurysm formation in PDGF-B-deficient mice. *Science* **1997**, *277*, 242–245. [CrossRef]
42. Nikolakopoulou, A.M.; Montagne, A.; Kisler, K.; Dai, Z.; Wang, Y.; Huuskonen, M.T.; Sagare, A.P.; Lazic, D.; Sweeney, M.D.; Kong, P.; et al. Pericyte loss leads to circulatory failure and pleiotrophin depletion causing neuron loss. *Nat. Neurosci.* **2019**, *22*, 1089–1098. [CrossRef]
43. Bhattacharya, A.; Kaushik, D.K.; Lozinski, B.M.; Yong, V.W. Beyond barrier functions: Roles of pericytes in homeostasis and regulation of neuroinflammation. *J. Neurosci. Res.* **2020**, *98*, 2390–2405. [CrossRef]
44. Vanlandewijck, M.; He, L.; Mäe, M.A.; Andrae, J.; Ando, K.; Del Gaudio, F.; Nahar, K.; Lebouvier, T.; Laviña, B.; Gouveia, L.; et al. A molecular atlas of cell types and zonation in the brain vasculature. *Nature* **2018**, *554*, 475–480. [CrossRef]
45. Attwell, D.; Mishra, A.; Hall, C.N.; O'Farrell, F.M.; Dalkara, T. What is a pericyte? *J. Cereb. Blood Flow Metab.* **2016**, *36*, 451–455. [CrossRef] [PubMed]
46. Marques, S.; van Bruggen, D.; Vanichkina, D.P.; Floriddia, E.M.; Munguba, H.; Väremo, L.; Giacomello, S.; Falcão, A.M.; Meijer, M.; Björklund, Å.K.; et al. Transcriptional Convergence of Oligodendrocyte Lineage Progenitors during Development. *Dev. Cell* **2018**, *46*, 504–517.e7. [CrossRef]
47. Bondjers, C.; He, L.; Takemoto, M.; Norlin, J.; Asker, N.; Hellström, M.; Lindahl, P.; Betsholtz, C. Microarray analysis of blood microvessels from PDGF-B and PDGF-Rbeta mutant mice identifies novel markers for brain pericytes. *FASEB J.* **2006**, *20*, 1703–1705. [CrossRef]
48. Iacobaeus, E.; Sugars, R.V.; Törnqvist Andrén, A.; Alm, J.J.; Qian, H.; Frantzen, J.; Newcombe, J.; Alkass, K.; Druid, H.; Bottai, M.; et al. Dynamic Changes in Brain Mesenchymal Perivascular Cells Associate with Multiple Sclerosis Disease Duration, Active Inflammation, and Demyelination. *Stem. Cells Transl. Med.* **2017**, *6*, 1840–1851. [CrossRef] [PubMed]
49. Zeisel, A.; Hochgerner, H.; Lönnerberg, P.; Johnsson, A.; Memic, F.; van der Zwan, J.; Häring, M.; Braun, E.; Borm, L.E.; La Manno, G.; et al. Molecular Architecture of the Mouse Nervous System. *Cell* **2018**, *174*, 999–1014.e22. [CrossRef]
50. Damisah, E.C.; Hill, R.A.; Tong, L.; Murray, K.N.; Grutzendler, J. A fluoro-Nissl dye identifies pericytes as distinct vascular mural cells during in vivo brain imaging. *Nat. Neurosci.* **2017**, *20*, 1023–1032. [CrossRef] [PubMed]
51. Sweeney, M.D.; Sagare, A.P.; Zlokovic, B.V. Blood-brain barrier breakdown in Alzheimer disease and other neurodegenerative disorders. *Nat. Rev. Neurol.* **2018**, *14*, 133–150. [CrossRef]

52. Navarro, R.; Compte, M.; Álvarez-Vallina, L.; Sanz, L. Immune Regulation by Pericytes: Modulating Innate and Adaptive Immunity. *Front. Immunol.* **2016**, *7*, 480. [CrossRef]
53. Nehmé, A.; Edelman, J. Dexamethasone inhibits high glucose-, TNF-alpha-, and IL-1beta-induced secretion of inflammatory and angiogenic mediators from retinal microvascular pericytes. *Investig. Ophthalmol. Vis. Sci.* **2008**, *49*, 2030–2038. [CrossRef]
54. Fabene, P.F.; Bramanti, P.; Constantin, G. The emerging role for chemokines in epilepsy. *J. Neuroimmunol.* **2010**, *224*, 22–27. [CrossRef] [PubMed]
55. Vezzani, A.; Aronica, E.; Mazarati, A.; Pittman, Q.J. Epilepsy and brain inflammation. *Exp. Neurol.* **2013**, *244*, 11–21. [CrossRef] [PubMed]
56. Glass, C.K.; Saijo, K.; Winner, B.; Marchetto, M.C.; Gage, F.H. Mechanisms underlying inflammation in neurodegeneration. *Cell* **2010**, *140*, 918–934. [CrossRef] [PubMed]
57. Kim, J.Y.; Kim, N.; Yenari, M.A. Mechanisms and potential therapeutic applications of microglial activation after brain injury. *CNS Neurosci. Ther.* **2015**, *21*, 309–319. [CrossRef]
58. Gutierrez, H.; Hale, V.A.; Dolcet, X.; Davies, A. NF-kappaB signalling regulates the growth of neural processes in the developing PNS and CNS. *Development* **2005**, *132*, 1713–1726. [CrossRef] [PubMed]
59. Bodnar, R.J.; Yang, T.; Rigatti, L.H.; Liu, F.; Evdokiou, A.; Kathju, S.; Satish, L. Pericytes reduce inflammation and collagen deposition in acute wounds. *Cytotherapy* **2018**, *20*, 1046–1060. [CrossRef]
60. Minutti, C.M.; Modak, R.V.; Macdonald, F.; Li, F.; Smyth, D.J.; Dorward, D.A.; Blair, N.; Husovsky, C.; Muir, A.; Giampazolias, E.; et al. A Macrophage-Pericyte Axis Directs Tissue Restoration via Amphiregulin-Induced Transforming Growth Factor Beta Activation. *Immunity* **2019**, *50*, 645–654.e6. [CrossRef]
61. Gaceb, A.; Özen, I.; Padel, T.; Barbariga, M.; Paul, G. Pericytes secrete pro-regenerative molecules in response to platelet-derived growth factor-BB. *J. Cereb. Blood Flow Metab.* **2018**, *38*, 45–57. [CrossRef]
62. Ishitsuka, K.; Ago, T.; Arimura, K.; Nakamura, K.; Tokami, H.; Makihara, N.; Kuroda, J.; Kamouchi, M.; Kitazono, T. Neurotrophin production in brain pericytes during hypoxia: A role of pericytes for neuroprotection. *Microvasc. Res.* **2012**, *83*, 352–359. [CrossRef] [PubMed]
63. Liwnicz, B.H.; Leach, J.L.; Yeh, H.S.; Privitera, M. Pericyte degeneration and thickening of basement membranes of cerebral microvessels in complex partial seizures: Electron microscopic study of surgically removed tissue. *Neurosurgery* **1990**, *26*, 409–420. [CrossRef]
64. Van Vliet, E.A.; da Costa Araújo, S.; Redeker, S.; van Schaik, R.; Aronica, E.; Gorter, J.A. Blood-brain barrier leakage may lead to progression of temporal lobe epilepsy. *Brain* **2007**, *130*, 521–534. [CrossRef]
65. Marchi, N.; Angelov, L.; Masaryk, T.; Fazio, V.; Granata, T.; Hernandez, N.; Hallene, K.; Diglaw, T.; Franic, L.; Najm, I.; et al. Seizure-promoting effect of blood-brain barrier disruption. *Epilepsia* **2007**, *48*, 732–742. [CrossRef]
66. Marchi, N.; Granata, T.; Ghosh, C.; Janigro, D. Blood-brain barrier dysfunction and epilepsy: Pathophysiologic role and therapeutic approaches. *Epilepsia* **2012**, *53*, 1877–1886. [CrossRef]
67. Uprety, A.; Kang, Y.; Kim, S.Y. Blood-brain barrier dysfunction as a potential therapeutic target for neurodegenerative disorders. *Arch. Pharm. Res.* **2021**, *44*, 487–498. [CrossRef] [PubMed]
68. Ivens, S.; Kaufer, D.; Flores, L.P.; Bechmann, I.; Zumsteg, D.; Tomkins, O.; Seiffert, E.; Heinemann, U.; Friedman, A. TGF-beta receptor-mediated albumin uptake into astrocytes is involved in neocortical epileptogenesis. *Brain* **2007**, *130*, 535–547. [CrossRef]
69. Weissberg, I.; Wood, L.; Kamintsky, L.; Vazquez, O.; Milikovsky, D.Z.; Alexander, A.; Oppenheim, H.; Ardizzone, C.; Becker, A.; Frigerio, F.; et al. Albumin induces excitatory synaptogenesis through astrocytic TGF-β/ALK5 signaling in a model of acquired epilepsy following blood-brain barrier dysfunction. *Neurobiol. Dis.* **2015**, *78*, 115–125. [CrossRef]
70. Pieper, C.; Marek, J.J.; Unterberg, M.; Schwerdtle, T.; Galla, H.J. Brain capillary pericytes contribute to the immune defense in response to cytokines or LPS in vitro. *Brain Res.* **2014**, *1550*, 1–8. [CrossRef] [PubMed]
71. Galea, I.; Bernardes-Silva, M.; Forse, P.A.; van Rooijen, N.; Liblau, R.S.; Perry, V.H. An antigen-specific pathway for CD8 T cells across the blood-brain barrier. *J. Exp. Med.* **2007**, *204*, 2023–2030. [CrossRef]
72. Fabene, P.F.; Mora, G.N.; Martinello, M.; Rossi, B.; Merigo, F.; Ottoboni, L.; Bach, S.; Angiari, S.; Benati, D.; Chakir, A.; et al. A role for leukocyte-endothelial adhesion mechanisms in epilepsy. *Nat. Med.* **2008**, *14*, 1377–1383. [CrossRef] [PubMed]
73. Ravizza, T.; Gagliardi, B.; Noe, F.; Boer, K.; Aronica, E.; Vezzani, A. Innate and adaptive immunity during epileptogenesis and spontaneous seizures: Evidence from experimental models and human temporal lobe epilepsy. *Neurobiol. Dis.* **2008**, *29*, 142–160. [CrossRef] [PubMed]
74. Marchi, N.; Teng, Q.; Ghosh, C.; Fan, Q.; Nguyen, M.T.; Desai, N.K.; Bawa, H.; Rasmussen, P.; Masaryk, T.K.; Janigro, D. Blood-brain barrier damage, but not parenchymal white blood cells, is a hallmark of seizure activity. *Brain Res.* **2010**, *1353*, 176–186. [CrossRef]
75. Varvel, N.H.; Neher, J.J.; Bosch, A.; Wang, W.; Ransohoff, R.M.; Miller, R.J.; Dingledine, R. Infiltrating monocytes promote brain inflammation and exacerbate neuronal damage after status epilepticus. *Proc. Natl. Acad. Sci. USA* **2016**, *113*, E5665–E5674. [CrossRef]
76. Broekaart, D.W.M.; Anink, J.J.; Baayen, J.C.; Idema, S.; de Vries, H.E.; Aronica, E.; Gorter, J.A.; van Vliet, E.A. Activation of the innate immune system is evident throughout epileptogenesis and is associated with blood-brain barrier dysfunction and seizure progression. *Epilepsia* **2018**, *59*, 1931–1944. [CrossRef] [PubMed]

77. Aronica, E.; Bauer, S.; Bozzi, Y.; Caleo, M.; Dingledine, R.; Gorter, J.A.; Henshall, D.C.; Kaufer, D.; Koh, S.; Loscher, W.; et al. Neuroinflammatory targets and treatments for epilepsy validated in experimental models. *Epilepsia* **2017**, *58* (Suppl. S3), 27–38. [CrossRef]
78. Feng, L.; Murugan, M.; Bosco, D.B.; Liu, Y.; Peng, J.; Worrell, G.A.; Wang, H.L.; Ta, L.E.; Richardson, J.R.; Shen, Y.; et al. Microglial proliferation and monocyte infiltration contribute to microgliosis following status epilepticus. *Glia* **2019**, *67*, 1434–1448. [CrossRef]
79. Yamanaka, G.; Takamatsu, T.; Morichi, S.; Yamazaki, T.; Mizoguchi, I.; Ohno, K.; Watanabe, Y.; Ishida, Y.; Oana, S.; Suzuki, S.; et al. Interleukin-1β in peripheral monocytes is associated with seizure frequency in pediatric drug-resistant epilepsy. *J. Neuroimmunol.* **2021**, *352*, 577475. [CrossRef] [PubMed]
80. Boer, K.; Spliet, W.G.; van Rijen, P.C.; Redeker, S.; Troost, D.; Aronica, E. Evidence of activated microglia in focal cortical dysplasia. *J. Neuroimmunol.* **2006**, *173*, 188–195. [CrossRef]
81. Swissa, E.; Serlin, Y.; Vazana, U.; Prager, O.; Friedman, A. Blood-brain barrier dysfunction in status epileptics: Mechanisms and role in epileptogenesis. *Epilepsy Behav.* **2019**, *101*, 106285. [CrossRef]
82. Logan, A.; Berry, M.; Gonzalez, A.M.; Frautschy, S.A.; Sporn, M.B.; Baird, A. Effects of transforming growth factor beta 1 on scar production in the injured central nervous system of the rat. *Eur. J. Neurosci.* **1994**, *6*, 355–363. [CrossRef] [PubMed]
83. Lindholm, D.; Castrén, E.; Kiefer, R.; Zafra, F.; Thoenen, H. Transforming growth factor-beta 1 in the rat brain: Increase after injury and inhibition of astrocyte proliferation. *J. Cell Biol.* **1992**, *117*, 395–400. [CrossRef] [PubMed]
84. Pierce, G.F.; Mustoe, T.A.; Lingelbach, J.; Masakowski, V.R.; Griffin, G.L.; Senior, R.M.; Deuel, T.F. Platelet-derived growth factor and transforming growth factor-beta enhance tissue repair activities by unique mechanisms. *J. Cell Biol.* **1989**, *109*, 429–440. [CrossRef]
85. Aronica, E.; van Vliet, E.A.; Mayboroda, O.A.; Troost, D.; da Silva, F.H.; Gorter, J.A. Upregulation of metabotropic glutamate receptor subtype mGluR3 and mGluR5 in reactive astrocytes in a rat model of mesial temporal lobe epilepsy. *Eur. J. Neurosci.* **2000**, *12*, 2333–2344. [CrossRef]
86. Dohgu, S.; Takata, F.; Yamauchi, A.; Nakagawa, S.; Egawa, T.; Naito, M.; Tsuruo, T.; Sawada, Y.; Niwa, M.; Kataoka, Y. Brain pericytes contribute to the induction and up-regulation of blood-brain barrier functions through transforming growth factor-beta production. *Brain Res.* **2005**, *1038*, 208–215. [CrossRef] [PubMed]
87. Bar-Klein, G.; Cacheaux, L.P.; Kamintsky, L.; Prager, O.; Weissberg, I.; Schoknecht, K.; Cheng, P.; Kim, S.Y.; Wood, L.; Heinemann, U.; et al. Losartan prevents acquired epilepsy via TGF-β signaling suppression. *Ann. Neurol.* **2014**, *75*, 864–875. [CrossRef] [PubMed]
88. Lim, D.S.; Lutucuta, S.; Bachireddy, P.; Youker, K.; Evans, A.; Entman, M.; Roberts, R.; Marian, A.J. Angiotensin II blockade reverses myocardial fibrosis in a transgenic mouse model of human hypertrophic cardiomyopathy. *Circulation* **2001**, *103*, 789–791. [CrossRef] [PubMed]
89. Lavoie, P.; Robitaille, G.; Agharazii, M.; Ledbetter, S.; Lebel, M.; Larivière, R. Neutralization of transforming growth factor-beta attenuates hypertension and prevents renal injury in uremic rats. *J. Hypertens.* **2005**, *23*, 1895–1903. [CrossRef]
90. Nadal, J.A.; Scicli, G.M.; Carbini, L.A.; Nussbaum, J.J.; Scicli, A.G. Angiotensin II and retinal pericytes migration. *Biochem. Biophys. Res. Commun.* **1999**, *266*, 382–385. [CrossRef] [PubMed]
91. Benicky, J.; Sánchez-Lemus, E.; Honda, M.; Pang, T.; Orecna, M.; Wang, J.; Leng, Y.; Chuang, D.M.; Saavedra, J.M. Angiotensin II AT1 receptor blockade ameliorates brain inflammation. *Neuropsychopharmacology* **2011**, *36*, 857–870. [CrossRef]
92. Bull, N.D.; Johnson, T.V.; Welsapar, G.; DeKorver, N.W.; Tomarev, S.I.; Martin, K.R. Use of an adult rat retinal explant model for screening of potential retinal ganglion cell neuroprotective therapies. *Investig. Ophthalmol. Vis. Sci.* **2011**, *52*, 3309–3320. [CrossRef]
93. Xiao, B.G.; Link, H. IFN-gamma production of adult rat astrocytes triggered by TNF-alpha. *Neuroreport* **1998**, *9*, 1487–1490. [CrossRef]
94. Wei, Y.P.; Kita, M.; Shinmura, K.; Yan, X.Q.; Fukuyama, R.; Fushiki, S.; Imanishi, J. Expression of IFN-gamma in cerebrovascular endothelial cells from aged mice. *J. Interferon Cytokine Res.* **2000**, *20*, 403–409. [CrossRef]
95. Lau, L.T.; Yu, A.C. Astrocytes produce and release interleukin-1, interleukin-6, tumor necrosis factor alpha and interferon-gamma following traumatic and metabolic injury. *J. Neurotrauma* **2001**, *18*, 351–359. [CrossRef]
96. Mount, M.P.; Lira, A.; Grimes, D.; Smith, P.D.; Faucher, S.; Slack, R.; Anisman, H.; Hayley, S.; Park, D.S. Involvement of interferon-gamma in microglial-mediated loss of dopaminergic neurons. *J. Neurosci.* **2007**, *27*, 3328–3337. [CrossRef] [PubMed]
97. Kreutzfeldt, M.; Bergthaler, A.; Fernandez, M.; Brück, W.; Steinbach, K.; Vorm, M.; Coras, R.; Blümcke, I.; Bonilla, W.V.; Fleige, A.; et al. Neuroprotective intervention by interferon-γ blockade prevents CD8+ T cell-mediated dendrite and synapse loss. *J. Exp. Med.* **2013**, *210*, 2087–2103. [CrossRef]
98. Li, T.; Zhai, X.; Jiang, J.; Song, X.; Han, W.; Ma, J.; Xie, L.; Cheng, L.; Chen, H.; Jiang, L. Intraperitoneal injection of IL-4/IFN-γ modulates the proportions of microglial phenotypes and improves epilepsy outcomes in a pilocarpine model of acquired epilepsy. *Brain Res.* **2017**, *1657*, 120–129. [CrossRef]
99. Vezzani, A.; French, J.; Bartfai, T.; Baram, T.Z. The role of inflammation in epilepsy. *Nat. Rev. Neurol.* **2011**, *7*, 31–40. [CrossRef] [PubMed]
100. Jyonouchi, H.; Geng, L. Intractable Epilepsy (IE) and Responses to Anakinra, a Human Recombinant IL-1 Receptor Agonist (IL-1ra): Case Reports. *J. Clin. Cell. Immunol.* **2016**, *7*. [CrossRef]

101. Kenney-Jung, D.L.; Vezzani, A.; Kahoud, R.J.; LaFrance-Corey, R.G.; Ho, M.L.; Muskardin, T.W.; Wirrell, E.C.; Howe, C.L.; Payne, E.T. Febrile infection-related epilepsy syndrome treated with anakinra. *Ann. Neurol.* **2016**, *80*, 939–945. [CrossRef]
102. Dilena, R.; Mauri, E.; Aronica, E.; Bernasconi, P.; Bana, C.; Cappelletti, C.; Carrabba, G.; Ferrero, S.; Giorda, R.; Guez, S.; et al. Therapeutic effect of Anakinra in the relapsing chronic phase of febrile infection-related epilepsy syndrome. *Epilepsia Open* **2019**, *4*, 344–350. [CrossRef] [PubMed]
103. Clarkson, B.D.S.; LaFrance-Corey, R.G.; Kahoud, R.J.; Farias-Moeller, R.; Payne, E.T.; Howe, C.L. Functional deficiency in endogenous interleukin-1 receptor antagonist in patients with febrile infection-related epilepsy syndrome. *Ann. Neurol.* **2019**, *85*, 526–537. [CrossRef]
104. Paglinawan, R.; Malipiero, U.; Schlapbach, R.; Frei, K.; Reith, W.; Fontana, A. TGFbeta directs gene expression of activated microglia to an anti-inflammatory phenotype strongly focusing on chemokine genes and cell migratory genes. *Glia* **2003**, *44*, 219–231. [CrossRef]
105. Lodge, P.A.; Sriram, S. Regulation of microglial activation by TGF-beta, IL-10, and CSF-1. *J. Leukoc. Biol.* **1996**, *60*, 502–508. [CrossRef]
106. Smith, A.M.; Graham, E.S.; Feng, S.X.; Oldfield, R.L.; Bergin, P.M.; Mee, E.W.; Faull, R.L.; Curtis, M.A.; Dragunow, M. Adult human glia, pericytes and meningeal fibroblasts respond similarly to IFNγ but not to TGFβ1 or M-CSF. *PLoS ONE* **2013**, *8*, e80463. [CrossRef]
107. Brionne, T.C.; Tesseur, I.; Masliah, E.; Wyss-Coray, T. Loss of TGF-beta 1 leads to increased neuronal cell death and microgliosis in mouse brain. *Neuron* **2003**, *40*, 1133–1145. [CrossRef]
108. Klein, P.; Friedman, A.; Hameed, M.Q.; Kaminski, R.M.; Bar-Klein, G.; Klitgaard, H.; Koepp, M.; Jozwiak, S.; Prince, D.A.; Rotenberg, A.; et al. Repurposed molecules for antiepileptogenesis: Missing an opportunity to prevent epilepsy? *Epilepsia* **2020**, *61*, 359–386. [CrossRef]
109. Stebbins, M.J.; Gastfriend, B.D.; Canfield, S.G.; Lee, M.S.; Richards, D.; Faubion, M.G.; Li, W.J.; Daneman, R.; Palecek, S.P.; Shusta, E.V. Human pluripotent stem cell-derived brain pericyte-like cells induce blood-brain barrier properties. *Sci. Adv.* **2019**, *5*, eaau7375. [CrossRef] [PubMed]

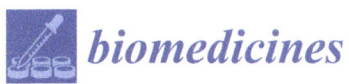

Review

Targeting the Ghrelin Receptor as a Novel Therapeutic Option for Epilepsy

An Buckinx [1], Dimitri De Bundel [1], Ron Kooijman [2] and Ilse Smolders [1],*

[1] Research Group Experimental Pharmacology, Department of Pharmaceutical Chemistry, Drug Analysis and Drug Information, Center for Neurosciences (C4N), Vrije Universiteit Brussel (VUB), 1090 Brussels, Belgium; an.buckinx@vub.be (A.B.); dimitri.de.bundel@vub.be (D.D.B.)

[2] Research Group Experimental Pharmacology, Center for Neurosciences (C4N), Vrije Universiteit Brussel (VUB), 1090 Brussels, Belgium; ron.kooijman@vub.be

* Correspondence: ilse.smolders@vub.be

Abstract: Epilepsy is a neurological disease affecting more than 50 million individuals worldwide. Notwithstanding the availability of a broad array of antiseizure drugs (ASDs), 30% of patients suffer from pharmacoresistant epilepsy. This highlights the urgent need for novel therapeutic options, preferably with an emphasis on new targets, since "me too" drugs have been shown to be of no avail. One of the appealing novel targets for ASDs is the ghrelin receptor (ghrelin-R). In epilepsy patients, alterations in the plasma levels of its endogenous ligand, ghrelin, have been described, and various ghrelin-R ligands are anticonvulsant in preclinical seizure and epilepsy models. Up until now, the exact mechanism-of-action of ghrelin-R-mediated anticonvulsant effects has remained poorly understood and is further complicated by multiple downstream signaling pathways and the heteromerization properties of the receptor. This review compiles current knowledge, and discusses the potential mechanisms-of-action of the anticonvulsant effects mediated by the ghrelin-R.

Keywords: epilepsy; ghrelin; ghrelin receptor

1. Introduction

Epilepsy is a neurological disease characterized by spontaneous and recurrent seizures [1]. With approximately 50 million patients, it is one of the most common neurological diseases worldwide [2]. Despite the availability of a wide range of antiseizure drugs (ASDs), up to 30% of patients suffer from pharmacoresistant epilepsy [2], of which a large proportion has temporal lobe epilepsy (TLE) [3,4]. This highlights the urgent need for the development of novel pharmacological treatment options.

One of these potential options is the orexigenic peptide, ghrelin. Ghrelin exerts both peripheral as well as central effects, and is primarily secreted by X/A-like cells in the stomach [5], but also, to less extents, in the small intestine, kidney, testis, pancreas, and the brain [5–10]. Peripherally, ghrelin plays an important role in gastric acid secretion, gastric emptying, and gastric motility [11–13], and it maintains glucose homeostasis via the inhibition of the insulin response to glucose administration [14]. Additionally, ghrelin is generally accepted to be a cardioprotective peptide [15,16].

In the central nervous system (CNS), ghrelin and its receptor are best known for their critical role in food intake, mediated by neuropeptide Y and agouti-related peptide [17–19] (reviewed in [20]). Additionally, ghrelin confers a regulatory role on growth hormone (GH) release [19], is implicated in learning and memory [21–23], modulates motivation and reward [24,25], and regulates the stress response (reviewed in [26]).

Soon after its discovery in 1999 [27], the interest in ghrelin within the context of epilepsy started to emerge. Ghrelin levels were shown to be altered in epilepsy patients, and ghrelin administration in preclinical seizure and epilepsy models is considered to be anticonvulsive [28–31]. However, up until now, the exact mechanism-of-action remains to be understood.

2. Ghrelin and Its Receptor

The main molecular form of ghrelin is a 28-amino acid (AA)-long peptide, with the active form containing a unique acylation on serine 3 [32]. Ghrelin is transcribed as a 117-AA-long preproghrelin. This is cleaved to render proghrelin, after which it undergoes acylation on serine 3, established by the membrane-bound enzyme, ghrelin O-acyltransferase (GOAT), which is distributed in a similar manner to ghrelin [33,34]. The acylation is either an octanoylation (eight-carbon fatty acid) or decanoylation (ten-carbon fatty acid) [33,34]. This action is followed by further processing of the 94-AA-long acylated pro-ghrelin by prohormone convertases 1/3 (PC1/3), which results in acylated ghrelin (AG), and also yields the mature peptide, obestatin [35]. Acylation on serine 3 was first believed to be imperative for the ability of ghrelin to bind to its receptor and to exert ghrelin's biological function [27]. Later, it became clear that desacyl ghrelin (DAG) is not completely devoid of physiological actions, as it was shown to also induce food intake, albeit through orexin neurons and not ghrelin receptor (ghrelin-R)-expressing neurons [36]. On the other hand, the anticonvulsant effects elicited by DAG required the presence of the ghrelin-R [37]. DAG shares some physiological functions similar to ghrelin but antagonizes others. Therefore, opposite effects might be mediated via a distinct receptor, and similar effects may be mediated by the ghrelin-R [38].

In human plasma, circulating esterases deacylate ghrelin, and 90% of total ghrelin consists of DAG, while only 10% consists of acylated ghrelin [39]. Ghrelin is rapidly cleared from plasma, with a plasma half-life ranging from 9–13 min for ghrelin, and 27–34 min for total ghrelin, including DAG [40,41]. Although the plasma concentration of DAG is much higher than that of ghrelin, its binding capacity to the ghrelin-R is substantially lower compared to ghrelin [38,42], which may explain why DAG was initially considered to be the "nonactive" variant of the peptide.

Recently, GOAT was shown to be expressed on the cell surface of mature bone marrow adipocytes, and to be necessary for DAG to promote adipogenesis in mice [43]. In line with this observation, GOAT was shown to be localized in the hilar border of dentate gyrus (DG) in the hippocampi of mice, and the incubation of live hippocampal slice cultures with DAG showed equal binding to the ghrelin-R as incubation with ghrelin, reliant on both the ghrelin-R and GOAT expression [44]. These data suggest that the local reacylation of DAG via GOAT expression at the cell surface may occur, and that it may be relevant for the biological functions of DAG mediated via the ghrelin-R.

2.1. Signaling Pathways and Heteromerization Complicate Ghrelin-R Signaling

Ghrelin establishes its numerous effects by interacting with its G-protein-coupled receptor (GPCR), of which two isoforms exist: the full-length (366 amino acids (AA) long) 7-transmembrane GPCR GHSR1a (a growth hormone secretagogue receptor, denoted as "ghrelin-R"), and a shorter (289 AA long) 3'-truncated variant, GHSR1b [27,45]. This nonsignaling short variant lacks the ability to exert biological effects in response to ghrelin and hampers the cell surface expression of the functional GHSR-1a variant, thus acting as a coregulator of ghrelin-R signaling [46,47].

The ghrelin-R is present in the brain and the periphery. The peripheral sites of ghrelin-R expression include the pancreas, spleen, bone tissue, cardiac tissue, the thyroid gland and immune cells, the adrenal glands, adipose tissue, and the vagal afferents [45,48].

Centrally, the ghrelin-R is widely expressed in a variety of brain areas and shows high expression levels in several nuclei of the hypothalamus, among which are the arcuate nucleus and the anterior hypothalamic nucleus. The receptor is further expressed in the olfactory bulb, the neocortex, in a variety of nuclei in the midbrain, in the pons, and in the medulla oblongata. These include the globus pallidus, the area postrema, the nucleus tractus solitarius, the substantia nigra, and the ventral tegmental area. In the hippocampus, the ghrelin-R was shown to be modestly expressed in the Cornu Ammonis (CA)1, compared to the higher expression levels in CA2, CA3, and DG of the mouse brain [45,49–51].

The expression of the ghrelin-R is highly dynamic, and depends on the developmental stage [52], the disease states [53,54], the metabolic state of the organism [55], or ghrelin availability [49]. Additionally, the receptor has a rich molecular pharmacology, with a multitude of signaling pathways associated with the receptor, and an ability to alter canonical ghrelin-R signaling via the formation of functional heteromeric complexes with other receptors. These factors contribute to diverse ghrelin-R signaling patterns.

The signaling pathways downstream of the ghrelin-R include $G\alpha_{q/11}$, $G\alpha_{i/o}$, and $G\alpha_{12/13}$ signaling, followed by β-arrestin recruitment [56–58]. The canonical $G\alpha_q$ protein activates the phospholipase C (PLC)—inositol 1,4,5-triphosphate (IP3)—diacylglycerol (DAG) pathway, which leads to an intracellular calcium (Ca^{2+}) increase [59,60]. $G\alpha_{i/o}$ activates phosphatidylinositol-3-kinase (PI3K) [61] and reduces cyclic AMP (cAMP) levels via reduced adenylyl cyclase (AC) activity [60]. $G\alpha_{12/13}$ signaling is associated with the activation of Ras homolog family member A (RhoA), other Rho guanine exchange factors, and their associated Rho kinases [62] (reviewed by [63]). Finally, G-protein-mediated signaling is halted via the recruitment of β-arrestin to the receptor [64], which not only vouches for the desensitization and internalization, but may also activate G-protein independent signaling pathways (reviewed in [65,66]). Recent studies have shown the ability of the β-arrestin-mediated activation of ERK1/2, mitogen-activated protein kinase (MAPK), the Akt/protein kinase B (PKB) pathways, and RhoA signaling [56,61,67] (Figure 1).

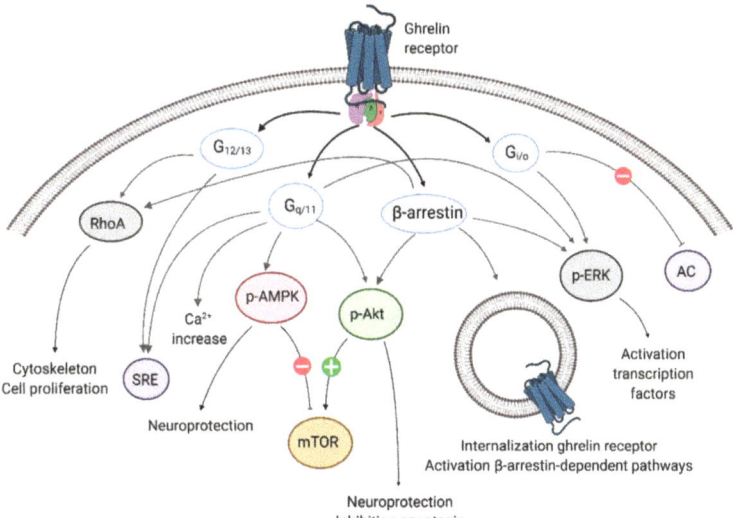

Figure 1. Signaling pathways associated with the ghrelin receptor. The ghrelin receptor employs $G\alpha_{q/11}$ signaling, $G\alpha_{i/o}$ signaling, and $G\alpha_{12/13}$ signaling, followed by β-arrestin recruitment. Each G-protein/β-arrestin is associated with physiological effects. AC: adenylyl cyclase; AMPK: adenosine-monophosphate-activated protein kinase; ERK: extracellular signal-regulated kinase; mTOR: mammalian target of rapamycin; p-: phosphorylated-; RhoA: Ras homolog family member A; SRE: serum response element. Created with BioRender.com.

The ghrelin-R confers extraordinarily high intracellular signaling in the absence of ghrelin or a ghrelin-R full agonist, signaling at approximately 50% of its maximal capacity [67,68]. Constitutive activity includes signaling via G-proteins, while it does not entail β-arrestin-mediated endocytosis [67–69].

2.2. What Is Known about Ghrelin's Central Availability?

Ghrelin, DAG, or synthetic compounds must access the brain to be centrally active. The transport of ghrelin across the blood–brain barrier (BBB) has been shown to occur via saturable mechanisms in mice [23,70], and does not depend on the expression of the ghrelin-R [71]. The notion that the BBB may be compromised in epilepsy should be taken into account, which would facilitate the availability of ghrelin to the CNS.

Additionally, systemically injected ghrelin was shown to cross the fenestrated capillaries in the circumventricular organs (CVO) via passive diffusion, and dose-dependently impacted more distant brain areas [72]. Finally, fluorescent ghrelin was shown to internalize in ependymal cells located in the choroid plexus and in β-type tanycytes, which constitute the foundation of the blood–cerebrospinal fluid (CSF) barrier (BCSFB). Fluorescent ghrelin was detected in periventricular hypothalamic tissue, and decreased with distance from the third ventricle [73]. The transport of ghrelin via the BCSFB depends predominantly on the presence of the ghrelin-R [74]. The kinetics of diffusion into the brain via the BCSFB is somewhat slower compared to the diffusion via the CVOs, with the CSF ghrelin concentrations peaking approximately 30 min after the ghrelin plasma concentration peak, depending on plasma ghrelin levels [75]. Additionally, an in vitro study showed that ghrelin was internalized in rat primary tanycytes via clathrin-coated vesicles [76].

Up until now, it has remained incompletely understood whether ghrelin is centrally available in areas more remote from the aforementioned barriers. It is possible that circulating ghrelin reaches certain permeable parts of the brain, and affects other areas indirectly, via the innervation of the nuclei located in the vicinity of accessible brain parts. This was shown in the case of the area postrema, which directly notes alterations in plasma ghrelin levels and innervates the nucleus tractus solitarius [72]. Additionally, central ghrelin expression may serve as an explanation for the high ghrelin-R expression in brain areas that are seemingly inaccessible to circulating ghrelin [9,27]. Indeed, central ghrelin messenger ribonucleic acid (mRNA) expression and immunoreactivity have been shown in multiple studies; however, there are also some studies refuting this notion (reviewed in [77]).

3. Studies in Humans

In humans, the majority of total circulating ghrelin consists of DAG, due to the deacylation of AG [39]. The acylation is located at the N-terminal part of the peptide, while the rest of the molecule is equivalent between AG and DAG. The studies outlined below do not always specify the portion of the peptide that is recognized by the used assays, nor is this information always available on the manufacturer's website. Failing to specify which isoform was measured may explain some of the observed interstudy variations. Most of the studies investigating AG or DAG levels assessed this peptide in plasma (in a small number of studies, the saliva and urine ghrelin levels were also assessed) after overnight fasting and were conducted in children and adolescents. Ghrelin levels are negatively correlated with age [78], and even pubertal children have significantly lower total plasma ghrelin levels compared to prepubertal children [79]. Therefore, in this review, a distinction is made between studies on adults and studies on children.

3.1. Adults

Up to now, there has been no general consensus regarding the differences in interictal ghrelin levels between adult epilepsy patients and healthy subjects. Three studies showed lower ghrelin levels in seizure-controlled epilepsy patients compared to healthy controls [80–82], while two studies did not detect differences in plasma ghrelin levels between epilepsy patients and controls [83,84]. One study demonstrated that patients with seizure-controlled epilepsy had significantly higher serum ghrelin compared to healthy controls [85]. Three studies demonstrated that patients suffering from focal epilepsy had higher ghrelin plasma levels compared to patients suffering from generalized seizures [80,81,85]. Two studies were not able to replicate this finding [84,86] (Table 1).

Table 1. Overview of interictal ghrelin levels in adults with focal and generalized epilepsy. AG: acyl ghrelin; ASD: antiseizure drug; CBZ: carbamazepine; DAG: desacyl ghrelin; DR-TLE: drug-resistant temporal lobe epilepsy; PHT: phenytoin; Ref: reference; TLE: temporal lobe epilepsy; VPA: valproic acid. * the different ghrelin levels in epilepsy patients versus controls. ** the differences in generalized epilepsy versus focal epilepsy.

ASD	Ghrelin Form	Controls (pg/mL)	*	Epilepsy Patients (pg/mL)		**	Ref
				Focal Seizures	Generalized Seizures		
VPA, PHT, CBZ	Total	93	↑	234	134	↓	[85]
VPA, PHT, CBZ	DAG AG	DAG: 585 AG: 46	↓	DAG: 439 AG: 35	DAG: 267 AG: 23	↓	[80]
VPA, PHT, CBZ	Total	700	↓	500	300	↓	[81]
VPA	N/A	381	=	364 (both types)		/	[83]
VPA, CBZ	DAG AG	DAG: 196 AG: 7	=	DAG: 207-239, AG: 7-22	DAG: 250 AG: 8	=	[84]
N/A	DAG AG	DAG 242 AG: 13	↑	DAG: 238 AG: 14.5	DAG: 245 AG: 19	↑	[86]
N/A	N/A	1320	↓	TLE: 1010	DR-TLE: 910	/	[82]

The AG/DAG ratio was significantly higher in epilepsy patients compared to controls, and it did not differ between different epilepsy types, or between refractory and nonrefractory epilepsy [84]. In females with Rett syndrome, the AG/total ghrelin ratio was significantly increased compared to epilepsy patients not diagnosed with Rett syndrome [87]. An assessment of the ratios of AG and DAG or total ghrelin may explain the difficult-to-reconcile observations in the ghrelin levels, and may appear as a good alternative read-out for these studies. However, measuring AG from plasma is technically challenging, and the best practices for handling AG plasma samples are, up to now, not entirely resolved [88]. Thus, the sensitivity of AG to sample handling can lead to large observed interstudy variations.

To elucidate the impact of ASD treatment or epilepsy disease progression on ghrelin levels, some studies have assessed the interictal ghrelin plasma levels before and after ASD treatment. After two years of successful valproic acid treatment, only patients that had developed obesity had significantly lower plasma ghrelin levels compared to controls, while this was not the case in patients that had not developed obesity [83]. The serum DAG levels did not differ after three months of ASD treatment, while the AG levels were decreased after three months [80]. Finally, ASD-responsive patients had increased ghrelin levels compared to nonresponders in two studies, but not in another study [82,86,89]. A significant positive correlation has been shown between both the AG and DAG levels and disease duration, which could be indicative of ghrelin resistance, but could also be related to ASD use [84].

One study assessed the alterations in plasma ghrelin immediately after seizures. The AG and DAG levels decreased as soon as five minutes after a generalized seizure, and were restored after 24 h [89]. Moreover, in the preclinical pentylenetetrazole (PTZ) model, AG, but not DAG, as well as total ghrelin plasma levels, decreased 30 min after the induction of a seizure (see further) [90]. Overall, most studies show lower ghrelin levels in patients with epilepsy compared to healthy controls, or a decrease in ghrelin levels after a seizure.

3.2. Children

The latter statement could be extrapolated to children, as total ghrelin levels were significantly lower in prepubertal children with epilepsy compared to healthy controls [91,92]. Another study assessed the AG and DAG plasma levels within six hours after a seizure in children not yet receiving treatment (pretreatment), three months after treatment (post-treatment), and in healthy controls. The AG levels were significantly lower in the pretreatment group compared to the post-treatment group and the controls [93]. DAG levels were significantly higher in the post-treatment group compared to the pretreatment group in urine and saliva, but not in serum [93] (Table 2). Within the epilepsy group, lean children on valproic acid had significantly higher total ghrelin plasma levels compared to children on carbamazepine [91], but not compared to children receiving topiramate [94].

Table 2. Overview of interictal ghrelin levels in children. AG: acylated ghrelin; ASD: antiseizure drug; CBZ: carbamazepine; TPM: topiramate; DAG: desacyl ghrelin; Ref: reference; VPA: valproic acid. * the different ghrelin levels in epilepsy patients versus controls. ** the difference in condition 2 versus condition 1 within epilepsy patients. Age denotes either the mean age of the patient groups rounded to the nearest integer, or the age range.

ASD	Ghrelin Form	Controls (pg/mL)	*	Epilepsy Patients (pg/mL)		**	Age (Years)	Ref
VPA, CBZ	Total	554	↓	VPA: 381	CBZ: 283	↓	5	[91]
VPA, TPM	N/A	267	=	VPA: 240	TPM: 267	=	6–15	[94]
VPA	DAG AG	DAG: 446 AG: 45	↓	Pretreatment: DAG: 420 AG: 36	Post-treatment: DAG: 459 AG: 51	↑	9	[93]
VPA	N/A	333	↓	Pretreatment: 355	Post-treatment: 263	↓	11	[92]

The majority of studies that assessed ghrelin levels related to disease progression did not detect significant differences between ghrelin levels measured over time (Table 3) [95–97]. One study showed that plasma ghrelin was significantly decreased after the initiation of valproic acid treatment in pubertal children, but not in prepubertal children, nor in children on oxcarbazepine. In the latter case, this may be due to the increased weight gain in the children receiving valproic acid [98].

Table 3. Overview of interictal ghrelin levels in children after ASD or KD intervention. AG: acylated ghrelin; ASD: antiseizure drug; CBZ: carbamazepine; d: day; DAG: desacyl ghrelin; Int: intervention; KD: ketogenic diet; LEV: levetiracetam; m: month; OXC: oxcarbazepine; PHT: phenytoin; Ref: reference; T: time; TPM: topiramate; VPA: valproic acid; y: year. * the different ghrelin levels in epilepsy patients over time. ± the concentrations derived from graphs.

Int.	Ghrelin Form	Baseline (pg/mL)	T1	T2	T3	T4	*	Age (Years)	Ref
OXC	N/A	327	6 m: 306	18 m: 320	/	/	=	9	[95]
OXC	N/A	310	6 m: 288	18 m: 345	/	/	=	13	[98]
VPA	N/A	18	6 m: 18	12 m: 18	/	/	=	9	[96]
VPA	N/A	334	6 m: 275	18 m: 245	/	/	↓	14	[98]
VPA	N/A	1.37	6 m: 2.19	/	/	/	↑	8	[99]
TPM	N/A	1121	3 m: 1184	6 m: 1292	/	/	=	8	[97]
LEV	N/A	1900	6 m: 2950	/	/	/	=	7	[100]
KD	DAG AG	DAG: ±160 AG: ±250	15 d: DAG: ±110 AG: ±210	30 d: DAG: ±100 AG: ±140	90 d: DAG: ±140 AG: ±110	/	↓	7	[101]
KD	AG	±400	15 d: ±250	30 d: ±200	90 d: ±200	1 y: ±200	↓	6	[102]
KD	N/A	20	6 m: 19	12 m: 19	/	/	/	8	[103]

The Ketogenic Diet

The ketogenic diet (KD) is an alternative treatment option for refractory epilepsy and has often been proven useful, particularly in children. It remains to be elucidated to what extent the alterations in AG or DAG may mediate some of the effects of the KD [104]. Both AG and DAG levels were shown to be decreased after the initiation of a KD in children with drug-resistant epilepsy [101]. Another study showed that AG plasma levels were decreased as soon as 30 days after the initiation of a KD in children with pharmacoresistant epilepsy [102]. One study did not detect alterations in ghrelin levels after the onset of a KD in drug-resistant epilepsy patients [103] (Table 3).

4. Preclinical Evidence for Ghrelin as a Potential Antiseizure Drug

Ghrelin, in both its acylated and deacylated form, as well as synthetic ligands, have been studied in rodent seizure and epilepsy models. The majority of these studies focus on the administration of ghrelin or ghrelin-R ligands to modulate seizures or epilepsy, while only a few studies have assessed plasma ghrelin levels in these models.

4.1. Ghrelin in Seizure and Status Epilepticus Rodent Models

Both systemic and intrahippocampal ghrelin administration were anticonvulsant in the acute rat PTZ model [105–108]. A longer pretreatment of 10 days with ghrelin elicited the same antiseizure effect [107]. One study showed that ghrelin administration in PTZ-treated rats enhanced cognitive capacity in terms of spatial memory [109], which is interesting in light of cognitive impairments as important comorbidities of epilepsy [110].

AG, but not DAG, and total ghrelin plasma levels were decreased 30 min after the induction of a seizure in the PTZ model [90]. This decrease was confirmed in another study, where total ghrelin serum and brain levels were lower in rats after acute PTZ injection, but also after chronic PTZ kindling [111]. Finally, the brain tissue and plasma total ghrelin levels were decreased in mice that exhibited seizures, which were elicited after 24 h of fasting, followed by scopolamine administration [112].

In a study conducted on a rat penicillin model performed under anesthesia, only 1 μg, but not 2 μg of ghrelin administered 30 min after penicillin significantly lowered the spike frequency. These data imply that ghrelin might not follow a linear dose–response curve [113]. There is one study that recently demonstrated ghrelin administration to be proconvulsive in a WAG/Rij rat model presenting with absence seizures, as ghrelin increased the number of spike–wave discharges and the total seizure duration one hour after administration [114].

Ghrelin has been assessed in various status epilepticus (SE) models. However, given the short duration of these experiments, they only reflect the effects of ghrelin on the phenomenon of SE, and not on the subsequent chronic recurrent seizures. Ghrelin was not anticonvulsant in SE models in rats [31,115], except for one study [116], while ghrelin exerted anticonvulsant effects in a pilocarpine tail infusion mouse model and an intrahippocampal kainic acid (IHKA) mouse model [29,116]. One explanation for these observations could be the short timing of ghrelin administration prior to the stimulus (only 10 min) in the rat models. Additionally, the doses that were used in these studies varied highly. Interestingly, it appears that the choice of species may be involved as well, as ghrelin (both at a dose of 0.08 mg/kg and 1.8 mg/kg) was anticonvulsant in mice, but not in the pilocarpine or KA rat model at a dose of 1.5 mg/kg. On the other hand, the effects exerted by ghrelin may not be strong enough to interfere with the development of SE (Table 4).

Table 4. Overview of effects of ghrelin in experimental epilepsy models. i.c.v.: intracerebroventricular; i.h.: intrahippocampal; IHKA: intrahippocampal kainic acid; i.p.: intraperitoneal; KA: kainic acid; min: minute; pen: penicillin; pilo: pilocarpine; PTZ: pentylenetetrazole; Ref: reference.

Dose	Administration Regimen	Anticonvulsant	Animal Model	Ref
0.02–0.08 mg/kg	i.p. 30 min prior to PTZ	yes	PTZ i.p. rat model	[105,117]
0.08 mg/kg	i.p. 30 min prior to PTZ	no	PTZ i.p. rat model	[118]
0.3 nmol/μL	i.h. infusion 1 x 30 min prior to PTZ or 10 days	yes	PTZ i.p. rat model	[106,107]
0.08 mg/kg	i.c.v. 30 min prior to PTZ	yes	PTZ i.p. rat model (female rats)	[108]
0.5, 1 and 2 μg	i.c.v. 30 min after pen	yes	Intracortical penicillin rat model	[113,119]
0.08 mg/kg	i.p., immediate assessment	no	WAG/Rij rat model	[114]
0.01–10 μM	i.h. infusion, 120 min prior to pilo	yes	Pilocarpine i.h. infusion rat model	[116]
1.5 mg/kg	i.p. 10 min prior to pilo	no	Pilocarpine i.p. rat model	[31,115]
1.5 mg/kg	i.p. 10 min prior to KA	no	KA i.p. rat model	[115]
0.08 mg/kg	i.p. 30 min prior to KA, and 24 h after KA	yes	KA i.p. mouse model	[29]
1.8 mg/kg	i.p. 30 min prior to pilo	yes	Pilocarpine tail infusion mouse model	[116]

Ghrelin's deacylated form, DAG, was anticonvulsant in the IHKA rat model, the intracerebroventricular pilocarpine rat model, and the pilocarpine tail infusion mouse model [37,115] (Table 5). While this was not the case with ghrelin, the administration of DAG only 10 min prior to a pilocarpine or IHKA stimulus was anticonvulsant [115]. A possible explanation may rely on the fact that DAG has a faster transport rate across the BBB in mice compared to ghrelin [71].

Table 5. Overview of effects of desacyl ghrelin in experimental epilepsy models. i.c.v.: intracerebroventricular; i.p.: intraperitoneal; KA: kainic acid; min: minute; pilo: pilocarpine; Ref: reference.

Desacyl Ghrelin				
Dose	Administration Regimen	Anticonvulsant	Animal Model	Ref
1.5 mg/kg	i.p. 10 min prior to pilo	yes/no ($p = 0.07$)	Pilocarpine i.p. rat model	[115]
1.5 mg/kg	i.p. 10 min prior to KA	yes	KA i.p. rat model	[115]
1–10 μM	i.c.v. 2 h prior to pilo	yes	Pilocarpine i.c.v. rat model	[37]
3/5 mg/kg	i.p. 30 min prior to pilo	yes	Pilocarpine tail infusion mouse model	[37]

Another possible explanation could be the presence of GOAT in the hippocampus, which may locally acylate extracellular DAG [44]. This leads to the compelling hypothesis that DAG may exert anticonvulsant effects via its superior brain availability compared to ghrelin, in combination with local acylation, to render AG in the hippocampus and exert anticonvulsant effects via the ghrelin-R. This mechanism would drastically improve ghrelin availability at such difficult-to-reach brain areas. Additionally, this hypothesis may fit into the notion that DAG was shown to require ghrelin-R expression to exert anticonvulsant effects [37].

All preclinical studies involving the effect of ghrelin on seizures or SE have been conducted in male rodents. There is one study that used female rats to investigate whether ghrelin administration differentially affects the incidence of seizures at various time points of the estrous cycle. The authors found that ghrelin was anticonvulsant during all phases of the estrous cycle; however, the effects were more outspoken during the luteal phase compared to the follicular phase [108].

4.2. Ghrelin Receptor Agonists

A large number of shorter ligands with binding affinity at the ghrelin-R have been synthesized, of which the ghrelin-R agonists, macimorelin, capromorelin, and hexarelin have been tested in animal models of seizures or epilepsy (Table 6).

The pseudotripeptide, macimorelin (H-Aib-(d)-Trp-(d)-gTrp-formyl, also known as "JMV-1843") was first synthesized in 2003 [120], and it is currently on the market for the diagnosis of GH deficiency [121,122]. It is a full agonist of the ghrelin-R and has a longer plasma half-life compared to the endogenous agonist [122,123]. Our group showed that macimorelin was anticonvulsant in both the acute 6-Hz mouse model and fully 6-Hz-kindled mice through the ghrelin-R [124], and in a dopamine 1 receptor (D1R)-mediated mouse kindling model [125]. Macimorelin did not exert anticonvulsant effects in the SE pilocarpine rat model [31,115], but was anticonvulsant in the IHKA mouse model [126]. These studies differed in the dose, the timing of the administration, and the species used, which may explain these conflicting findings.

As ghrelin or macimorelin were shown to exert neuroprotective [28–31] and anti-inflammatory effects [31,121,122] in seizure models (see further), our group recently studied whether macimorelin was able to interfere with epileptogenesis. The prevention or attenuation of the development of epilepsy could drastically reduce morbidity and the socioeconomic costs associated with refractory epilepsy. However, we found that macimorelin was anticonvulsive, but not antiepileptogenic, in the IHKA mouse model [126].

Capromorelin is a ghrelin-R full agonist with a high affinity for its receptor [127], and it is currently FDA-approved for veterinary use for increasing food intake [128,129]. Capromorelin was intrahippocampally infused two hours prior to intrahippocampal pilocarpine infusion in rats and decreased the total seizure severity score [116].

The hexapeptide, hexarelin, was developed as a GH secretagogue prior to the discovery of ghrelin [130]. Its potential anticonvulsant effects were assessed in both the pilocarpine rat model and the IHKA rat model. While a low dose (0.33 mg/kg) was anticonvulsant in the pilocarpine rat model, the same administration regimen was not anticonvulsant in the IHKA rat model [115]. This once more underscores the variation between the models and the species used in the discovery of novel potential ASDs, and advocates for the use of multiple seizure or epilepsy models in the discovery of potential new ASDs.

4.3. Administration of Other Ghrelin Receptor Ligands

Neutral antagonists prevent the activation of a receptor by blocking the agonist binding to the receptor, but do not affect its basal constitutive activity. Three ghrelin-R antagonists have been investigated in a variety of epilepsy models, of which the neutral antagonist, JMV-2959, was without effects in the pilocarpine rat model, in acute 6-Hz- or fully kindled mice, and in the D1R-mediated kindling model [115,124,125]. The hexapeptide, EP-80317 (Haic-D-Mrp-D-Lys-Trp-D-Phe-Lys-NH2), was anticonvulsive in the pilocarpine SE model and the 6-Hz-kindled mouse model [115,131,132] (Table 6). Interestingly, resistance to the initial anticonvulsant effects of EP-80317 treatment were observed with seizure progression in the 6-Hz-kindling model [131,132]. Its anticonvulsant effects were shown to be dependent on the peroxisome-proliferator-activated receptor, S-gamma (PPAR-γ), presumably via the cluster of differentiation (CD)36 receptor [131,132]. By contrast, one recent study showed that the ghrelin-R antagonist, D-Lys-3-GHRP-6, induced spontaneous seizures in an amygdala-kindled rat model, [133].

Intrahippocampal infusion of the inverse agonists, A778193 and [D-Arg1, D-Phe5, D-Trp7,9, Leu11]-substance P, were anticonvulsant in the intrahippocampal pilocarpine infusion rat model. Inverse agonists are typified by their ability to block the intracellular signaling of a receptor, including basal constitutive signaling, which resembles an absence of the receptor. In line with this notion, ghrelin-R knock-out (KO) mice were shown to be protected from seizures [116,124], which suggests that the absence of ghrelin-R signaling is anticonvulsant. In agreement with this, the biased agonist, YIL671, a $G\alpha_q$ and $G\alpha_{12}$ selective biased ligand of the ghrelin-R that is not able to recruit β-arrestin, increased the seizure burden in the D1R-mediated kindling model [125].

Table 6. Overview of anticonvulsant effects of ghrelin-R ligands in experimental epilepsy models. D1R: Dopamine 1 receptor; i.v.: intravenous; i.h.: intrahippocampal; IHKA: intrahippocampal kainic acid; i.p.: intraperitoneal; KA: kainic acid; min: minute; pilo: pilocarpine; Ref: reference; SP: [D-Arg1,D-Phe5,D-Trp7,9,Leu11]substance P.

Compound	Dose	Administration Regimen	Anticonvulsant	Animal Model	Ref
Agonists					
Macimorelin	0.33 mg/kg	i.p 10 min prior to pilo	no	Pilocarpine i.p. rat model	[31,115]
Macimorelin	5 mg/kg	i.p., 20 min prior to stimulus	yes	Acute 6-Hz mouse model	[124]
Macimorelin	5 mg/kg	i.v. infusion	yes	Fully kindled 6-Hz mouse model	[124]
Macimorelin	5 mg/kg	30 min prior to SKF	yes	D1R-mediated kindling mouse model	[125]
Macimorelin	5 mg/kg	14 days, 2×/day	yes	IHKA mouse model	[126]
Capromorelin	0.01–10 μM	i.h. infusion 120 min prior to pilo	yes	Pilocarpine i.h. infusion rat model	[116]
Hexarelin	0.33 mg/kg	i.p. 10 min prior to pilo	yes	Pilocarpine i.p. rat model	[115]
Hexarelin	0.33 mg/kg	i.p. 10 min prior to KA	no	KA i.p. rat model	[115]

Table 6. Cont.

Compound	Dose	Administration Regimen	Anticonvulsant	Animal Model	Ref
Antagonists					
EP-80317	0.33 mg/kg	i.p. 10 min prior to pilo	yes/no	Pilocarpine i.p. rat model	[115]
EP-80317	0.33 mg/kg	i.p. 10 min prior to KA	no	KA i.p. rat model	[115]
EP-80317	0.33 mg/kg	i.p. 10–15 min prior to stimulus	yes	6-Hz repeated mouse model	[131]
JMV-2959	0.33 mg/kg	i.p. 10 min prior to pilo	no	Pilocarpine i.p. rat model	[115]
JMV-2959	10 mg/kg	i.p. 20 min prior to stimulus	no	Acute 6-Hz mouse model	[124]
JMV-2959	10 mg/kg	i.v. infusion	no	6-Hz fully kindled mice	[124]
JMV-2959	5 mg/kg	i.p. 30 min prior to SKF	no	D1R-mediated kindling mouse model	[125]
D-Lys-3-GHRP-6	1–100 µg	i.c.v. 30 min prior to stimulus	no	Amygdala kindling rat model	[133]
Inverse Agonists					
A778193	0.01–10 µM	i.h. infusion 120 min prior to pilo	yes	Pilocarpine i.h. infusion rat model	[116]
SP	0.01–10 µM	i.h. infusion 120 min prior to pilo	yes	Pilocarpine i.h. infusion rat model	[116]
Biased Agonists					
YIL781	5 mg/kg	i.p. 30 min prior to SKF	no	D1R-mediated kindling mouse model	[125]

5. Molecular Mechanisms-of-Action

5.1. Mechanisms of Ghrelin's Anticonvulsant Action

Ghrelin-R expression is dynamic and may be influenced by the presence of a disease state, or may depend on exposure to ghrelin [54,55,134], which are both relevant in the context of ghrelin administration in seizure and epilepsy models. Neither ghrelin nor pilocarpine altered hippocampal ghrelin-R mRNA expression in the pilocarpine rat model [28], while another group showed a decrease in the hippocampal ghrelin-R mRNA expression in pilocarpine-treated rats, which was restored upon ghrelin administration [30].

Hippocampal Akt signaling was decreased in a pilocarpine rat model, which could be restored by ghrelin administration [28,30]. Akt is a downstream target of the ghrelin-R, which can be activated both by $G\alpha_q$ signaling and β-arrestin recruitment. The ghrelin-R antagonist, EP-80317, restored the increased hippocampal phosphorylation levels of the other canonical downstream target ERK in the 6-Hz mouse model [131].

Up until now, the exact signaling pathways responsible for anticonvulsant effects downstream of ghrelin-R have remained elusive, but a few possibilities exist, on the basis of previous findings. Not only ghrelin-R agonists, but also ghrelin-R inverse agonists exerted anticonvulsant effects, and ghrelin-R KO mice were protected from seizures [116,124]. The truncated ghrelin variant, ghrelin (1–5) amide, shows similar EC_{50} values compared to ghrelin with regard to the ghrelin-R signaling pathways, but is unable to internalize the ghrelin receptor, and was not able to exert anticonvulsant effects [116]. Because of these intuitively irreconcilable observations, a novel concept emerged, hypothesizing that the absence of the ghrelin-R on the cell surface was responsible for exerting ghrelin's anticonvulsant effect [116]. We showed that a $G\alpha_q$ and $G\alpha_{12}$ selective biased ligand of the ghrelin-R, YIL781, increased seizure severity in a kindling model [125]. Given these observations, β-arrestin recruitment remains the most probable pathway involved in ghrelin-R-mediated anticonvulsive effects and it requires further investigation.

However, we cannot completely exclude that G-protein-dependent signaling may be required for ghrelin-R-mediated anticonvulsant effects, as Akt and ERK activation have been described [30,32,135]. However, this would not fit with the notions of ghrelin-R KO mice being protected from seizures, and inverse agonists exerting anticonvulsant effects; in these cases, there is no G-protein-dependent signaling downstream of the ghrelin-R. Finally, one could hypothesize that the possibility exists that the signaling pathways downstream of β-arrestin may be responsible for ghrelin's anticonvulsant effects. Indeed, Akt and ERK are mediators that can also be activated via β-arrestin-dependent signaling. Nonetheless, and also here, the data obtained from the experiments with ghrelin-R KO mice and inverse agonists [116] suggest otherwise, and point towards an absence of signaling, which is imperative for ghrelin's anticonvulsant effects.

5.2. Mechanisms of Neuroprotection

Ghrelin increased the number of surviving neurons in the CA1 and CA3 hippocampal regions in the pilocarpine rat model [28]. Pilocarpine reduced the apoptotic repressor, B-cell lymphoma 2 (Bcl-2), increased the proapoptotic member Bcl-2-associated X protein (Bax), and increased cleaved caspase-3, crucial in apoptosis. Ghrelin was able to restore these markers, and may thus exert neuroprotection through antiapoptotic effects [28].

This latter finding was confirmed in the i.p. KA mouse model, in which ghrelin decreased cleaved caspase-3 immunoreactivity in pyramidal CA1 and CA3 neurons, and restored neuronal loss in CA1 and CA3 [29]. Terminal deoxynucleotidyl transferase dUTP nick end labeling (TUNEL)-positive cells were abundantly present in vehicle-treated KA mice, but no TUNEL-positive cells could be observed in ghrelin-treated KA mice. All of the above described effects were dependent on ghrelin-R, as they were reversed by the concurrent administration of a ghrelin-R antagonist [29]. A study conducted by Zhang and colleagues confirmed the necessity of ghrelin-R availability in order for ghrelin to exert its neuroprotective effects [30]. Ghrelin significantly rescued neuronal cell loss in CA3, and inhibited cleaved caspase-3 activation, mediated via the phosphorylation of Akt [30].

A two-week-long administration of the ghrelin-R agonist, macimorelin, in the IHKA mouse model, exerted anticonvulsant effects on spontaneous recurrent seizures, but did not increase neuronal survival in the CA1, CA3, and DG of the hippocampus. This could be due to the omission of pretreatment, as the onset of the treatment commenced 24 h after SE induction, or due to the additional two-week wash-out in this study [126]. A lower dose of macimorelin, administered prior to SE, was found to increase neuronal survival and decrease apoptosis in the DG in the pilocarpine rat model, but not in CA1 [31]. Additionally, this study was able to demonstrate neuroprotective effects exerted by macimorelin, but not anticonvulsant effects against the pilocarpine-induced SE.

The possibility should be considered that ghrelin exerts neuroprotective effects via the activation of a variety of signaling pathways mediated through the employment of G-proteins, whereas the rapid and subsequent internalization via β-arrestin signaling may be responsible for anticonvulsant effects. Unraveling which ghrelin-R downstream signaling pathway is responsible for a particular effect may be obtained by doing further experiments in genetic models, or by using biased ligands that selectively activate a subset of pathways while leaving others untouched.

5.3. Inflammation

Inflammation is a major hallmark of epileptogenesis, seizures, and chronic epilepsy. This ranges from infiltration of the inflammatory cells and the release of proinflammatory mediators to widespread gliosis [134–137]. Given the fact that inflammation is known to progress the development of epilepsy [138], one of the presumed mechanisms-of-action of ghrelin may rely on its ability to attenuate inflammation, stemming from both direct central actions, and through peripheral anti-inflammatory effects [139].

Ghrelin significantly reduced the elevated plasma calcitonin gene-related peptide (CGRP), substance P, interleukin (IL)-6, tumor necrosis factor (TNF)-α, and IL-1β in the

PTZ rat model [117,118]. Additionally, ghrelin inhibited KA-induced increases in TNF-α, IL-1β and cyclooxygenase-2 (COX2) mRNA levels in CA1 and CA3 in the i.p. KA mouse model, mediated via the ghrelin-R [29]. Ghrelin restored KA-induced increased matrix metalloproteinase 3 levels, which is an important mediator of inflammation and neuronal cell death [29]. Additionally, KA-induced increases in microglia and glial fibrillary acidic protein (GFAP) immunoreactivity in CA1 and CA3 three days after SE were inhibited by ghrelin [29]. This was not detectable after a two-week wash-out following macimorelin administration in the IHKA mouse model, in which macimorelin was administered after KA, and not as a pretreatment [126]. Another study showed that ghrelin administration decreased cortical TNF-α and NF-κB expression in the pilocarpine rat model [140]. However, ghrelin did not alter serum levels of galanin, fibroblast growth factor (FGF-2), IL-6, TNF-α, and IL-1β in the Wag/Rij rat model with nonconvulsive absence seizures [114].

5.4. Oxidative Stress

Seizures induce oxidative stress, which, in turn, exacerbates seizures (reviewed by [141]). Ghrelin prevented the PTZ-induced decrease in the catalase activity in both the CNS and erythrocytes, and prevented the augmentation in thiobarbituric acid reactive substances levels, a measure for lipid peroxidation [142]. Additionally, ghrelin normalized superoxide dismutase levels, an enzyme responsible for clearing superoxide anion in the erythrocytes, brain, and liver [142]. These data suggest that ghrelin protects against oxidative stress caused by PTZ. It remains unclear whether the effects of ghrelin on decreasing oxidative stress are caused directly, or because ghrelin is anticonvulsant, and the lower number of seizures leads to decreased oxidative stress. However, in the WAG/Rij rat model with nonconvulsive absence seizures, ghrelin was not anticonvulsant, but it still reduced the malondialdehyde [114].

6. Functional Implications of Diminished Ghrelin-R Signaling in the Context of Excitability

While several molecular mechanisms-of-action have been described, it remains unknown how these contribute to the anticonvulsant effects of ghrelin, and how they lead to an overall decrease in the brain excitability. The heteromerization of the ghrelin-R with other receptors can lead to the preferential recruitment of other noncanonical signaling pathways [143]. Ghrelin, as well as other signaling molecules, may exploit this phenomenon for inducing ghrelin-R-mediated anticonvulsant effects.

Ghrelin-R activation results in intracellular Ca^{2+} increases through the canonical $G\alpha_q$ protein [59,60]. One possible mechanism-of-action would be a decrease in intracellular Ca^{2+} in ghrelin-R-expressing neurons. Elevated levels of intracellular Ca^{2+} are associated with epileptiform activity and epileptogenesis [144,145]. Therefore, a reduction in intracellular Ca^{2+} may be an interesting putative mechanism for seizure suppression in the absence of ghrelin-R signaling. Various studies have shown the differential effects of ghrelin on neuronal excitability and synaptic transmission, which all support that ghrelin acts in a brain-region-specific manner [146–148].

The ghrelin-R is expressed in both excitatory neurons, as well as in inhibitory interneurons in the dorsal CA1. It was recently shown that a selective increased expression of the ghrelin-R in excitatory neurons was detrimental for learning and memory in mice, while an increased expression of the ghrelin-R in interneurons had a beneficial effect [149]. It remains to be uncovered if a dual effect on excitability also exists by, for instance, decreasing $G\alpha_q$ signaling in excitatory neurons via β-arrestin, while increasing $G\alpha_q$ signaling in inhibitory interneurons. Indeed, while GPCRs may be associated with several signaling pathways, these signaling pathways are not always all operative in the same cell. Thus far, the knowledge concerning the cell-specific expression of signaling pathways downstream of the ghrelin-R is lacking and requires further studies.

7. Conclusions and Future Perspectives

Ghrelin is increasingly recognized as a potential important player in seizures and epilepsy. Most studies show lower ghrelin levels in patients suffering from epilepsy, or lower ghrelin levels after a seizure. The exact implications of plasma ghrelin level alterations in epilepsy have remained, up until now, unknown, and should be further investigated in light of its treatments as well, including the KD. It is increasingly evident that there may be important differences between AG and DAG. This may advocate for future investigations of both isoforms of ghrelin in epilepsy, or for studying further whether the contributions of GOAT expression and the local reacylation of DAG are relevant for seizure control.

With only a few exceptions, ghrelin and synthetic agonists of the ghrelin-R are anticonvulsant in seizure, epilepsy, and SE models. The notion that both agonists and inverse agonists were anticonvulsant stirred up the discussion concerning the signaling pathways responsible for ghrelin-R-mediated anticonvulsant effects. The hypothesis that β-arrestin recruitment is involved should be more thoroughly investigated to confirm the relevance of this pathway. Overall, the complexity of ghrelin-R signaling, and the extensive list of other factors possibly influencing it, highlight the need for further investigations into the mechanism behind ghrelin-induced anticonvulsant effects.

Author Contributions: Conceptualization, A.B., D.D.B., R.K. and I.S.; Investigation, A.B.; Resources, D.D.B., R.K. and I.S.; Writing—Original Draft Preparation, A.B.; Writing—Review & Editing, A.B., D.D.B., R.K. and I.S.; Visualization, A.B.; Supervision, D.D.B., R.K. and I.S.; Project Administration, A.B.; Funding Acquisition, A.B., D.D.B., R.K. and I.S. All authors have read and agreed to the published version of the manuscript.

Funding: This research was supported by the scientific Willy Gepts fund of the UZ Brussel, the Queen Elizabeth Medical Foundation (ING prize), and the strategic research program of the Vrije Universiteit Brussel (SRP49). A Buckinx is a research fellow of the Fund for Scientific Research, Flanders (SB-FWO grant no. 1S84218N).

Conflicts of Interest: The authors declare no conflict of interest. The funders had no role in the design of the study; in the collection, analyses, or interpretation of data; in the writing of the manuscript; or in the decision to publish the results.

References

1. Fisher, R.S.; Cross, J.H.; French, J.A.; Higurashi, N.; Hirsch, E.; Jansen, F.E.; Lagae, L.; Moshé, S.L.; Peltola, J.; Roulet Perez, E.; et al. Operational classification of seizure types by the International League Against Epilepsy: Position Paper of the ILAE Commission for Classification and Terminology. *Epilepsia* **2017**, *58*, 522–530. [CrossRef]
2. World Health Organization. *Epilepsy: A Public Health Imperative. Licence: CC BY-NC-SA 3.0 IGO*; World Health Organization: Geneva, Switzerland, 2019.
3. Nayak, C.S.; Bandyopadhyay, S. *Mesial Temporal Lobe Epilepsy*; Updated 5 June 2020; StatPearls Publishing: Treasure Island, FL, USA, 2020.
4. Téllez-Zenteno, J.F.; Hernández-Ronquillo, L. A review of the epidemiology of temporal lobe epilepsy. *Epilepsy Res. Treat.* **2012**, *2012*, 630853. [CrossRef]
5. Date, Y.; Kojima, M.; Hosoda, H.; Sawaguchi, A.; Mondal, M.S.; Suganuma, T.; Matsukura, S.; Kangawa, K.; Nakazato, M. Ghrelin, a novel growth hormone-releasing acylated peptide, is synthesized in a distinct endocrine cell type in the gastrointestinal tracts of rats and humans. *Endocrinology* **2000**, *141*, 4255–4261. [CrossRef] [PubMed]
6. Tanaka, M.; Hayashida, Y.; Nakao, N.; Nakai, N.; Nakashima, K. Testis-specific and developmentally induced expression of a ghrelin gene-derived transcript that encodes a novel polypeptide in the mouse. *Biochim. Biophys. Acta* **2001**, *1522*, 62–65. [CrossRef]
7. Mori, K.; Yoshimoto, A.; Takaya, K.; Hosoda, K.; Ariyasu, H.; Yahata, K.; Mukoyama, M.; Sugawara, A.; Hosoda, H.; Kojima, M.; et al. Kidney produces a novel acylated peptide, ghrelin. *FEBS Lett.* **2000**, *486*, 213–216. [CrossRef]
8. Volante, M.; Allìa, E.; Gugliotta, P.; Funaro, A.; Broglio, F.; Deghenghi, R.; Muccioli, G.; Ghigo, E.; Papotti, M. Expression of ghrelin and of the GH secretagogue receptor by pancreatic islet cells and related endocrine tumors. *J. Clin. Endocrinol. Metab.* **2002**, *87*, 1300–1308. [CrossRef] [PubMed]
9. Cowley, M.A.; Smith, R.G.; Diano, S.; Tschöp, M.; Pronchuk, N.; Grove, K.L.; Strasburger, C.J.; Bidlingmaier, M.; Esterman, M.; Heiman, M.L.; et al. The distribution and mechanism of action of ghrelin in the CNS demonstrates a novel hypothalamic circuit regulating energy homeostasis. *Neuron* **2003**, *37*, 649–661. [CrossRef]

10. Lu, S.; Guan, J.L.; Wang, Q.P.; Uehara, K.; Yamada, S.; Goto, N.; Date, Y.; Nakazato, M.; Kojima, M.; Kangawa, K.; et al. Immunocytochemical observation of ghrelin-containing neurons in the rat arcuate nucleus. *Neurosci. Lett.* **2002**, *321*, 157–160. [CrossRef]
11. Masuda, Y.; Tanaka, T.; Inomata, N.; Ohnuma, N.; Tanaka, S.; Itoh, Z.; Hosoda, H.; Kojima, M.; Kangawa, K. Ghrelin stimulates gastric acid secretion and motility in rats. *Biochem. Biophys. Res. Commun.* **2000**, *276*, 905–908. [CrossRef]
12. Dornonville de la Cour, C.; Lindström, E.; Norlén, P.; Håkanson, R. Ghrelin stimulates gastric emptying but is without effect on acid secretion and gastric endocrine cells. *Regul. Pept.* **2004**, *120*, 23–32. [CrossRef]
13. Colldén, G.; Tschöp, M.H.; Müller, T.D. Therapeutic Potential of Targeting the Ghrelin Pathway. *Int. J. Mol. Sci.* **2017**, *18*, 798. [CrossRef] [PubMed]
14. Reimer, M.K.; Pacini, G.; Ahrén, B. Dose-dependent inhibition by ghrelin of insulin secretion in the mouse. *Endocrinology* **2003**, *144*, 916–921. [CrossRef] [PubMed]
15. Soeki, T.; Kishimoto, I.; Schwenke, D.O.; Tokudome, T.; Horio, T.; Yoshida, M.; Hosoda, H.; Kangawa, K. Ghrelin suppresses cardiac sympathetic activity and prevents early left ventricular remodeling in rats with myocardial infarction. *Am. J. Physiol. Heart Circ. Physiol.* **2008**, *294*, H426–H432. [CrossRef]
16. Khatib, M.N.; Shankar, A.; Kirubakaran, R.; Agho, K.; Simkhada, P.; Gaidhane, S.; Saxena, D.; Unnikrishnan, B.; Gode, D.; Gaidhane, A.; et al. Effect of ghrelin on mortality and cardiovascular outcomes in experimental rat and mice models of heart failure: A systematic review and meta-analysis. *PLoS ONE* **2015**, *10*, e0126697. [CrossRef]
17. Dickson, S.L.; Leng, G.; Robinson, I.C. Systemic administration of growth hormone-releasing peptide activates hypothalamic arcuate neurons. *Neuroscience* **1993**, *53*, 303–306. [CrossRef]
18. Dickson, S.L.; Luckman, S.M. Induction of c-fos messenger ribonucleic acid in neuropeptide Y and growth hormone (GH)-releasing factor neurons in the rat arcuate nucleus following systemic injection of the GH secretagogue, GH-releasing peptide-6. *Endocrinology* **1997**, *138*, 771–777. [CrossRef] [PubMed]
19. Sun, Y.; Wang, P.; Zheng, H.; Smith, R.G. Ghrelin stimulation of growth hormone release and appetite is mediated through the growth hormone secretagogue receptor. *Proc. Natl. Acad. Sci. USA* **2004**, *101*, 4679–4684. [CrossRef] [PubMed]
20. Perello, M.; Dickson, S.L. Ghrelin signalling on food reward: A salient link between the gut and the mesolimbic system. *J. Neuroendocrinol.* **2015**, *27*, 424–434. [CrossRef]
21. Chen, L.; Xing, T.; Wang, M.; Miao, Y.; Tang, M.; Chen, J.; Li, G.; Ruan, D.Y. Local infusion of ghrelin enhanced hippocampal synaptic plasticity and spatial memory through activation of phosphoinositide 3-kinase in the dentate gyrus of adult rats. *Eur. J. Neurosci.* **2011**, *33*, 266–275. [CrossRef]
22. Zhao, Z.; Liu, H.; Xiao, K.; Yu, M.; Cui, L.; Zhu, Q.; Zhao, R.; Li, G.D.; Zhou, Y. Ghrelin administration enhances neurogenesis but impairs spatial learning and memory in adult mice. *Neuroscience* **2014**, *257*, 175–185. [CrossRef]
23. Diano, S.; Farr, S.A.; Benoit, S.C.; McNay, E.C.; da Silva, I.; Horvath, B.; Gaskin, F.S.; Nonaka, N.; Jaeger, L.B.; Banks, W.A.; et al. Ghrelin controls hippocampal spine synapse density and memory performance. *Nat. Neurosci.* **2006**, *9*, 381–388. [CrossRef] [PubMed]
24. Prieto-Garcia, L.; Egecioglu, E.; Studer, E.; Westberg, L.; Jerlhag, E. Ghrelin and GHS-R1A signaling within the ventral and laterodorsal tegmental area regulate sexual behavior in sexually naïve male mice. *Psychoneuroendocrinology* **2015**, *62*, 392–402. [CrossRef]
25. Menzies, J.R.; Skibicka, K.P.; Leng, G.; Dickson, S.L. Ghrelin, reward and motivation. *Endocr. Dev.* **2013**, *25*, 101–111. [CrossRef] [PubMed]
26. Spencer, S.J.; Xu, L.; Clarke, M.A.; Lemus, M.; Reichenbach, A.; Geenen, B.; Kozicz, T.; Andrews, Z.B. Ghrelin regulates the hypothalamic-pituitary-adrenal axis and restricts anxiety after acute stress. *Biol. Psychiatry* **2012**, *72*, 457–465. [CrossRef]
27. Kojima, M.; Hosoda, H.; Date, Y.; Nakazato, M.; Matsuo, H.; Kangawa, K. Ghrelin is a growth-hormone-releasing acylated peptide from stomach. *Nature* **1999**, *402*, 656–660. [CrossRef]
28. Xu, J.; Wang, S.; Lin, Y.; Cao, L.; Wang, R.; Chi, Z. Ghrelin protects against cell death of hippocampal neurons in pilocarpine-induced seizures in rats. *Neurosci. Lett.* **2009**, *453*, 58–61. [CrossRef]
29. Lee, J.; Lim, E.; Kim, Y.; Li, E.; Park, S. Ghrelin attenuates kainic acid-induced neuronal cell death in the mouse hippocampus. *J. Endocrinol.* **2010**, *205*, 263–270. [CrossRef]
30. Zhang, R.; Yang, G.; Wang, Q.; Guo, F.; Wang, H. Acylated ghrelin protects hippocampal neurons in pilocarpine-induced seizures of immature rats by inhibiting cell apoptosis. *Mol. Biol. Rep.* **2013**, *40*, 51–58. [CrossRef] [PubMed]
31. Lucchi, C.; Curia, G.; Vinet, J.; Gualtieri, F.; Bresciani, E.; Locatelli, V.; Torsello, A.; Biagini, G. Protective but not anticonvulsant effects of ghrelin and JMV-1843 in the pilocarpine model of *Status epilepticus*. *PLoS ONE* **2013**, *8*, e72716. [CrossRef] [PubMed]
32. Zhu, X.; Cao, Y.; Voogd, K.; Voodg, K.; Steiner, D.F. On the processing of proghrelin to ghrelin. *J. Biol. Chem.* **2006**, *281*, 38867–38870. [CrossRef]
33. Yang, J.; Brown, M.S.; Liang, G.; Grishin, N.V.; Goldstein, J.L. Identification of the acyltransferase that octanoylates ghrelin, an appetite-stimulating peptide hormone. *Cell* **2008**, *132*, 387–396. [CrossRef]
34. Gutierrez, J.A.; Solenberg, P.J.; Perkins, D.R.; Willency, J.A.; Knierman, M.D.; Jin, Z.; Witcher, D.R.; Luo, S.; Onyia, J.E.; Hale, J.E. Ghrelin octanoylation mediated by an orphan lipid transferase. *Proc. Natl. Acad. Sci. USA* **2008**, *105*, 6320–6325. [CrossRef] [PubMed]

35. Zhang, J.V.; Ren, P.G.; Avsian-Kretchmer, O.; Luo, C.W.; Rauch, R.; Klein, C.; Hsueh, A.J. Obestatin, a peptide encoded by the ghrelin gene, opposes ghrelin's effects on food intake. *Science* **2005**, *310*, 996–999. [CrossRef] [PubMed]
36. Toshinai, K.; Yamaguchi, H.; Sun, Y.; Smith, R.G.; Yamanaka, A.; Sakurai, T.; Date, Y.; Mondal, M.S.; Shimbara, T.; Kawagoe, T.; et al. Des-acyl ghrelin induces food intake by a mechanism independent of the growth hormone secretagogue receptor. *Endocrinology* **2006**, *147*, 2306–2314. [CrossRef]
37. Portelli, J.; Coppens, J.; Demuyser, T.; Smolders, I. Des-acyl ghrelin attenuates pilocarpine-induced limbic seizures via the ghrelin receptor and not the orexin pathway. *Neuropeptides* **2015**, *51*, 1–7. [CrossRef] [PubMed]
38. Gauna, C.; van de Zande, B.; van Kerkwijk, A.; Themmen, A.P.; van der Lely, A.J.; Delhanty, P.J. Unacylated ghrelin is not a functional antagonist but a full agonist of the type 1a growth hormone secretagogue receptor (GHS-R). *Mol. Cell. Endocrinol.* **2007**, *274*, 30–34. [CrossRef]
39. Patterson, M.; Murphy, K.G.; le Roux, C.W.; Ghatei, M.A.; Bloom, S.R. Characterization of ghrelin-like immunoreactivity in human plasma. *J. Clin. Endocrinol. Metab.* **2005**, *90*, 2205–2211. [CrossRef]
40. Tong, J.; Dave, N.; Mugundu, G.M.; Davis, H.W.; Gaylinn, B.D.; Thorner, M.O.; Tschöp, M.H.; d'Alessio, D.; Desai, P.B. The pharmacokinetics of acyl, des-acyl, and total ghrelin in healthy human subjects. *Eur. J. Endocrinol.* **2013**, *168*, 821–828. [CrossRef]
41. Akamizu, T.; Takaya, K.; Irako, T.; Hosoda, H.; Teramukai, S.; Matsuyama, A.; Tada, H.; Miura, K.; Shimizu, A.; Fukushima, M.; et al. Pharmacokinetics, safety, and endocrine and appetite effects of ghrelin administration in young healthy subjects. *Eur. J. Endocrinol.* **2004**, *150*, 447–455. [CrossRef]
42. Docanto, M.M.; Yang, F.; Callaghan, B.; Au, C.C.; Ragavan, R.; Wang, X.; Furness, J.B.; Andrews, Z.B.; Brown, K.A. Ghrelin and des-acyl ghrelin inhibit aromatase expression and activity in human adipose stromal cells: Suppression of cAMP as a possible mechanism. *Breast Cancer Res. Treat* **2014**, *147*, 193–201. [CrossRef]
43. Hopkins, A.L.; Nelson, T.A.; Guschina, I.A.; Parsons, L.C.; Lewis, C.L.; Brown, R.C.; Christian, H.C.; Davies, J.S.; Wells, T. Unacylated ghrelin promotes adipogenesis in rodent bone marrow via ghrelin O-acyl transferase and GHS-R. *Sci. Rep.* **2017**, *7*, 45541. [CrossRef]
44. Murtuza, M.I.; Isokawa, M. Endogenous ghrelin-O-acyltransferase (GOAT) acylates local ghrelin in the hippocampus. *J. Neurochem.* **2018**, *144*, 58–67. [CrossRef]
45. Guan, X.M.; Yu, H.; Palyha, O.C.; McKee, K.K.; Feighner, S.D.; Sirinathsinghji, D.J.; Smith, R.G.; van der Ploeg, L.H.; Howard, A.D. Distribution of mRNA encoding the growth hormone secretagogue receptor in brain and peripheral tissues. *Brain Res. Mol. Brain Res.* **1997**, *48*, 23–29. [CrossRef]
46. Leung, P.K.; Chow, K.B.; Lau, P.N.; Chu, K.M.; Chan, C.B.; Cheng, C.H.; Wise, H. The truncated ghrelin receptor polypeptide (GHS-R1b) acts as a dominant-negative mutant of the ghrelin receptor. *Cell. Signal.* **2007**, *19*, 1011–1022. [CrossRef] [PubMed]
47. Howard, A.D.; Feighner, S.D.; Cully, D.F.; Arena, J.P.; Liberator, P.A.; Rosenblum, C.I.; Hamelin, M.; Hreniuk, D.L.; Palyha, O.C.; Anderson, J.; et al. A receptor in pituitary and hypothalamus that functions in growth hormone release. *Science* **1996**, *273*, 974–977. [CrossRef]
48. Gnanapavan, S.; Kola, B.; Bustin, S.A.; Morris, D.G.; McGee, P.; Fairclough, P.; Bhattacharya, S.; Carpenter, R.; Grossman, A.B.; Korbonits, M. The tissue distribution of the mRNA of ghrelin and subtypes of its receptor, GHS-R, in humans. *J. Clin. Endocrinol. Metab.* **2002**, *87*, 2988. [CrossRef]
49. Xiao, X.; Bi, M.; Jiao, Q.; Chen, X.; Du, X.; Jiang, H. A new understanding of GHSR1a–independent of ghrelin activation. *Ageing Res. Rev.* **2020**, *64*, 101187. [CrossRef]
50. Mani, B.K.; Walker, A.K.; Lopez Soto, E.J.; Raingo, J.; Lee, C.E.; Perelló, M.; Andrews, Z.B.; Zigman, J.M. Neuroanatomical characterization of a growth hormone secretagogue receptor-green fluorescent protein reporter mouse. *J. Comp. Neurol.* **2014**, *522*, 3644–3666. [CrossRef]
51. Zigman, J.M.; Jones, J.E.; Lee, C.E.; Saper, C.B.; Elmquist, J.K. Expression of ghrelin receptor mRNA in the rat and the mouse brain. *J. Comp. Neurol.* **2006**, *494*, 528–548. [CrossRef] [PubMed]
52. Katayama, M.; Nogami, H.; Nishiyama, J.; Kawase, T.; Kawamura, K. Developmentally and regionally regulated expression of growth hormone secretagogue receptor mRNA in rat brain and pituitary gland. *Neuroendocrinology* **2000**, *72*, 333–340. [CrossRef]
53. Kim, K.; Arai, K.; Sanno, N.; Osamura, R.Y.; Teramoto, A.; Shibasaki, T. Ghrelin and growth hormone (GH) secretagogue receptor (GHSR) mRNA expression in human pituitary adenomas. *Clin. Endocrinol.* **2001**, *54*, 759–768. [CrossRef] [PubMed]
54. Nakata, S.; Yoshino, Y.; Okita, M.; Kawabe, K.; Yamazaki, K.; Ozaki, Y.; Mori, Y.; Ochi, S.; Iga, J.I.; Ueno, S.I. Differential expression of the ghrelin-related mRNAs GHS-R1*a*, GHS-R1*b*, and MBOAT4 in Japanese patients with schizophrenia. *Psychiatry Res.* **2019**, *272*, 334–339. [CrossRef]
55. Kim, M.S.; Yoon, C.Y.; Park, K.H.; Shin, C.S.; Park, K.S.; Kim, S.Y.; Cho, B.Y.; Lee, H.K. Changes in ghrelin and ghrelin receptor expression according to feeding status. *Neuroreport* **2003**, *14*, 1317–1320. [CrossRef] [PubMed]
56. Evron, T.; Peterson, S.M.; Urs, N.M.; Bai, Y.; Rochelle, L.K.; Caron, M.G.; Barak, L.S. G Protein and β-arrestin signaling bias at the ghrelin receptor. *J. Biol. Chem.* **2014**, *289*, 33442–33455. [CrossRef]
57. Sivertsen, B.; Lang, M.; Frimurer, T.M.; Holliday, N.D.; Bach, A.; Els, S.; Engelstoft, M.S.; Petersen, P.S.; Madsen, A.N.; Schwartz, T.W.; et al. Unique interaction pattern for a functionally biased ghrelin receptor agonist. *J. Biol. Chem.* **2011**, *286*, 20845–20860. [CrossRef]

58. Damian, M.; Marie, J.; Leyris, J.P.; Fehrentz, J.A.; Verdié, P.; Martinez, J.; Banères, J.L.; Mary, S. High constitutive activity is an intrinsic feature of ghrelin receptor protein: A study with a functional monomeric GHS-R1a receptor reconstituted in lipid discs. *J. Biol. Chem.* **2012**, *287*, 3630–3641. [CrossRef] [PubMed]
59. McKee, K.K.; Palyha, O.C.; Feighner, S.D.; Hreniuk, D.L.; Tan, C.P.; Phillips, M.S.; Smith, R.G.; van der Ploeg, L.H.; Howard, A.D. Molecular analysis of rat pituitary and hypothalamic growth hormone secretagogue receptors. *Mol. Endocrinol.* **1997**, *11*, 415–423. [CrossRef]
60. Hedegaard, M.A.; Holst, B. The Complex Signaling Pathways of the Ghrelin Receptor. *Endocrinology* **2020**, *161*, bqaa020. [CrossRef]
61. Camiña, J.P.; Lodeiro, M.; Ischenko, O.; Martini, A.C.; Casanueva, F.F. Stimulation by ghrelin of p42/p44 mitogen-activated protein kinase through the GHS-R1a receptor: Role of G-proteins and beta-arrestins. *J. Cell. Physiol.* **2007**, *213*, 187–200. [CrossRef]
62. Offermanns, S.; Mancino, V.; Revel, J.P.; Simon, M.I. Vascular system defects and impaired cell chemokinesis as a result of Galpha13 deficiency. *Science* **1997**, *275*, 533–536. [CrossRef] [PubMed]
63. Suzuki, N.; Hajicek, N.; Kozasa, T. Regulation and physiological functions of G12/13-mediated signaling pathways. *Neurosignals* **2009**, *17*, 55–70. [CrossRef]
64. Bouzo-Lorenzo, M.; Santo-Zas, I.; Lodeiro, M.; Nogueiras, R.; Casanueva, F.F.; Castro, M.; Pazos, Y.; Tobin, A.B.; Butcher, A.J.; Camiña, J.P. Distinct phosphorylation sites on the ghrelin receptor, GHSR1a, establish a code that determines the functions of β-arrestins. *Sci. Rep.* **2016**, *6*, 22495. [CrossRef]
65. Gurevich, V.V.; Gurevich, E.V. The structural basis of arrestin-mediated regulation of G-protein-coupled receptors. *Pharmacol. Ther.* **2006**, *110*, 465–502. [CrossRef]
66. Wootten, D.; Christopoulos, A.; Marti-Solano, M.; Babu, M.M.; Sexton, P.M. Mechanisms of signalling and biased agonism in G protein-coupled receptors. *Nat. Rev. Mol. Cell Biol.* **2018**, *19*, 638–653. [CrossRef] [PubMed]
67. Holst, B.; Cygankiewicz, A.; Jensen, T.H.; Ankersen, M.; Schwartz, T.W. High constitutive signaling of the ghrelin receptor–identification of a potent inverse agonist. *Mol. Endocrinol.* **2003**, *17*, 2201–2210. [CrossRef] [PubMed]
68. Holliday, N.D.; Holst, B.; Rodionova, E.A.; Schwartz, T.W.; Cox, H.M. Importance of constitutive activity and arrestin-independent mechanisms for intracellular trafficking of the ghrelin receptor. *Mol. Endocrinol.* **2007**, *21*, 3100–3112. [CrossRef]
69. Holst, B.; Holliday, N.D.; Bach, A.; Elling, C.E.; Cox, H.M.; Schwartz, T.W. Common structural basis for constitutive activity of the ghrelin receptor family. *J. Biol. Chem.* **2004**, *279*, 53806–53817. [CrossRef] [PubMed]
70. Banks, W.A.; Tschöp, M.; Robinson, S.M.; Heiman, M.L. Extent and direction of ghrelin transport across the blood-brain barrier is determined by its unique primary structure. *J. Pharmacol. Exp. Ther.* **2002**, *302*, 822–827. [CrossRef] [PubMed]
71. Rhea, E.M.; Salameh, T.S.; Gray, S.; Niu, J.; Banks, W.A.; Tong, J. Ghrelin transport across the blood-brain barrier can occur independently of the growth hormone secretagogue receptor. *Mol. Metab.* **2018**, *18*, 88–96. [CrossRef] [PubMed]
72. Cabral, A.; Valdivia, S.; Fernandez, G.; Reynaldo, M.; Perello, M. Divergent neuronal circuitries underlying acute orexigenic effects of peripheral or central ghrelin: Critical role of brain accessibility. *J. Neuroendocrinol.* **2014**, *26*, 542–554. [CrossRef] [PubMed]
73. Uriarte, M.; de Francesco, P.N.; Fernandez, G.; Cabral, A.; Castrogiovanni, D.; Lalonde, T.; Luyt, L.G.; Trejo, S.; Perello, M. Evidence Supporting a Role for the Blood-Cerebrospinal Fluid Barrier Transporting Circulating Ghrelin into the Brain. *Mol. Neurobiol.* **2019**, *56*, 4120–4134. [CrossRef]
74. Uriarte, M.; de Francesco, P.N.; Fernández, G.; Castrogiovanni, D.; d'Arcangelo, M.; Imbernon, M.; Cantel, S.; Denoyelle, S.; Fehrentz, J.A.; Praetorius, J.; et al. Circulating ghrelin crosses the blood-cerebrospinal fluid barrier via growth hormone secretagogue receptor dependent and independent mechanisms. *Mol. Cell. Endocrinol.* **2021**, *538*, 111449. [CrossRef]
75. Grouselle, D.; Chaillou, E.; Caraty, A.; Bluet-Pajot, M.T.; Zizzari, P.; Tillet, Y.; Epelbaum, J. Pulsatile cerebrospinal fluid and plasma ghrelin in relation to growth hormone secretion and food intake in the sheep. *J. Neuroendocrinol.* **2008**, *20*, 1138–1146. [CrossRef] [PubMed]
76. Collden, G.; Balland, E.; Parkash, J.; Caron, E.; Langlet, F.; Prevot, V.; Bouret, S.G. Neonatal overnutrition causes early alterations in the central response to peripheral ghrelin. *Mol. Metab.* **2015**, *4*, 15–24. [CrossRef] [PubMed]
77. Edwards, A.; Abizaid, A. Clarifying the Ghrelin System's Ability to Regulate Feeding Behaviours Despite Enigmatic Spatial Separation of the GHSR and Its Endogenous Ligand. *Int. J. Mol. Sci.* **2017**, *18*, 859. [CrossRef]
78. Nass, R.; Farhy, L.S.; Liu, J.; Pezzoli, S.S.; Johnson, M.L.; Gaylinn, B.D.; Thorner, M.O. Age-dependent decline in acyl-ghrelin concentrations and reduced association of acyl-ghrelin and growth hormone in healthy older adults. *J. Clin. Endocrinol. Metab.* **2014**, *99*, 602–608. [CrossRef]
79. Whatmore, A.J.; Hall, C.M.; Jones, J.; Westwood, M.; Clayton, P.E. Ghrelin concentrations in healthy children and adolescents. *Clin. Endocrinol.* **2003**, *59*, 649–654. [CrossRef] [PubMed]
80. Aydin, S.; Dag, E.; Ozkan, Y.; Erman, F.; Dagli, A.F.; Kilic, N.; Sahin, I.; Karatas, F.; Yoldas, T.; Barim, A.O.; et al. Nesfatin-1 and ghrelin levels in serum and saliva of epileptic patients: Hormonal changes can have a major effect on seizure disorders. *Mol. Cell. Biochem.* **2009**, *328*, 49–56. [CrossRef]
81. Dag, E.; Aydin, S.; Ozkan, Y.; Erman, F.; Dagli, A.F.; Gurger, M. Alteration in chromogranin A, obestatin and total ghrelin levels of saliva and serum in epilepsy cases. *Peptides* **2010**, *31*, 932–937. [CrossRef]
82. Erkec, O.E.; Milanlıoğlu, A.; Komuroglu, A.U.; Kara, M.; Huyut, Z.; Keskin, S. Evaluation of serum ghrelin, nesfatin-1, irisin, and vasoactive intestinal peptide levels in temporal lobe epilepsy patients with and without drug resistance: A cross-sectional study. *Rev. Assoc. Med. Bras.* **2021**, *67*, 207–212. [CrossRef]

83. Greco, R.; Latini, G.; Chiarelli, F.; Iannetti, P.; Verrotti, A. Leptin, ghrelin, and adiponectin in epileptic patients treated with valproic acid. *Neurology* **2005**, *65*, 1808–1809. [CrossRef]
84. Varrasi, C.; Strigaro, G.; Sola, M.; Falletta, L.; Moia, S.; Prodam, F.; Cantello, R. Interictal ghrelin levels in adult patients with epilepsy. *Seizure* **2014**, *23*, 852–855. [CrossRef] [PubMed]
85. Berilgen, M.S.; Mungen, B.; Ustundag, B.; Demir, C. Serum ghrelin levels are enhanced in patients with epilepsy. *Seizure* **2006**, *15*, 106–111. [CrossRef]
86. Mohamed, W.S.; Nageeb, R.S.; Elsaid, H.H. Serum and urine ghrelin in adult epileptic patients. *Egypt. J. Neurol. Psychiatry Neurosurg.* **2019**, *55*, 82. [CrossRef]
87. Hara, M.; Nishi, Y.; Yamashita, Y.; Hirata, R.; Takahashi, S.; Nagamitsu, S.; Hosoda, H.; Kangawa, K.; Kojima, M.; Matsuishi, T. Relation between circulating levels of GH, IGF-1, ghrelin and somatic growth in Rett syndrome. *Brain Dev.* **2014**, *36*, 794–800. [CrossRef]
88. Deschaine, S.L.; Leggio, L. Understanding plasma treatment effect on human acyl-ghrelin concentrations. *Eur. Rev. Med. Pharmacol. Sci.* **2020**, *24*, 1585–1589. [CrossRef] [PubMed]
89. Aydin, S.; Dag, E.; Ozkan, Y.; Arslan, O.; Koc, G.; Bek, S.; Kirbas, S.; Kasikci, T.; Abasli, D.; Gokcil, Z.; et al. Time-dependent changes in the serum levels of prolactin, nesfatin-1 and ghrelin as a marker of epileptic attacks young male patients. *Peptides* **2011**, *32*, 1276–1280. [CrossRef]
90. Ataie, Z.; Golzar, M.G.; Babri, S.; Ebrahimi, H.; Mohaddes, G. Does ghrelin level change after epileptic seizure in rats? *Seizure* **2011**, *20*, 347–349. [CrossRef]
91. Prodam, F.; Bellone, S.; Casara, G.; de Rienzo, F.; Grassino, E.C.; Bonsignori, I.; Demarchi, I.; Rapa, A.; Radetti, G.; Bona, G. Ghrelin levels are reduced in prepubertal epileptic children under treatment with carbamazepine or valproic acid. *Epilepsia* **2010**, *51*, 312–315. [CrossRef]
92. Cansu, A.; Serdaroglu, A.; Camurdan, O.; Hirfanoglu, T.; Cinaz, P. Serum Insulin, Cortisol, Leptin, Neuropeptide Y, Galanin and Ghrelin Levels in Epileptic Children Receiving Valproate. *Horm. Res. Paediatr.* **2011**, *76*, 65–71. [CrossRef]
93. Taskin, E.; Atli, B.; Kiliç, M.; Sari, Y.; Aydin, S. Serum, urine, and saliva levels of ghrelin and obestatin pre- and post-treatment in pediatric epilepsy. *Pediatr. Neurol.* **2014**, *51*, 365–369. [CrossRef] [PubMed]
94. Çiçek, N.P.; Kamaşak, T.; Serin, M.; Okten, A.; Alver, A.; Cansu, A. The effects of valproate and topiramate use on serum insulin, leptin, neuropeptide Y and ghrelin levels in epileptic children. *Seizure* **2018**, *58*, 90–95. [CrossRef]
95. Cansu, A.; Serdaroglu, A.; Cinaz, P. Serum insulin, cortisol, leptin, neuropeptide Y, galanin and ghrelin levels in epileptic children receiving oxcarbazepine. *Eur. J. Paediatr. Neurol.* **2011**, *15*, 527–531. [CrossRef]
96. Tokgoz, H.; Aydin, K.; Oran, B.; Kiyici, A. Plasma leptin, neuropeptide Y, ghrelin, and adiponectin levels and carotid artery intima media thickness in epileptic children treated with valproate. *Childs Nerv. Syst.* **2012**, *28*, 1049–1053. [CrossRef] [PubMed]
97. Ozcelik, A.A.; Serdaroglu, A.; Bideci, A.; Arhan, E.; Soysal, Ş.; Demir, E.; Gücüyener, K. The effect of topiramate on body weight and ghrelin, leptin, and neuropeptide-Y levels of prepubertal children with epilepsy. *Pediatr. Neurol.* **2014**, *51*, 220–224. [CrossRef]
98. Cansu, A.; Yesilkaya, E.; Serdaroglu, A.; Camurdan, O.; Hirfanoglu, T.L.; Karaoglu, A.; Bideci, A.; Cinaz, P. The Effects of Oxcarbazepine and Valproate Therapies on Growth in Children with Epilepsy. *Endocr. Res.* **2012**, *37*, 163–174. [CrossRef]
99. Gungor, S.; Yücel, G.; Akinci, A.; Tabel, Y.; Ozerol, I.H.; Yologlu, S. The role of ghrelin in weight gain and growth in epileptic children using valproate. *J. Child Neurol.* **2007**, *22*, 1384–1388. [CrossRef]
100. Hasaneen, B.; Salem, N.A.; El Sallab, S.; Elgaml, D.; Elhelaly, R. Body weight, body composition, and serum ghrelin in epileptic children receiving levetiracetam monotherapy. *Egypt. Pediatr. Assoc. Gaz.* **2016**, *64*, 154–159. [CrossRef]
101. Marchiò, M.; Roli, L.; Giordano, C.; Trenti, T.; Guerra, A.; Biagini, G. Decreased ghrelin and des-acyl ghrelin plasma levels in patients affected by pharmacoresistant epilepsy and maintained on the ketogenic diet. *Clin. Nutr.* **2019**, *38*, 954–957. [CrossRef] [PubMed]
102. Marchiò, M.; Roli, L.; Lucchi, C.; Costa, A.M.; Borghi, M.; Iughetti, L.; Trenti, T.; Guerra, A.; Biagini, G. Ghrelin Plasma Levels After 1 Year of Ketogenic Diet in Children With Refractory Epilepsy. *Front. Nutr.* **2019**, *6*, 112. [CrossRef]
103. De Amicis, R.; Leone, A.; Lessa, C.; Foppiani, A.; Ravella, S.; Ravasenghi, S.; Trentani, C.; Ferraris, C.; Veggiotti, P.; de Giorgis, V.; et al. Long-Term Effects of a Classic Ketogenic Diet on Ghrelin and Leptin Concentration: A 12-Month Prospective Study in a Cohort of Italian Children and Adults with GLUT1-Deficiency Syndrome and Drug Resistant Epilepsy. *Nutrients* **2019**, *11*, 1716. [CrossRef] [PubMed]
104. Giordano, C.; Marchiò, M.; Timofeeva, E.; Biagini, G. Neuroactive peptides as putative mediators of antiepileptic ketogenic diets. *Front. Neurol.* **2014**, *5*, 63. [CrossRef]
105. Obay, B.D.; Tasdemir, E.; Tümer, C.; Bilgin, H.M.; Sermet, A. Antiepileptic effects of ghrelin on pentylenetetrazole-induced seizures in rats. *Peptides* **2007**, *28*, 1214–1219. [CrossRef]
106. Ghahramanian Golzar, M.; Babri, S.; Ataie, Z.; Ebrahimi, H.; Mirzaie, F.; Mohaddes, G. NPY Receptors Blockade Prevents Anticonvulsant Action of Ghrelin in the Hippocampus of Rat. *Adv. Pharm. Bull.* **2013**, *3*, 265–271. [CrossRef] [PubMed]
107. Ataie, Z.; Babri, S.; Ghahramanian Golzar, M.; Ebrahimi, H.; Mirzaie, F.; Mohaddes, G. GABAB Receptor Blockade Prevents Antiepileptic Action of Ghrelin in the Rat Hippocampus. *Adv. Pharm. Bull.* **2013**, *3*, 353–358. [CrossRef]
108. Zendehdel, M.; Kaboutari, J.; Ghadimi, D.; Hassanpour, S. The Antiepileptic Effect of Ghrelin during Different Phases of the Estrous Cycle in PTZ-Induced Seizures in Rat. *Int. J. Pept. Res. Ther.* **2014**, *20*, 511–517. [CrossRef]

109. Babri, S.; Amani, M.; Mohaddes, G.; Mirzaei, F.; Mahmoudi, F. Effects of intrahippocampal injection of ghrelin on spatial memory in PTZ-induced seizures in male rats. *Neuropeptides* **2013**, *47*, 355–360. [CrossRef]
110. Keezer, M.R.; Sisodiya, S.M.; Sander, J.W. Comorbidities of epilepsy: Current concepts and future perspectives. *Lancet Neurol.* **2016**, *15*, 106–115. [CrossRef]
111. Ergul Erkec, O.; Algul, S.; Kara, M. Evaluation of ghrelin, nesfatin-1 and irisin levels of serum and brain after acute or chronic pentylenetetrazole administrations in rats using sodium valproate. *Neurol. Res.* **2018**, *40*, 923–929. [CrossRef] [PubMed]
112. Turkmen, A.Z.; Nurten, A. Investigation of Ghrelin Levels in Antimuscarinic Induced Convulsions in Fasted Animals after Food Intake. *Bezmialem Sci.* **2020**, *8*, 138–143. [CrossRef]
113. Aslan, A.; Yildirim, M.; Ayyildiz, M.; Güven, A.; Agar, E. The role of nitric oxide in the inhibitory effect of ghrelin against penicillin-induced epileptiform activity in rat. *Neuropeptides* **2009**, *43*, 295–302. [CrossRef]
114. Oztas, B.; Sahin, D.; Kir, H.; Kuskay, S.; Ates, N. Effects of leptin, ghrelin and neuropeptide y on spike-wave discharge activity and certain biochemical parameters in WAG/Rij rats with genetic absence epilepsy. *J. Neuroimmunol.* **2021**, *351*, 577454. [CrossRef]
115. Biagini, G.; Torsello, A.; Marinelli, C.; Gualtieri, F.; Vezzali, R.; Coco, S.; Bresciani, E.; Locatelli, V. Beneficial effects of desacyl-ghrelin, hexarelin and EP-80317 in models of status epilepticus. *Eur. J. Pharmacol.* **2011**, *670*, 130–136. [CrossRef]
116. Portelli, J.; Thielemans, L.; ver Donck, L.; Loyens, E.; Coppens, J.; Aourz, N.; Aerssens, J.; Vermoesen, K.; Clinckers, R.; Schallier, A.; et al. Inactivation of the constitutively active ghrelin receptor attenuates limbic seizure activity in rodents. *Neurotherapeutics* **2012**, *9*, 658–672. [CrossRef]
117. Oztas, B.; Sahin, D.; Kir, H.; Eraldemir, F.C.; Musul, M.; Kuskay, S.; Ates, N. The effect of leptin, ghrelin, and neuropeptide-Y on serum Tnf-A, Il-1β, Il-6, Fgf-2, galanin levels and oxidative stress in an experimental generalized convulsive seizure model. *Neuropeptides* **2017**, *61*, 31–37. [CrossRef]
118. Kilinc, E.; Gunes, H. Modulatory effects of neuropeptides on pentylenetetrazol-induced epileptic seizures and neuroinflammation in rats. *Rev. Assoc. Med. Bras.* **2019**, *65*, 1188–1192. [CrossRef]
119. Arslan, G.; Ayyildiz, M.; Agar, E. The interaction between ghrelin and cannabinoid systems in penicillin-induced epileptiform activity in rats. *Neuropeptides* **2014**, *48*, 345–352. [CrossRef] [PubMed]
120. Guerlavais, V.; Boeglin, D.; Mousseaux, D.; Oiry, C.; Heitz, A.; Deghenghi, R.; Locatelli, V.; Torsello, A.; Ghé, C.; Catapano, F.; et al. New active series of growth hormone secretagogues. *J. Med. Chem.* **2003**, *46*, 1191–1203. [CrossRef] [PubMed]
121. Garcia, J.M.; Biller, B.M.K.; Korbonits, M.; Popovic, V.; Luger, A.; Strasburger, C.J.; Chanson, P.; Medic-Stojanoska, M.; Schopohl, J.; Zakrzewska, A.; et al. Macimorelin as a Diagnostic Test for Adult GH Deficiency. *J. Clin. Endocrinol. Metab.* **2018**, *103*, 3083–3093. [CrossRef] [PubMed]
122. Klaus, B.; Sachse, R.; Ammer, N.; Kelepouris, N.; Ostrow, V. Safety, tolerability, pharmacokinetics, and pharmacodynamics of macimorelin in healthy adults: Results of a single-dose, randomized controlled study. *Growth Horm. IGF Res.* **2020**, *52*, 101321. [CrossRef] [PubMed]
123. M'Kadmi, C.; Leyris, J.P.; Onfroy, L.; Galés, C.; Saulière, A.; Gagne, D.; Damian, M.; Mary, S.; Maingot, M.; Denoyelle, S.; et al. Agonism, Antagonism, and Inverse Agonism Bias at the Ghrelin Receptor Signaling. *J. Biol. Chem.* **2015**, *290*, 27021–27039. [CrossRef]
124. Coppens, J.; Aourz, N.; Walrave, L.; Fehrentz, J.A.; Martinez, J.; de Bundel, D.; Portelli, J.; Smolders, I. Anticonvulsant effect of a ghrelin receptor agonist in 6Hz corneally kindled mice. *Epilepsia* **2016**, *57*, e195–e199. [CrossRef] [PubMed]
125. Buckinx, A.; van den Herrewegen, Y.; Pierre, A.; Cottone, E.; Ben Haj Salah, K.; Fehrentz, J.A.; Kooijman, R.; de Bundel, D.; Smolders, I. Differential Effects of a Full and Biased Ghrelin Receptor Agonist in a Mouse Kindling Model. *Int. J. Mol. Sci.* **2019**, *20*, 2480. [CrossRef] [PubMed]
126. Buckinx, A.; Pierre, A.; van den Herrewegen, Y.; Guenther, E.; Gerlach, M.; van Laethem, G.; Kooijman, R.; de Bundel, D.; Smolders, I. Translational potential of the ghrelin receptor agonist macimorelin for seizure suppression in pharmacoresistant epilepsy. *Eur. J. Neurol.* **2021**, *28*, 3100–3112. [CrossRef] [PubMed]
127. Carpino, P.A.; Lefker, B.A.; Toler, S.M.; Pan, L.C.; Hadcock, J.R.; Murray, M.C.; Cook, E.R.; DiBrino, J.N.; DeNinno, S.L.; Chidsey-Frink, K.L.; et al. Discovery and biological characterization of capromorelin analogues with extended half-lives. *Bioorg. Med. Chem. Lett.* **2002**, *12*, 3279–3282. [CrossRef]
128. Zollers, B.; Rhodes, L.; Heinen, E. Capromorelin oral solution (ENTYCE®) increases food consumption and body weight when administered for 4 consecutive days to healthy adult Beagle dogs in a randomized, masked, placebo controlled study. *BMC Vet. Res.* **2017**, *13*, 10. [CrossRef]
129. Rhodes, L.; Zollers, B.; Wofford, J.A.; Heinen, E. Capromorelin: A ghrelin receptor agonist and novel therapy for stimulation of appetite in dogs. *Vet. Med. Sci.* **2018**, *4*, 3–16. [CrossRef]
130. Deghenghi, R.; Cananzi, M.M.; Torsello, A.; Battisti, C.; Muller, E.E.; Locatelli, V. GH-releasing activity of Hexarelin, a new growth hormone releasing peptide, in infant and adult rats. *Life Sci.* **1994**, *54*, 1321–1328. [CrossRef]
131. Giordano, C.; Costa, A.M.; Lucchi, C.; Leo, G.; Brunel, L.; Fehrentz, J.A.; Martinez, J.; Torsello, A.; Biagini, G. Progressive Seizure Aggravation in the Repeated 6-Hz Corneal Stimulation Model Is Accompanied by Marked Increase in Hippocampal p-ERK1/2 Immunoreactivity in Neurons. *Front. Cell. Neurosci.* **2016**, *10*, 281. [CrossRef]
132. Lucchi, C.; Costa, A.M.; Giordano, C.; Curia, G.; Piat, M.; Leo, G.; Vinet, J.; Brunel, L.; Fehrentz, J.A.; Martinez, J.; et al. Involvement of PPARγ in the Anticonvulsant Activity of EP-80317, a Ghrelin Receptor Antagonist. *Front. Pharmacol.* **2017**, *8*, 676. [CrossRef] [PubMed]

133. Azimzadeh, M.; Beheshti, S. Antagonism of the ghrelin receptor type 1a in the rat brain induces status epilepticus in an electrical kindling model of epilepsy. *Psychopharmacology* **2021**, *238*, 1–9. [CrossRef]
134. Barker-Haliski, M.; White, H.S. Glutamatergic Mechanisms Associated with Seizures and Epilepsy. *Cold Spring Harb. Perspect. Med.* **2015**, *5*, a022863. [CrossRef]
135. Viviani, B.; Bartesaghi, S.; Gardoni, F.; Vezzani, A.; Behrens, M.M.; Bartfai, T.; Binaglia, M.; Corsini, E.; di Luca, M.; Galli, C.L.; et al. Interleukin-1beta enhances NMDA receptor-mediated intracellular calcium increase through activation of the Src family of kinases. *J. Neurosci.* **2003**, *23*, 8692–8700. [CrossRef] [PubMed]
136. Vezzani, A.; French, J.; Bartfai, T.; Baram, T.Z. The role of inflammation in epilepsy. *Nat. Rev. Neurol.* **2011**, *7*, 31–40. [CrossRef] [PubMed]
137. Takeuchi, H.; Jin, S.; Wang, J.; Zhang, G.; Kawanokuchi, J.; Kuno, R.; Sonobe, Y.; Mizuno, T.; Suzumura, A. Tumor necrosis factor-alpha induces neurotoxicity via glutamate release from hemichannels of activated microglia in an autocrine manner. *J. Biol. Chem.* **2006**, *281*, 21362–21368. [CrossRef]
138. Rana, A.; Musto, A.E. The role of inflammation in the development of epilepsy. *J. Neuroinflamm.* **2018**, *15*, 144. [CrossRef] [PubMed]
139. Chang, L.; Zhao, J.; Yang, J.; Zhang, Z.; Du, J.; Tang, C. Therapeutic effects of ghrelin on endotoxic shock in rats. *Eur. J. Pharmacol.* **2003**, *473*, 171–176. [CrossRef]
140. Han, K.; Wang, Q.Y.; Wang, C.X.; Luan, S.Y.; Tian, W.P.; Wang, Y.; Zhang, R.Y. Ghrelin improves pilocarpine-induced cerebral cortex inflammation in epileptic rats by inhibiting NF-κB and TNF-α. *Mol. Med. Rep.* **2018**, *18*, 3563–3568. [CrossRef] [PubMed]
141. Shin, E.J.; Jeong, J.H.; Chung, Y.H.; Kim, W.K.; Ko, K.H.; Bach, J.H.; Hong, J.S.; Yoneda, Y.; Kim, H.C. Role of oxidative stress in epileptic seizures. *Neurochem. Int.* **2011**, *59*, 122–137. [CrossRef] [PubMed]
142. Obay, B.D.; Taşdemir, E.; Tümer, C.; Bilgin, H.; Atmaca, M. Dose dependent effects of ghrelin on pentylenetetrazole-induced oxidative stress in a rat seizure model. *Peptides* **2008**, *29*, 448–455. [CrossRef] [PubMed]
143. Kern, A.; Mavrikaki, M.; Ullrich, C.; Albarran-Zeckler, R.; Brantley, A.F.; Smith, R.G. Hippocampal Dopamine/DRD1 Signaling Dependent on the Ghrelin Receptor. *Cell* **2015**, *163*, 1176–1190. [CrossRef] [PubMed]
144. Pisani, A.; Bonsi, P.; Martella, G.; de Persis, C.; Costa, C.; Pisani, F.; Bernardi, G.; Calabresi, P. Intracellular calcium increase in epileptiform activity: Modulation by levetiracetam and lamotrigine. *Epilepsia* **2004**, *45*, 719–728. [CrossRef] [PubMed]
145. Pal, S.; Sun, D.; Limbrick, D.; Rafiq, A.; DeLorenzo, R.J. Epileptogenesis induces long-term alterations in intracellular calcium release and sequestration mechanisms in the hippocampal neuronal culture model of epilepsy. *Cell Calcium* **2001**, *30*, 285–296. [CrossRef] [PubMed]
146. Cavalier, M.; Crouzin, N.; Ben Sedrine, A.; de Jesus Ferreira, M.C.; Guiramand, J.; Cohen-Solal, C.; Fehrentz, J.A.; Martinez, J.; Barbanel, G.; Vignes, M. Involvement of PKA and ERK pathways in ghrelin-induced long-lasting potentiation of excitatory synaptic transmission in the CA1 area of rat hippocampus. *Eur. J. Neurosci.* **2015**, *42*, 2568–2576. [CrossRef] [PubMed]
147. Cruz, M.T.; Herman, M.A.; Cote, D.M.; Ryabinin, A.E.; Roberto, M. Ghrelin increases GABAergic transmission and interacts with ethanol actions in the rat central nucleus of the amygdala. *Neuropsychopharmacology* **2013**, *38*, 364–375. [CrossRef] [PubMed]
148. Mir, J.F.; Zagmutt, S.; Lichtenstein, M.P.; García-Villoria, J.; Weber, M.; Gracia, A.; Fabriàs, G.; Casas, J.; López, M.; Casals, N.; et al. Ghrelin Causes a Decline in GABA Release by Reducing Fatty Acid Oxidation in Cortex. *Mol. Neurobiol.* **2018**, *55*, 7216–7228. [CrossRef]
149. Li, N.; Xu, F.; Yu, M.; Qiao, Z.; Zhou, Y. Selectively increasing GHS-R1a expression in dCA1 excitatory/inhibitory neurons have opposite effects on memory encoding. *Mol. Brain* **2021**, *14*, 157. [CrossRef] [PubMed]

MDPI
St. Alban-Anlage 66
4052 Basel
Switzerland
Tel. +41 61 683 77 34
Fax +41 61 302 89 18
www.mdpi.com

Biomedicines Editorial Office
E-mail: biomedicines@mdpi.com
www.mdpi.com/journal/biomedicines

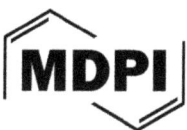

www.ingramcontent.com/pod-product-compliance
Lightning Source LLC
LaVergne TN
LVHW070425100526
838202LV00014B/1527